Atlas of Knee Arthroscopy

Radu Prejbeanu
Editor

Atlas of Knee Arthroscopy

Springer

Editor
Radu Prejbeanu
1st Orthopaedics and Tramatology Clinic
University of Medicine and Pharmacy
Victor Babes Timisoara
Timisoara, Romania

ISBN 978-1-4471-6592-7 ISBN 978-1-4471-6593-4 (eBook)
DOI 10.1007/978-1-4471-6593-4
Springer London Heidelberg New York Dordrecht

Library of Congress Control Number: 2014954744

Printed on acid-free paper

Springer is part of Springer Science+Business Media (www.springer.com)

Preface

Arthroscopy is minimal invasive surgery that is gaining more and more ground in favor of traditional approaches. The rapid postoperative recovery, reduced pain and accelerated return to physical activity makes it the ideal treatment is sports medicine.

This book summarizes the authors experience gained after performing thousands of knee arthroscopy and anterior cruciate ligament reconstructions over the last 10 years. We achieved international recognition of our educational programs when we became an ESSKA (European Society of Sports traumatology, Knee Surgery and Arthroscopy) Centre of Excellence in knee arthroscopy. Such an approach should bring an interesting blend of rigorous western methodology into a cross-cultural adaptation for Eastern Europe.

Our concise atlas of knee arthroscopy is intended as a practical start up guide for residents and young orthopedic surgeons alike. In addition, it provides detailed explanations on performing anterior cruciate ligament reconstruction, as well as potential pitfalls.

What we hope will make our material stand out from the abundance of available literature is the simple but comprehensive way in which it was structured and written. It should make it straight forward for anyone interested in knee arthroscopy and ACL reconstruction to access a lot of current data in a concise manner. The expert opinions are backed up by with many pictures and case examples, some of which were documented during our annual instructional courses.

Timisoara, Romania　　　　Radu Prejbeanu

Contents

Contributors

Dan Crisan, MD Department of Orthopedics and Trauma, University of Medicine and Pharmacy 'Victor Babes' Timisoara, Timisoara, Romania

I-st Clinic of Orthopedics and Trauma, Emergency Clinical County Hospital Timisoara, Timisoara, Romania

Horia Haragus, MD, PhD Department of Orthopedics and Trauma, University of Medicine and Pharmacy 'Victor Babes' Timisoara, Timisoara, Romania

I-st Clinic of Orthopedics and Trauma, Emergency Clinical County Hospital Timisoara, Timisoara, Romania

Radu Prejbeanu, MD, PhD Department of Orthopedics and Trauma, University of Medicine and Pharmacy 'Victor Babes' Timisoara, Timisoara, Romania

I-st Clinic of Orthopedics and Trauma, Emergency Clinical County Hospital Timisoara, Timisoara, Romania

Florin Ramadani, MD, PhD Unfallchirurgie Klinikum Wels-Grieskirchen, Wels, Austria

University of Medicine and Pharmacy 'Victor Babes' Timisoara, Timisoara, Romania

Dinu Vermesan, MD, PhD Department of Orthopedics and Trauma, University of Medicine and Pharmacy 'Victor Babes' Timisoara, Timisoara, Romania

I-st Clinic of Orthopedics and Trauma, Emergency Clinical County Hospital Timisoara, Timisoara, Romania

1 Operating Setup and Normal Anatomy

Dinu Vermesan and Radu Prejbeanu

1.1 Operating Setup

1.1.1 Historical Perspective

Arthroscopy of the knee is the most common orthopedic procedure performed in the United States. Given the frequency of this procedure, it is hard to fathom that knee arthroscopy did not enter into the mainstream of orthopedic surgery until the 1970s [1].

The first attempts to inspect the knee via endoscopy have been made as early as 1912 by Severin Nordentoft from Denmark and 1919 by Kenji Takaji in Japan but Eugene Bircher is considered to be the parent of knee arthroscopy because of his pioneering work between 1920 and 1930 [2]. These were mostly diagnostic procedures; Masaki Watanabe and his student Richard Connor are seen as the parents of interventional arthroscopy. Arthroscopic procedures have expanded since the 1970s and 1980s mostly due to important advances in arthroscopic technology such as fiber optics and color intraoperative imaging. While the first instruments used 7.3 mm cystoscopes (Takagi) or thoracoscopes (Bircher), the standard optical unit nowadays is 4 mm in diameter and has a 30° angle of the lens. From a local perspective, in our centre the first arthroscopic interventions took place in the early 90s, and were the first arthroscopic surgeries in the west of the country, in a time when resources were scarce and public acceptance of new procedures limited.

D. Vermesan, MD, PhD • R. Prejbeanu, MD, PhD (✉)
Department of Orthopedics and Trauma,
University of Medicine and Pharmacy 'Victor Babes' Timisoara,
2 Eftimie Murgu Square, 300041 Timisoara, Romania

I-st Clinic of Orthopedics and Trauma,
Emergency Clinical County Hospital Timisoara,
10 Iosif Bulbuca Blvd, 300736 Timisoara, Romania
e-mail: vermesan@gmail.com; raduprejbeanu@gmail.com

In the beginning, diagnostic arthroscopy was fairly common, but nowadays, with the advent of knee MRI as a routine investigation, there is a clear shift towards interventional use. Common procedures performed during arthroscopic surgery are meniscectomies and meniscal sutures, ACL reconstructions, cartilage debridement and less frequently PCL or multiligament reconstructions, patellar subluxations and cartilage repairs (ACI, MACI).

The success of this procedure worldwide pertains to a combination of factors, such as the excellent detailed visualization of articular structures and the relative ease in accessing areas that were impossible to visualize trough classic arthrotomy. The posterior horn of the medial meniscus is a classic example. The minimally invasive character of the procedure makes for an excellent patient compliance because of the rapid postoperative healing and recovery, the lack of extensive postoperative scars and the shortened hospital stay. Some of these reasons are of definite value to the surgeon as well such as the reduced hospitalization time and with it, the diminished cost of this procedure. Also notable are the large (and continuously increasing) number of procedures that can be accomplished using standard arthroscopic approaches. Arthroscopic exploration and intervention is now surgically feasible in all large joints, being a frequent surgical intervention on the shoulder, ankle and hip for various types of intra and extraarticular pathology. Recent progress has been made in the arthroscopic evaluation of smaller joints such as the elbow and the radiocarpus, with various levels of postoperative success. This is all in the global trend for more minimally invasive, patient oriented surgery. However, knee arthroscopy remains by far the most frequent arthroscopic procedure that is performed worldwide. This is due, in part, to its historical longevity and the large number of well trained surgeons, as well as the extensive amount of knee pathology that can be addressed arthroscopically and the ease of access to the articular structures, compared to other joints.

R. Prejbeanu (ed.), *Atlas of Knee Arthroscopy*,
DOI 10.1007/978-1-4471-6593-4_1, © Springer-Verlag London 2015

1.1.2 Instruments

The primary goal at the start of the arthroscopic era was to inspect the interior of joints as clearly and accurately as possible. But even in the age of the arthroscopic surgery, high performance optical systems that provide optimum image quality cannot be taken for granted and great care must be taken in assembling an effective arthroscopic system.

The heart of arthroscopic system is the arthroscope (telescope) itself. It consists of an eyepiece, an attachment for the light cable, a series of lenses, and optical for transmitting light into the joint. The lens's fiberoptics and metal casing constitute the arthroscopic barrel. Older arthroscopes used achromatic lens systems that provided only a relatively small visual field. Modern arthroscopes are based on the Hopkins rod lens system, which combines a smaller overall diameter with a substantially larger visual field and brighter field. Arthroscopes are available with various view angles: O (forward-view scope) 30 wide-angle and 70 wide-angle.

Arthroscopes are available in various barrel lengths, depending on the manufacturer, A barrel length of 18 cm is recommended for knee arthroscopy. Some manufacturers offer shorter scopes for use in the knee, but these instruments make it difficult to inspect posterior areas such as the posterior horn of the medial meniscus in large knee joints or in patients with a thick subcutaneous tissue layer. Also portions of the posterior cruciate ligament (PCL) cannot be adequately visualized with a short scope.

The diameter of the arthroscope is determined by the dimensions of the lens system, the fiber optics and the metal barrel. Arthroscopes are available in various diameters. Standard arthroscopes designed for use in various joints have diameters ranging from 1.7 to 4 mm. The 4-mm arthroscope has become the standard for knee arthroscopy, and generally is no need to use smaller scopes in the knee. Even pediatric and adolescent knees can be diagnosed and treated with a 4-mm scope. Only very small knee joints in children under 5 years of age would require the use of a 2.4-mm scope. Barrel length, however, is a more important consideration in smaller joints than scope diameter. When using a long arthroscope, the surgeon is forced to work nearly freehanded because he cannot steady himself by bracing a finger or hand against the patient's knee to improve the control, and coordination of fine arthroscope movements.

Image quality is an important criterion that, unfortunately, is frequently neglected and is difficult to evaluate. In the majority of cases, arthroscopes are selected solely on the basis of viewing angle and outer diameter. When scopes from different manufacturer are compared, however it is common to find significant differences in their optical quality. The image transmitted by the scope should have sharp edges (if the camera is properly focused) and adequate brightness. The scope should have satisfactory resolution, i.e., it should be able to discriminate fine surface details.

Historically, arthroscopes had to be sterilized by gas. Today this method is no longer used due to environment concerns, and arthroscopes are sterilized in steam autoclaves (at 134 C). Scopes cannot be adequately sterilized with a disinfectant solution. The standard instrument recommended for knee arthroscopy is the 30 wide-angle arthroscope. The 70 scope is a useful adjunct, but it can be dispensed with by using arthroscopic mirrors or by switching the 30 scope to different portal. Since the indications for the 70 scopes are limited, this instrument should be only added, if at all, after an adequate number of 30 scopes have been obtained.

To fully utilize the physical properties of the oblique arthroscope, it is necessary to maneuver the scope within the joint and, if necessary, adjust the position of the joint. Thus a distinction is drawn between scope movements and joints movements.

The sheath, with a blunt obturator inserted, is introduced into the joint in preparation for arthroscopy. We do not recommend using a sharp trocar, as it may plunge into the joint space causing irreversible damage to the articular cartilage. Once the sheath has entered the joint, the obturator is replaced by the arthroscope. The sheath consists of three parts: Coupler (for securing the obturator or scope), spigot plane (for connecting the inflow and outflow tubing), sheath barrel – with suction openings, and an inflow channel for the distention medium.

To illuminate the joint interior, light from a light source is transmitted into the joint through a light cable and through glass fibers that are integrated into the arthroscope. Either a cold light source or xenon source may be used. The light provide to the arthroscope is transmitted to the arthroscope through a light cable (lightcord). Either a fiberoptic or fluid type cable may be used.

The basic elements of the video system are the video camera and the monitor. Digital video offers the added option of digital image processing and picture-in-a-picture (Digivideo, Karl Storz, Germany) is a feature that permits adjacent images to be displayed and compared. The system can be expanded by adding recording devices such as a VCR, video printer, or digital still-image recorder.

Arthroscopic surgery may involve procedures on the meniscus, ligaments or bone. Often it is necessary to detach tissue fragments and extract them from the joint. Mechanical instruments for knee arthroscopy have a relatively uniform design consisting of jaws, shaft, and handle. Manual action of the handle transmits the cutting or grasping force to the instrument jaws. The shaft may be straight or curved. The jaws may be straight or angled in relation to the shaft. The basket forceps, known also as a punch or cutting forceps is the most commonly used mechanical instrument. Various types and degrees of angulations are available, but straight or up-angled instruments are most often used. Basket forceps with an approximately 10° up-curved shaft and 10° up-angled jaws are useful to cut the posterior horn of the medial meniscus. In a very tight medial compartment, it can be extremely difficult to reach the posterior horn of the medial meniscus with a straight instrument, particularly since the medial tibial plateau is convex and the medial meniscus occupies a relatively high position on the back of the plateau.

Cutting with basket forceps is initiated at an accessible tissue margin, such as the free edge on the size and shape of the jaws. The tissue fragments remain in the joint initially, and they are removed from the joint with a shaver or large-bore irrigation cannula at the end of the resection. Special types of basket forceps are: **suction punch** – which is a basket forceps connected to a vacuum suction, virtually eliminates the intraarticular retention of tissue fragments from the joint as they are excised. This requires considerably larger shaft diameter than ordinary basket forceps; **retrograde basket forceps** – tissue structures located just below or adjacent to the instrument portal are difficult to reach with forward-cutting basket forceps. In a bucket – handle tear, for example, the anterior attachment of the fragment may be inadequately detached with a basket forceps passed through medial instrument portal. This problem can be solved using a retrograde or back-biting basket forceps.

The basic instrument for arthroscopic surgery is a narrow, angled grasping forceps, which combines the advantages of small size and tip angulations. It is introduced in the closed position, advanced to the target structure, and is it slightly rotated and opened for grasping the detached tissue fragment. Grasping forceps are required for the removal of: meniscal fragments (partially detached), loose bodies, cartilage flaps, osteophytes, retrieving a synovial biopsy, grasping the sutures for arthroscopic repairs and reconstruction (cruciate ligament reconstruction, reefing the medial retinaculum, meniscal repairs).

Arthroscopic scissors were used in the early days of arthroscopic surgery for detaching meniscal fragments. The problem with scissors is that considerable force must be applied in order to divide hard or scarred areas such as meniscal tissue. As a result scissors are rarely nowadays and have been superseded by electrocautery hooks or slender basket forceps.

Mechanical knives were widely used in the early days of arthroscopic surgery, and some surgeons still recommend them today. Knives should definitely not be used in tight posterior joint areas, as in surgeries on the posterior horn of the medial meniscus. Careless manipulations may cause the knife tip to break off in the joint, or the knife may advance farther posterior than intended.

Motorized instruments or shavers have become a standard and established part of the arthroscopic surgical routine. A motorized instrument set is comprised of: control unit, connecting cable between the handpiece and control unit, handpiece, blades, suction. Because the shaver is an expensive and complex instrument, it is advisable to use the drive for other powered devices such as saws and drills. This expands the applications of the system not just to other joints but to a variety of surgical procedures.

Electrosurgical instruments have been used for decades in urology and general surgery. They are commonly used to achieve hemostasis in parenchymatous organs. Starting in 1981, electrocautery devices were adapted for use in arthroscopic surgery. Electrosurgical techniques are based entirely on the thermal effect produced by electric current. Electrosurgical instruments, or electrocautery devices, may be operated in the coagulation mode or the cutting mode.

A number of arthroscopic surgeries require specialized instruments. A large assortment of these instruments is available on the market, and a variety of different surgical techniques have been developed for their use. In many cases, slight modifications of traditional instruments may be adapted for use in arthroscopic surgery, making it unnecessary to procure costly devices.

Chisels. Traditional chisels are difficult to insert into joints and may accidentally gouge the articular cartilage, producing deep chondral lesions. A chisel with rounded edges not only protects the cartilage but is much easier to pass since sharp edges tend to "hang up" on or in the instrument portal during insertion. Besides the rounded chisel, a curved chisel is a very useful instrument for notch plasty. Following the removal of osteophytes or other bone tissue, the resection side should be smoothed to create a homogeneous surface.

Curettes. Sharp spoons, are commonly used for debriding bone tunnels. This is a tedious process, however, and it is easier to smooth and round off bone tunnels with curettes that have a special bone bevel. These instruments can also be used to debride bone surfaces covered with soft tissue or scar tissue.

Arthroscopic operating room instrumentation (Figs. 1.1, 1.2, 1.3, and 1.4):

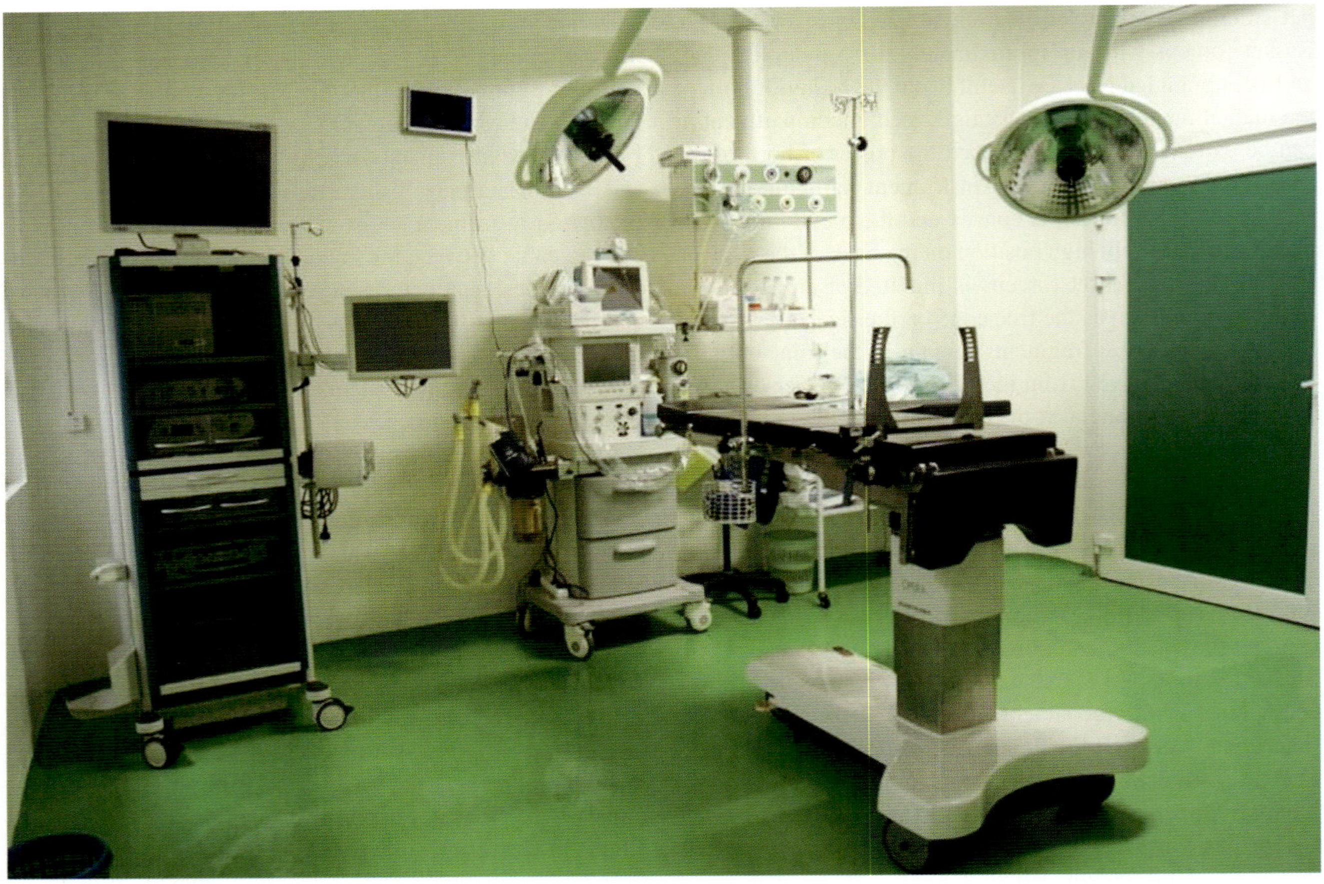

Fig. 1.1 Operating room dedicated for arthroscopic intervention, equipped with arthroscopic tower, anesthetic device, operating table with "leg holder" device which allows patient position with the knee in variable flexion. The arthroscopic tower incorporates equipement for data archiving

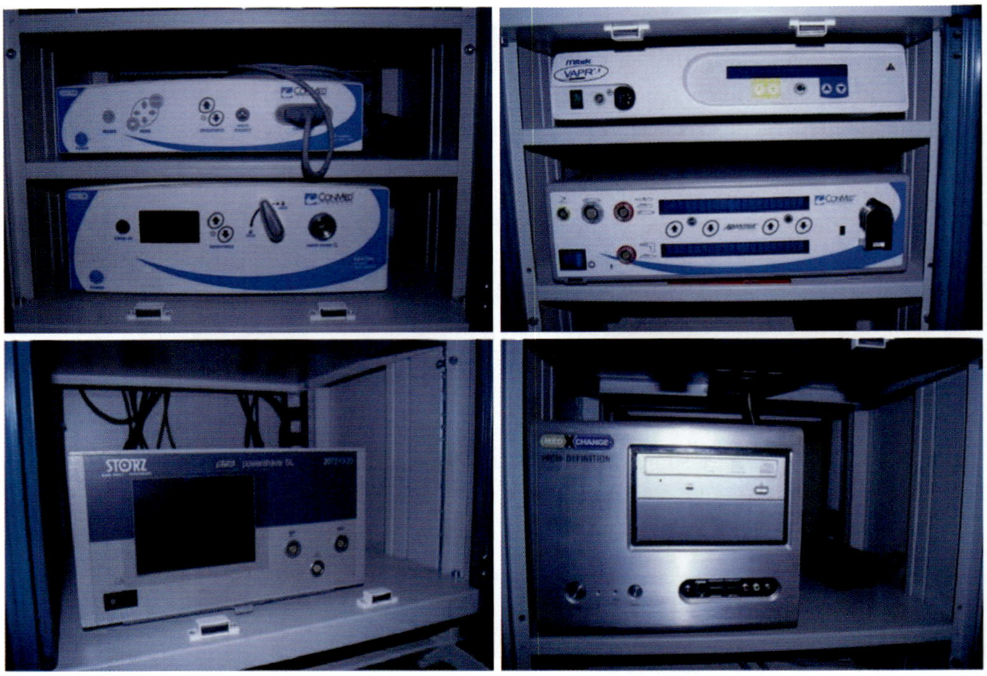

Fig. 1.2 Typical camera, light source, shaver and electro frequency

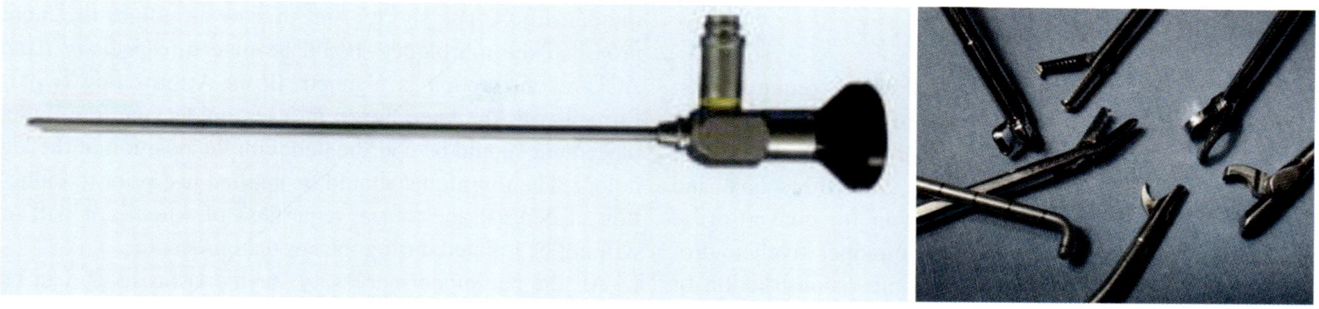

Fig. 1.3 Optical piece (telescope) at 30°, 4 mm (Hopkins). Forceps, pointed probes and arthroscopic punches

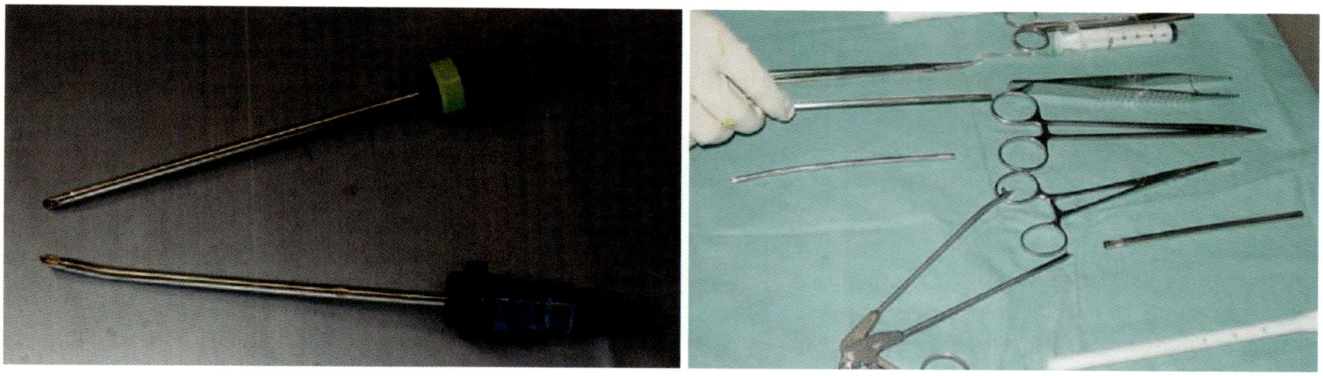

Fig. 1.4 Shaver pieces for soft tissue and miscellaneous instruments (No. 11 scalpel blade)

1.1.3 Positioning

Positioning has to fulfill the following requirements: **Accessibility of all joint compartments** – the position should permit access to all joint compartments. It should also provide easy access for establishing the arthroscopic and instrument portals; **convenience**, option for converting to open surgery – if the surgeon decides intraoperatively to proceed with a more complex arthroscopic reconstruction or with open surgery, this should be possible without a change of setup or time-consuming repositioning of the leg. For example, if the leg must be moved to apposition of 90° knee flexion, this should be possible without breaching sterility; **simple devices** – the device used to hold or position the leg for arthroscopy should be simple and economical. The simpler the positioning device, the faster it can be mounted on the operating table and the shorter the learning curve for operating room personnel; **free tourniquet access** – there should be unrestricted access to perform surgery with the deflated tourniquet in place and for inflating the tourniquet as needed during the operation. Either a straight-leg of flexed-leg position may be used.

The straight leg position for arthroscopic surgery meets all the requirements for a simple, fast, and secure technique. A simple side post is mounted on the operating table on the lateral side of the thigh. The side post is positioned about a handwidth proximal to the base of the patella. One advantage of this position is that allows the surgeon to be seated during the procedure. Sitting is not only comfortable but is also convenient for applying varus/valgus stresses to open the joint compartments, allowing the surgeon to concentrate on manual manipulation of the arthroscope and operating instruments.

Flexed-Knee Position. In this position the knee is flexed 90° in a padded leg holder. This provides a medial fulcrum so that both varus and valgus stresses can be applied to the knee joint. This positioning technique is disadvantageous in that extra equipment is needed (leg holder), and that the surgeon must stand during the procedure in order to apply varus/valgus stresses to the joint. It is more difficult to control these forces than in the straight-leg position.

Tourniquet. Tourniquet control and limb exsanguinations are controversial issues in arthroscopic surgery. A bloodless field provides the best intraarticular image quality. All surgical manipulation in the knee joint can be done without significant image clouding, and troublesome bleeding is eliminated. IF surgery is performed without a tourniquet, bleeding can seriously obscure vision. This not means, however, that tourniquet inflation or exsanguinations is necessary for every arthroscopic surgery. A discriminating approach is required. The pneumatic tourniquet is placed on the proximal third of the thigh or the junction of the proximal and middle thirds. The shorter and thicker the thigh, the more proximal the tourniquet should be placed, especially if an ACL reconstruction is planned. IF an Arthroscopy is performed with the knee flexed in a leg holder, the tourniquet placement should be coordinated with the position of the leg holder. The tourniquet should be applied just prior to induction of general anesthesia, regardless of whether it will or will not be inflated during the surgical procedure.

All the equipment necessary for the arthroscopy can be arranged separately positioned in a logical order around the operating table, but it is more efficient to place all the devices on a dedicated arthroscopy cart or trolley. The equipment should be arranged in a way that the surgeon can see all important control devices and can quickly detect any malfunctions or faulty settings. The monitor should be at the surgeon's eye level, so its placement will depend on whether the surgeon works in a sitting or standing position (Fig. 1.5).

In tight joints or cases where difficult surgical conditions are anticipated, whether in the knee or in other joints, optimum muscle relaxation is essential, which can only be accomplished by general anesthesia. It is more easily controlled in terms of onset and muscle relaxation. Even in ambulatory settings, general anesthesia is better for achieving rapid and complete post procedure recovery. Ultra short–acting anesthetics with a short half life are excellent choice under these circumstances.

Spinal or epidural anesthesia can be used for arthroscopic surgery. Spinal anesthesia has a more predictable onset of action, but there is a potential for adverse circulatory effects and for postoperative spinal headache and bladder dysfunction.

Local anesthesia can be administrated by the surgeon himself although a standby anesthesiologist should be available. The preoperative preparations are the same as for other anesthetic techniques. Because local anesthesia does not produce muscle relaxation, difficulties may be encountered in the visualizing the posterior horn of the medial meniscus, for example, or in tight joints. Although local anesthesia is acceptable in theory for most arthroscopic surgeries, it is recommended only for selective cases.

Technique: Infiltration with local anesthetic – once the optimum site for the arthroscope portal has been selected, it can be infiltrated with a local anesthetic (bupivacaine 0.25 %) containing 1:200,000 epinephrine. Approximately 5 ml of solution is sufficient. The injection needle can be advanced into the joint cavity without injecting a large amount of local anesthetic into the joint. An important advantage of local anesthetic is that it prevents minor bleeding from the arthroscope portal in a non – bloodless field. It also numbs the pain – sensitive synovial membrane, so that the patients rarely complain of postoperative pain in the area of the arthroscope portal.

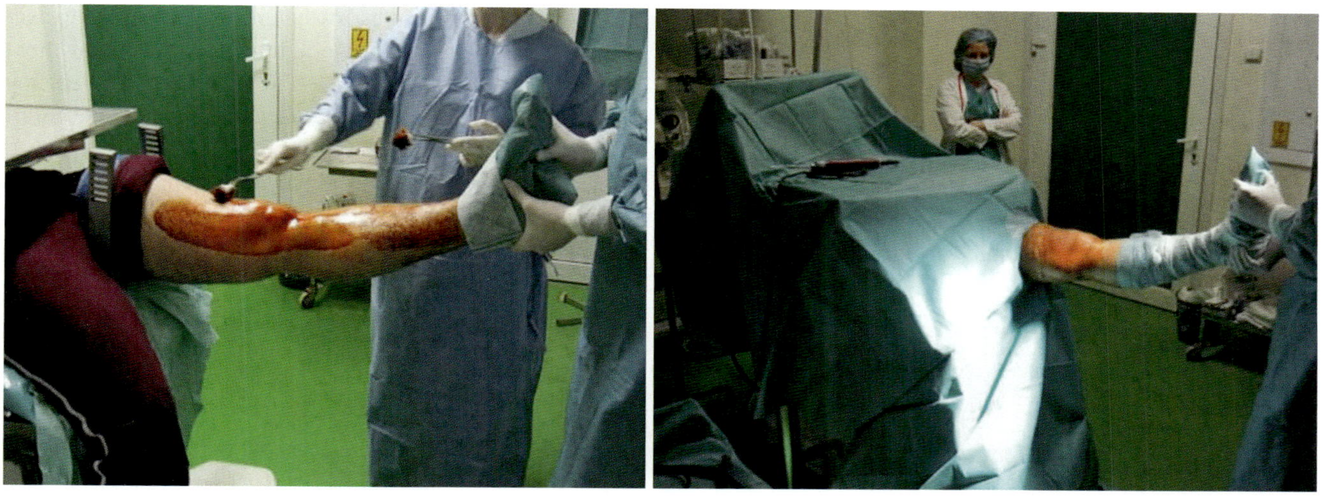

Fig. 1.5 Patient positioned on the operating table during sterile draping

1.1.4 ACL Reconstruction

After anesthesia is performed, the patient is positioned supine on the table with the leg part removed and the feet hanging down. The unoperated leg is placed in a proclivity holder. Alternatively, a normal table can be used. The thigh is placed in the leg holder over the Tourniquet band. Over the patient we use a Mayo table to support the instruments during surgery. It is mandatory that the knee be flexed to over 120° in order to drill the femoral tunnel. Alternatively, flexible reamers can be used [3]. A standard HD arthroscopy tower and ACL instrument set (reamers, guides and graft bench) are prepared (see Sect. 3.5.2.1). We use a shaver, reamer, chair and a second Mayo table compared to when performing arthroscopy alone. We do not routinely use a fluid pump (Fig. 1.6).

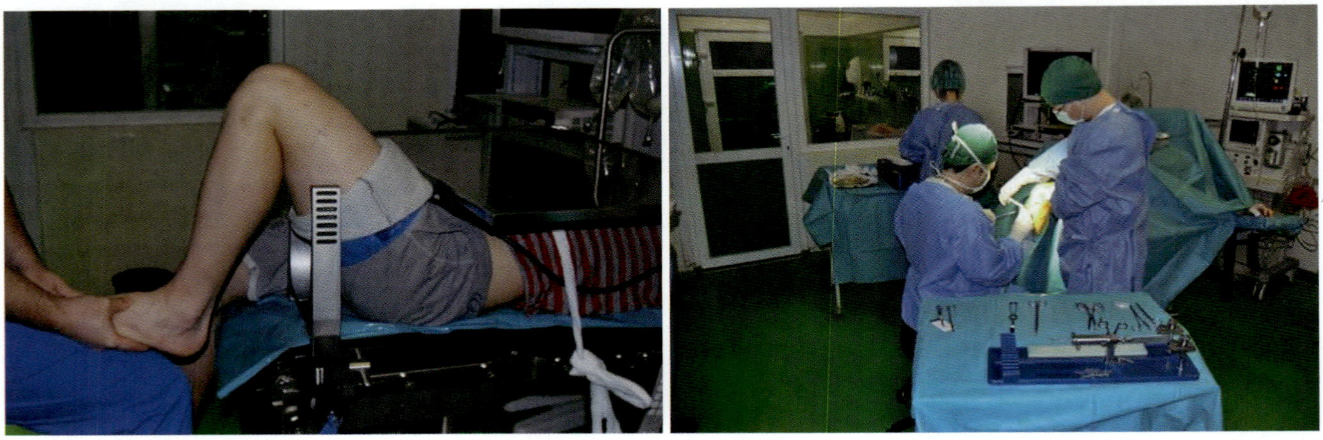

Fig. 1.6 Application of the leg holder on the thigh so that the knee can be flexed over 120°. A standard setup for ACL reconstruction with 2 back tables, the surgeon sited, helped by a scrub technician and a resident in training

1.2 Normal Anatomy

1.2.1 The Menisci

The menisci are two semilunar biconcave disks that reside within the medial and lateral tibio-femoral joints. They are fibro cartilaginous C-shape disc interposed between femoral and tibial condyles with strong attachments to bone and poor vascularization throughout its inner 2/3. Once thought as a vestige of leg muscle, they are now considered a vital structure with various functions: chondroprotection through weight distribution by enlarging the contact area between the femur and the tibia, weight bearing, joint stabilization, joint lubrication, articular cartilage nutrition, and proprioception [4].

1.2.1.1 Medial Meniscus

The medialmeniscus is somewhat semicircular in appearance. It is approximately 3.5 cm in length in the anteroposterior dimension and considerably wider posterior than it is anterior. Its radius of curvature varies, giving it greater length in the sagittal plane than in the coronal plane. The anterior horn is attached to the tibial plateau in the area of the anterior intercondylar fossa, 6–7 mm in front of the ACL insertion. An intermeniscal, or "transverse" ligament is present in 64 % of individuals; this connects the anterior horn (posterior fibers) of the medialmeniscus and the anterior horn (anterior fibers) of the lateral meniscus. The posterior horn attaches to the posterior intercondylar fossa between the attachments of the lateral meniscus and the posterior cruciate ligament (PCL). The medialmeniscus is continuously attached to the joint capsule along the entire periphery. The coronary ligament represents the tibial portion of this capsular attachment. At its midpoint, the medialmeniscus is firmly attached to the femur and tibia through a robust thickening in the capsule known as the deep medial collateral ligament [5].

The medial meniscus' posterior horn is smaller (28.5 mm^2) than the anterior horn (61.4 mm^2) but has a more stable implantation area. The anterior horn has a variable implantation area on the tibial plateau and is more prone to avulsions than the posterior horn. The types of anterior horn attachment have been described by Berlet and Fowler [6]. In cadaveric studies it has been shown that the posterior horn of the medial meniscus can be attached to the PCL's insertion while the anterior horn relates to the insertion of the ACL by means of an intermeniscal ligament or other soft tissues. The remaining large portion of the meniscus is attached to the joint capsule and the capsular ligaments. The body of the medial meniscus is also attached to the deep medial collateral ligament, which is a thickening of the medial capsular attachments that reaches from the tibia to the femur (Figs. 1.7 and 1.8).

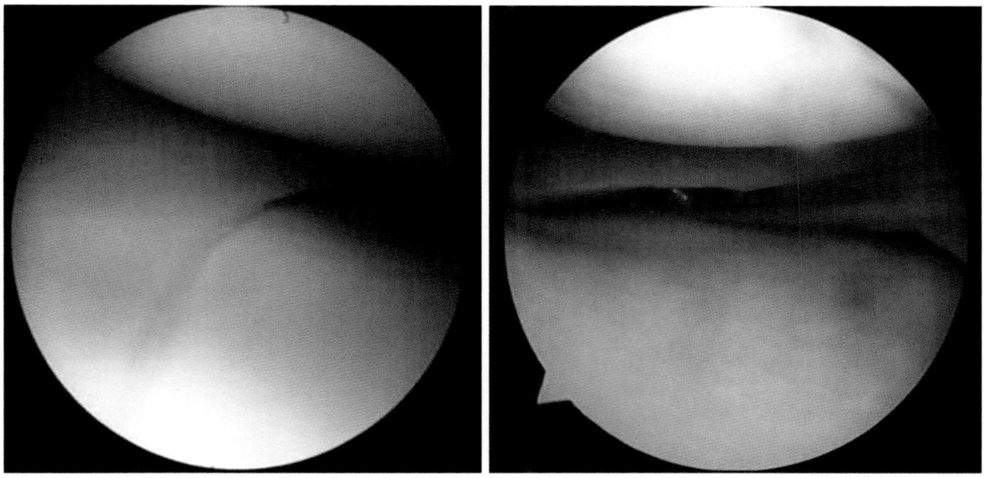

Fig. 1.7 Arthroscopic views of a normal medial meniscus through the antero medial and lateral portals respectively

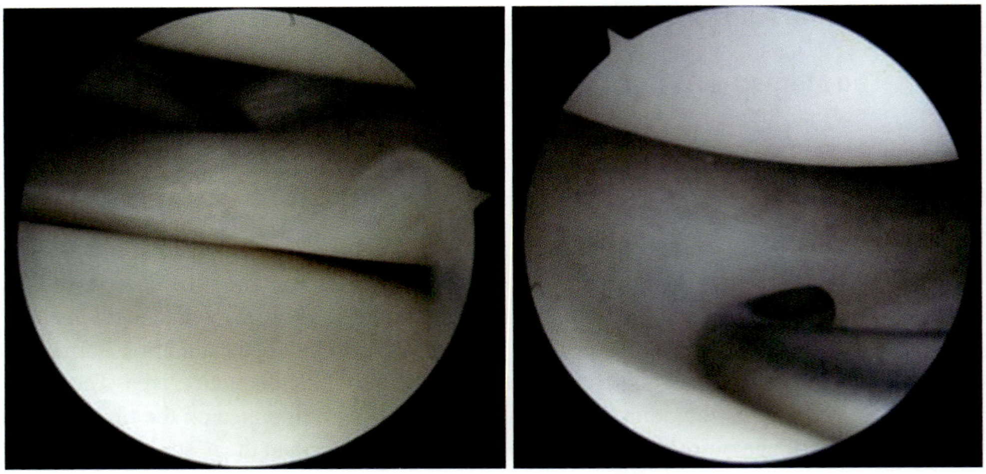

Fig. 1.8 View of a normal lateral meniscus. The physiological lack of capsular adherences can be noticed surrounding the intra-articular portion of the popliteal tendon. An anatomic variation of the lateral meniscus – discoid meniscus, checked for inconsistencies with a probe

1.2.1.2 Lateral Meniscus

The lateral meniscus covers a larger portion of the tibial surface than does the medialmeniscus. Its radius of curvature remains fairly constant, giving the lateral meniscus an almost circular appearance. The anterior horn is attached anterior to the intercondylar eminence, just posterior and lateral to the ACL attachment with which it partially blends. The posterior horn attaches posterior to the intercondylar eminence.

In 50 % of individuals, anterior fibers of the posterior enthesis extend to the lateral aspect of the medial femoral condyle, forming the anterior meniscofemoral ligament (ligament of Humphry). In 76 % of cases, the posterior fibers of the posterior horn cross posterior to the PCL and attach to the intercondylar fossa of the medial femoral condyle, forming the posterior meniscofemoral ligament (ligament of Wrisberg). The lateral meniscus has only a loose peripheral attachment to the capsule, which is interrupted by the popliteus tendon. Lateral meniscal variants, including the most recognized discoid meniscus, have a reported prevalence as high as 16.6 % [7].

The anterior and posterior horns are attached closer to each other on the tibia. These attachments can also act as visual and anatomic landmarks during ACL reconstruction. The posterior horn is positioned posterior to the lateral tibial eminence and is attached to the PCL and the femur through the anterior meniscofemoral ligament (described by Humphrey). One particularity about the lateral meniscus is a portion that lies near the part that comes in contact with the popliteal tendon. It is called the popliteal hiatus and it represents a part of the meniscus where it has no attachment neither to the femur nor to the tibia [8]. Thompson et al. [9] have shown with the aid of 3D MRI, that the lateral meniscus has a greater excursion (11.2 mm on average) than the medial meniscus (5.2 mm on average) through the knee range of motion.

1.2.2 The Cruciate Ligaments (ACL, PCL)

The ACL and PCL are two of the most important stabilizers of the knee joint. They are placed in the middle of the knee inside the intercondylar notch extending from anteromedial to posterolateral (ACL) and from the posterior tibia to anteromedially (PCL).

The anterior cruciate ligament (ACL) can be viewed as a band reaching from the anteromedial aspect of the tibia, just in front of the tibial spine, to the internal aspect of the posterior portion of the lateral femoral condyle [10, 11]. There have been several studies performed to determine the structure of the ACL. The most accepted model nowadays is the double-bundle one [10, 12, 13]. Thus, the ACL has been divided in the anteromedial bundle (AM) and the posterolateral bundle (PL). These two bundles act in different ways during the flexion-extension movement of the knee. They are parallel during full extension, with the AM bundle being longer (34 mm/22.5 mm) and very loose while the PL bundle is tight [14]. This configuration changes in knee flexion, were the AM becomes tight while the PL bundle is loose. The flexion of the knee also causes the two bundles to be wrapped around each other.

The posterior cruciate ligament (PCL) extends from the posterior aspect of the tibia to the medial femoral condyle and medial aspect of the intercondylar notch. It is longer, thicker, stronger and has bigger implantation areas than the ACL [15]. The PCL is also made up of two bundles – the anterolateral (AL) and the posteromedial (PM) [10, 16, 17]. The AL bundle is larger and stronger than the PM bundle, and has a curved shape in knee extension. During flexion, the PCL extends and becomes tight, preventing posterior tibial translation.

1.2.3 Arthroscopy Portals

Usually, there are two main portals that are used for knee arthroscopy – the anterolateral and the anteromedial ones. They serve as access for the arthroscopic piece (light and irrigation) as well as the punches used for meniscectomy or exploratory instruments. These two portals are placed on both sides of the patellar tendon at the level of the inferior patellar pole. Two "soft-spots" can be felt when palpating this area, and they act as a landmark when beginning the surgery (Figs. 1.9 and 1.10).

Besides these two standard portals, there is also a number of other accessory portals that can be performed, depending on the scheduled procedure and the surgeon's technique. The superomedial portal is made with the knee in extension and is usually used for irrigation, while the superolateral portal can be used as an aspiration or injection site.

Accessory anterior portals may be needed, depending on the pathology encountered. The accessory medial and lateral portals are created under direct visualization. The accessory medial portal is more medial and inferior to the standard portal, whereas the accessory lateral portal is more lateral and inferior to the standard portal [18].

Posterior portals are used for visualizing the posterior horn of the meniscus and the posterior cruciate ligament and are used in its reconstruction procedure. The posteromedial portal is located 1 cm above the joint line behind the medial collateral ligament. The posterolateral portal is made 1 cm above the joint line between the lateral collateral ligament and the biceps femoralis insertion tendon. In order to safely create a posterior portal, Kim et al. conducted a study with the aid of the MRI (90° knee flexion). They simulated the knee's position during arthroscopy and aimed to determine the dimensions and structures located in the posterior compartment, specifically the popliteal artery. They concluded that injury to the popliteal artery can be avoided by penetrating the posterior septum lateral to medial [19]. On the same note, McGinnis et al. aimed to establish a safe zone located on the posteromedial aspect of the knee, which could be used for creating arthroscopic portals without causing any neurovascular lesions. They concluded that at least two posteromedial portals could be placed at once in the knee during the complex arthroscopy of the posterior compartment [20].

Another portal described is the transpatellar tendon portal. This is located 1 cm distal to the patella, splitting the tendon in half longitudinally. It can be used in isolated meniscectomy procedures that involve bucket-handle or other complex tears. This portal can act as an aid in performing arthroscopy, and can reduce the time of the procedure. Some side effects on using the transpatellar portal could be recurrent anterior knee pain and patellar tendon shortening.

The standard technique used for creating the arthroscopy portals:

- **Position** – the knee joint is flexed approximately 70° and the foot or lower leg is placed on the thigh of the seated surgeon to maintain a constant flexion angle.
- **Identification of anatomical structures** – first the patellar apex, patellar tendon, and lateral femoral condyle, are identified by palpation. The lateral triangle, bounded, by the lateral border of the patellar tendon, the medial circumference of the lateral femoral condyle, and distally by the superior rim of the anterior horn of the lateral meniscus, is palpated. The patellar apex provides a key landmark for placement of the arthroscope portal.
- **Portal site** – The optimum site for the arthroscope portal is determined by reference to the palpable anatomic structures and any anatomic peculiarities that are present. Difficulties may result from a low-ridding patella (patella infera) or high-ridding patella (patella alta), previous surgery, scars, or prior unhealed arthroscope portals in revision surgery. The high anterolateral portal is considered the standard viewing portal in arthroscopic knee surgery.
- **High anterolateral portal** – this portal is placed adjacent to the lateral border of the patella tendon of the level of the patellar apex. It is placed slightly higher if the patella is low-riding and slightly lower if the patella is high-riding (determined by lateral x-ray film)
- **Skin incision** – a transverse skin incision approximately 6 mm long is made with scalpel (No. 11 or No. 15 blade). The knife is the rotated 90° and a vertical incision about 4–5 mm long is made in the lateral capsule. Finally the scalpel is partially withdrawn and, on reaching the skin level, is again rotated 90° to avoid making a cruciate incision
- **Insertion of the sheath** – the arthroscope sheath armed with a blunt obturator is introduced into the joint. The blunt obturator should securely locked in place at this stage to avoid capsular damage during insertion or, if plunging occurs, damage to the synovial ACL covering or even-punched-out defects or local elevations of the hyaline cartilage. The sheath is inserted with a careful rotary motion, initially directing the sheath toward the ACL. A rotary motion is important to uniformly reduce the tissue resistance at the skin and capsular incisions. At first there is a gradual increase in tissue resistance, but this subsides when the obturator has penetrated the joint capsule.
- **Extension of the knee joint** – when the sheath and blunt obturator have penetrated the fibrous capsule and tissue resistance declines, the knee joint is extended, and the sheath is carefully advanced into the medial portion of the superior recess. If the sheath can be moved slightly in the medial and lateral directions, the examiner may be certain that it has entered the intraarticular space.

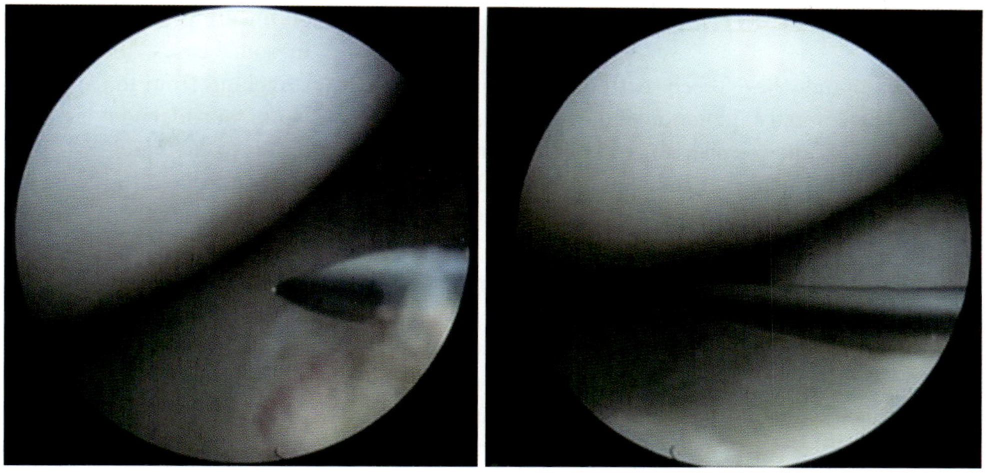

Fig. 1.9 Intra-articular view from the anterolateral portal; determination of the anteromedial portal insertion point. Fig. – Intra-articular view from the anterolateral portal; the trajectory of tools passed through the anteromedial portal

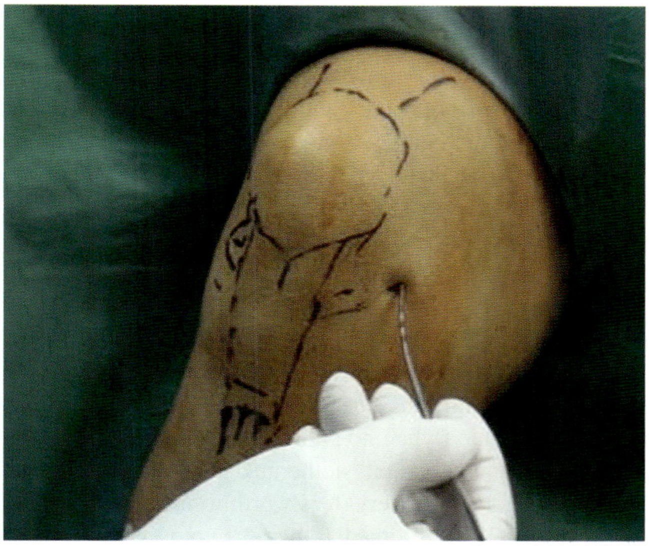

Fig. 1.10 Anatomical landmarks and main portals (anterolateral and anteromedial) drawings on a knee before the arthroscopy begins

1.2.4 Exploration

Once the portals have been performed, the surgeon can proceed to the initial exploration of the knee. The joint will be thoroughly checked for pathology in its structures, following a systematic pattern. After inserting the optical piece inside the joint through the medial portal, the medial meniscus can be seen once the tibia is externally rotated with valgus stress. Afterwards, with the knee fully extended, the exploration continues in the medial gutter and the suprapatellar pouch where the surgeon can find loose bodies, synovitis or certain plicae.

By twisting the optical chord with 180° we can inspect the patellofemoral joint. Cartilage damage can be assessed and the surgeon can also evaluate the patellar tracking on the trochlear groove. Patellar maltracking is a serious issue that can lead to chronic patellar subluxation and anterior knee pain (Figs. 1.11, 1.12, 1.13, and 1.14).

The exploration continues with the exploration of the lateral gutter, checking the popliteus tendon's insertion and for eventual plicae. Moving on to the lateral compartment, we can visualize the anterior horn of the lateral meniscus and a small portion of the lateral tibiofemoral joint. The integrity of the meniscus is tested out with a probe.

We flex the knee at 90° and we inspect the medial compartment. The medial meniscus, and the medial tibiofemoral joint can be thoroughly checked for pathology. Existing medial meniscal tears can be diagnosed and resected, as well as obtaining a proper evaluation of the cartilage damage. This is usually the area of the knee were the surgeon spends the most time during arthroscopic interventions. By moving the arthroscope towards the middle of the joint, in the intercondylar notch, the ACL and PCL can be checked for consistency and strength. Their integrity is checked by pulling on them with a probe in order to see if they come lose at any point. The anterior drawer can be also performed during arthroscopic surveillance, for an increased specificity. In some cases, the ligamentum mucosum can be viewed stretching from the superior edge of the notch towards the Hoffa fat pad, and it is often excised due to the impairment it brings to ACL and PCL visualization (Figs. 1.15 and 1.16).

By advancing with the scope through the notch and facing the light medially, the surgeon can also evaluate the posteromedial corner. In order to achieve a good visualization we recommend using a 70° scope placed as before, through the intercondylar notch (modified Gillquist view).

Finally, for a good view of the lateral compartment as well as the posterior horn of the lateral meniscus, the knee will be brought in the so-called figure-four position (90° flexion, adduction, maximum external rotation). This opens up the lateral compartment allowing the surgeon to inspect the entire lateral meniscus, the popliteal hiatus, as well as the entire lateral tibiofemoral joint to search for chondral damage.

After finishing the procedure, the knee must be cleaned. The surgeon must be sure that there are no remaining loose bodies left over from meniscectomy or other procedures that were carried out (synovectomy, plica removal, Hoffa fat pad). These loose bodies may be the cause of latter chronic pains and can lead to a bad patient outcome. Before the procedure is over and suture is done, opening the tourniquet helps us see if there is no important active bleeding inside the joint.

Follow-up visits are very important in achieving a good result. The patient must be encouraged to bend the knee throughout the full range of motion, walk with full load on the operated limb (when no chondral reparatory procedures were made) and attend physiotherapy sessions according to protocol until full recovery. It is worth to mention that usually the follow-up for a medial meniscectomy is shorter and the physical recovery is obtained easier than in the case of lateral meniscectomy [21].

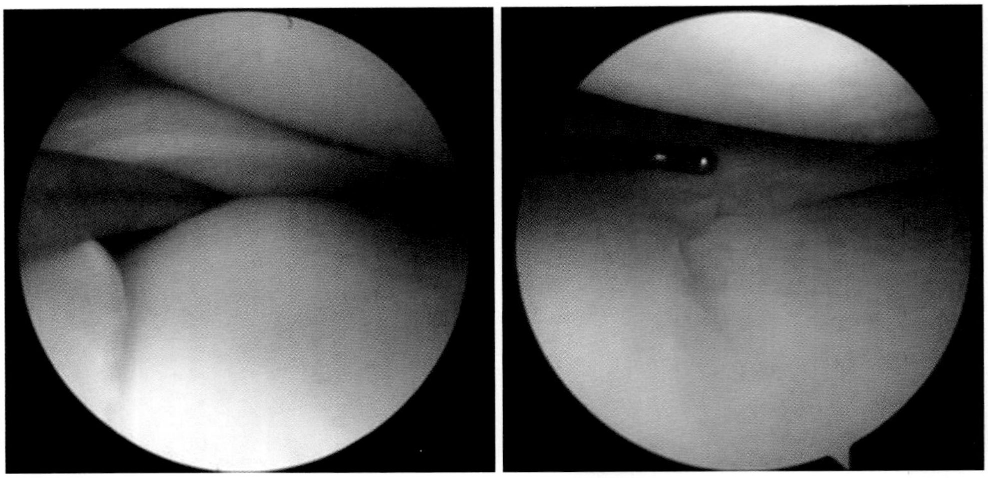

Fig. 1.11 Probing of the medial meniscus on it's tibial and femoral surfaces

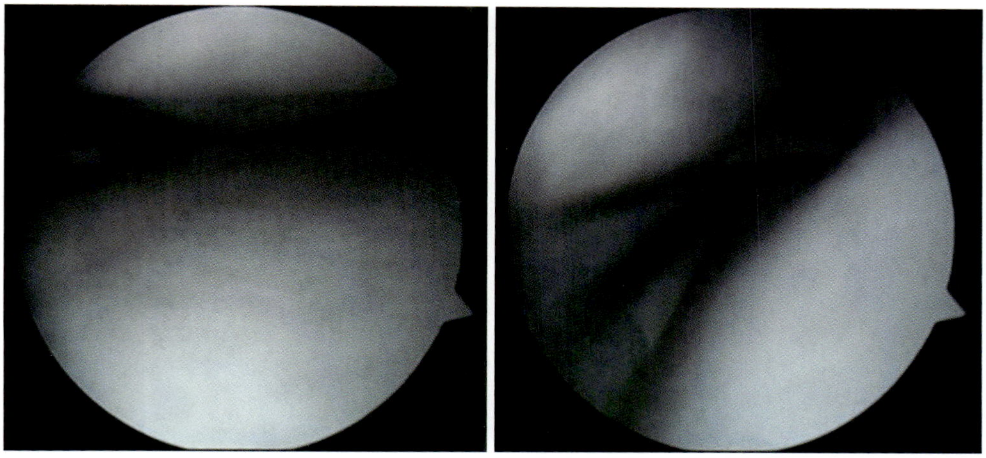

Fig. 1.12 The inspection of the posterior horn and insertion point of the medial meniscus with the probe

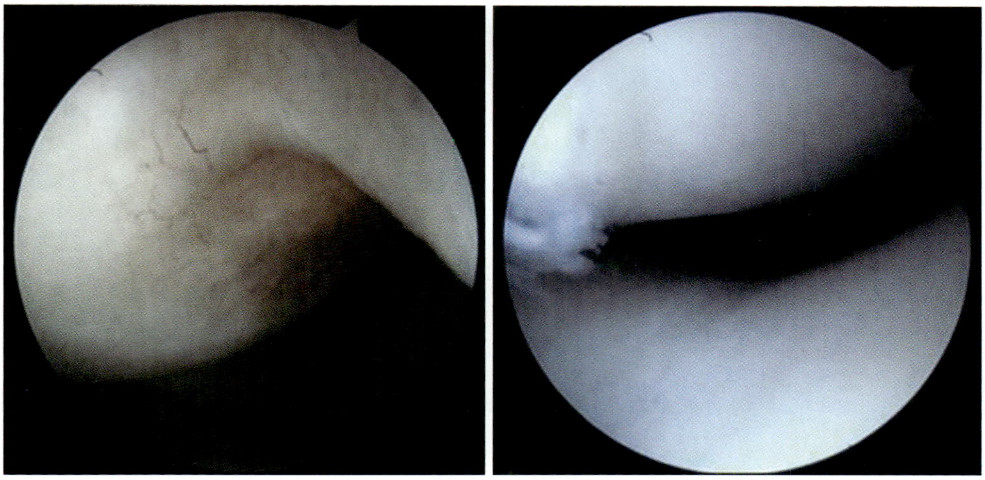

Fig. 1.13 Arthroscopic view of the medial gutter seen through the anteromedial portal. Arthroscopic views of the patellofemoral joint; checking for chondral damage and patellar tracking

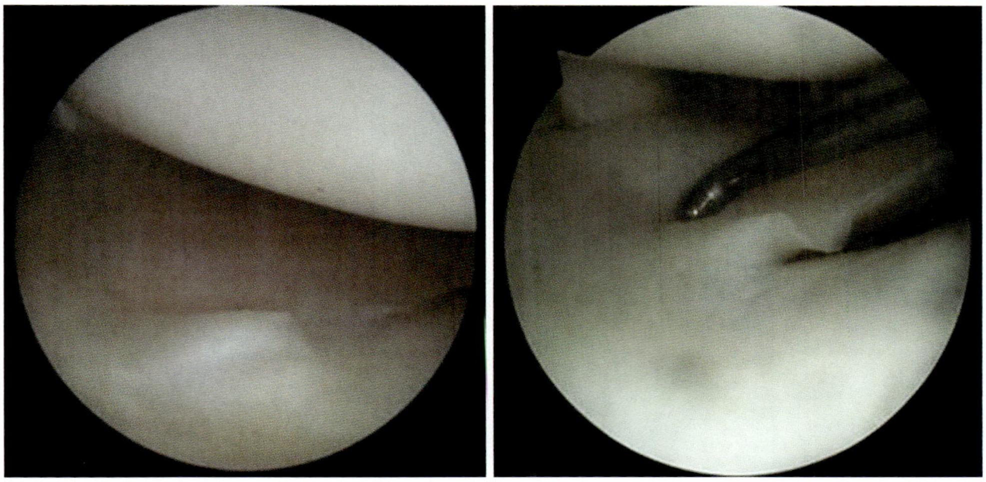

Fig. 1.14 View of the anterior horn of the lateral meniscus; the popliteal tendon can be viewed in the posterior aspect of the external rim of the meniscus. Checking the superior surface of the lateral meniscus for inconsistencies with the probe

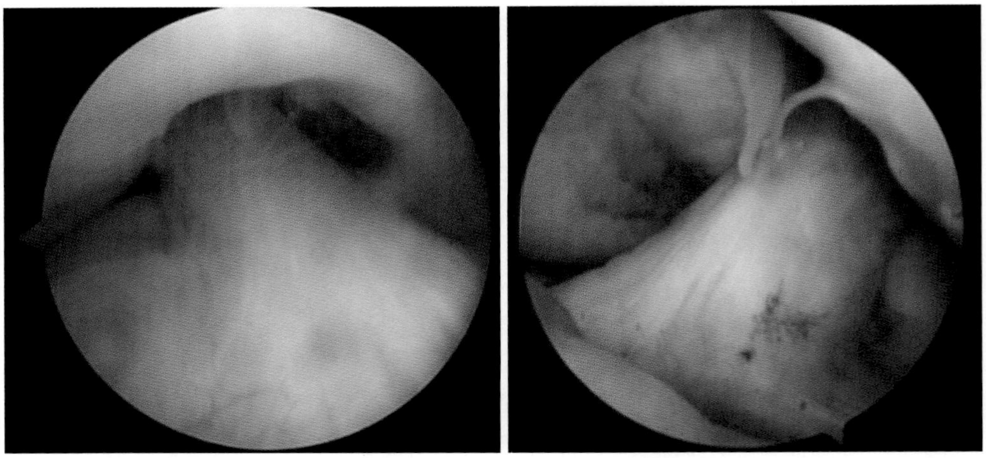

Fig. 1.15 The intercondylar notch viewed from the anterolateral and medial portals respectively, normal ACL with the knee close to extension and 90° of flexion

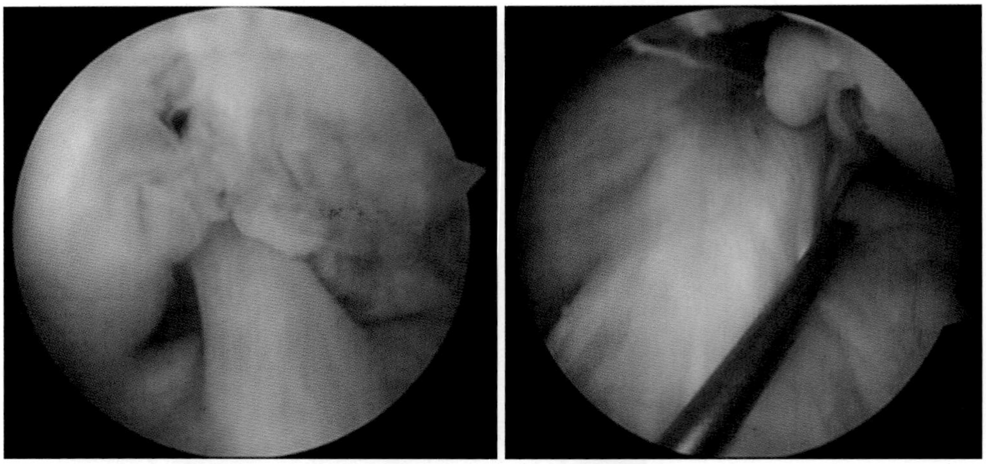

Fig. 1.16 Synovitis surrounding normal and well structured ACLs; view from the anterolateral and medial portals respectively. The integrity of the ACL is done by pulling it with the aid of a probe

References

1. Garrett WE, Swiontkowski MF, Weinstein JN, Callaghan J, Rosier RN, Berry DJ, Harrast J, Derosa GP. American Board of Orthopaedic Surgery Practice of the Orthopaedic Surgeon: part II, certification examination case mix. J Bone Joint Surg Am. 2006;88:660–7.
2. Takagi K. Practical experience using Takagi's arthroscope. J Jpn Orthop Assoc. 1933;8:132.
3. Silver AG, Kaar SG, Grisell MK, Reagan JM, Farrow LD. Comparison between rigid and flexible systems for drilling the femoral tunnel through an anteromedial portal in anterior cruciate ligament reconstruction. Arthroscopy. 2010;26(6):790–5.
4. Seedhom BB, Dowson D, Wright V. Proceedings: functions of the menisci. A preliminary study. Ann Rheum Dis. 1974;33:111.
5. Renstrom P, Johnson RJ. Anatomy and biomechanics of the menisci. Clin Sports Med. 1990;9:523–38.
6. Berlet GC, Fowler PJ. The anterior horn of the medial meniscus: an anatomic study of its insertion. Am J Sports Med. 1998;26:540–3.
7. Vandermeer RD, Cunningham FK. Arthroscopic treatment of the discoid lateral meniscus: results of longterm follow-up. Arthroscopy. 1989;5:101–9.
8. Simonian PT, Sussmann PS, van Trommel M, et al. Popliteomeniscal fasciculi and lateral meniscal stability. Am J Sports Med. 1997;25:849–53.
9. Thompson WO, Thaete FL, Fu FH, Dye SF. Tibial meniscal dynamics using three-dimensional reconstruction of magnetic resonance images. Am J Sports Med. 1991;19:210–6.
10. Girgis FG, Marshall JL, Monajem A. The cruciate ligaments of the knee joint. Anatomical, functional and experimental analysis. Clin Orthop Relat Res. 1975;106:216–31.
11. Arnoczky SP. Anatomy of the anterior cruciate ligament. Clin Orthop Relat Res. 1983;172:19–25.
12. Palmer I. On the injuries to the ligaments of the knee joint: a clinical study. Acta Chir Scand. 1938;91:1–282.
13. Smith BA, Livesay GA, Woo SL. Biology and biomechanics of the anterior cruciate ligament. Clin Sports Med. 1993;12(4):637–70.
14. Hollis JM, Takai S, Adams DJ, et al. The effects of knee motion and external loading on the length of the anterior cruciate ligament (ACL): a kinematic study. J Biomech Eng. 1991;113(2):208–14.
15. Harner CD, Baek GH, Vogrin TM, et al. Quantitative analysis of human cruciate ligament insertions. Arthroscopy. 1999;15(7):741–9.
16. Amis AA, Bull AM, Gupte CM, et al. Biomechanics of the PCL and related structures: posterolateral, posteromedial and meniscofemoral ligaments. Knee Surg Sports Traumatol Arthrosc. 2003;11(5):271–81.
17. Van Dommelen BA, Fowler PJ. Anatomy of the posterior cruciate ligament. A review. Am J Sports Med. 1989;17(1):24–9.
18. Kusayama T, Harner CD, Carlin GJ, Xerogeanes JW, Smith BA. Anatomical and biomechanical characteristics of human meniscofemoral ligaments. Knee Surg Sports Traumatol Arthrosc. 1994;2:234–7.
19. Kim SJ, Song HT, Moon HK, Chun YM, Chang WH. The safe establishment of a transseptal portal in the posterior knee. Knee Surg Sports Traumatol Arthrosc. 2011;19(8):1320–5. doi:10.1007/s00167-011-1429-9.
20. McGinnis MD, Gonzalez R, Nyland J, Caborn DN. The posteromedial knee arthroscopy portal: a cadaveric study defining a safety zone for portal placement. Arthroscopy. 2011;27(8):1090–5. doi:10.1016/j.arthro.2011.02.031.
21. Panisset JC, Neyret P. Méniscectomie sous arthroscopie. Encycl Med Chir. Techniques chirurgicales-Orthopédie-traumatologie. 2002;44–765:12

The Menisci

2

Radu Prejbeanu and Dinu Vermesan

2.1 Meniscal Ruptures

2.1.1 Epidemiology

There are over 636,000 knee arthroscopies performed annually in the USA and arthroscopic treatments of meniscal injuries are among the most common orthopedic procedures performed, constituting 10–20 % of all surgeries at some centers [1]. Surgery is increasingly the choice management for younger patients, athletes, and acute tears. Operative treatments for meniscal injuries have evolved in tandem with understanding of the structure, function, and biology of the meniscus [2]. The lesions of the menisci are often associated with lesions such as ligamentary ruptures and condral defects. The incidence of meniscal tears is 6/1,000, the male:female ratio being 4:2.5 [3].

A systematic review conducted by Snoeker et al. in 2013 analyzed a total of 7,358 participants enrolled in several studies from 1950 to 2012. They found strong evidence that several risk factors may lead up to meniscal tears (degenerative or traumatic). Results showed that degenerative meniscal tears were influenced by age (over 60 years old), gender (male), work-related kneeling and climbing stairs. Traumatic tears incidence was related to several sports such as rugby or soccer. Also delaying a torn ACL's reconstruction with more than 12 months greatly increased the risk of developing a medial meniscal tear [4].

A similar study performed by Sri-Ram et al. on 5,086 patients, analyzed the incidence of secondary pathologies related to ACL reconstruction delay. They found a link between the time that passes between an ACL rupture repair and the risk of developing future internal knee injuries. Increased intervals until ACL reconstruction determined medial meniscal lesions and chondral defects – 5 months of delay resulted in a doubled chance of requiring meniscal surgery. In patients that are less than 17 years old this effect is doubled [5].

2.1.2 Clinical Findings

Meniscal injuries are very common especially for the medial one. In young people they are usually due to sport activity in an older one due to fatigue of material. The medial meniscus is longer in the anterior-posterior direction than in the medial-lateral direction. It is attached to the deep medial collateral ligament, which renders it less mobile than the lateral meniscus and more prone to tears. It is a secondary stabilizer of the knee against anterior instability, and thus is commonly torn in anterior cruciate ligament deficient knees. The lateral meniscus has a more circular shape. It is more mobile than its medial counterpart, and it covers a greater portion of the articular cartilage. The lateral meniscus is more commonly torn in association with acute anterior cruciate ligament ruptures [6].

Patients may present with symptoms such as snapping, clicking, intermittent locking, sharp pain (acute injuries), joint effusion and chronic pain (degenerative lesions). The clinical evaluation of the knee is a very important step in diagnosing a meniscal tear, given that it can be performed accurately. Careful clinical examination can prove to be better than MRI in diagnosing medial meniscal tears and equally efficient as MRI when diagnosing lateral meniscal tears and ACL injuries.

The most commonly met clinical signs are joint line tenderness, joint effusion, an extension deficit, a positive McMurray test and the Steinmann sign. These must be correlated by an experienced practician in order for the diagnosis to be accurate. Ercin et al. found that a clinical examination performed by an experienced knee surgeon has better specificity (90–60 %), positive predictive value (95–83 %), negative predictive value (90–86 %) and diagnostic accuracy (93–83 %) than the MRI regarding medial meniscal tears, and very small differences regarding lateral meniscal tears [7].

R. Prejbeanu, MD, PhD • D. Vermesan, MD, PhD (✉)
Department of Orthopedics and Trauma,
University of Medicine and Pharmacy 'Victor Babes' Timisoara,
2 Eftimie Murgu Square, Timisoara 300041, Romania

I-st Clinic of Orthopedics and Trauma,
Emergency Clinical County Hospital Timisoara,
10 Iosif Bulbuca Blvd, Timisoara 300736, Romania
e-mail: raduprejbeanu@gmail.com; vermesan@gmail.com

R. Prejbeanu (ed.), *Atlas of Knee Arthroscopy*,
DOI 10.1007/978-1-4471-6593-4_2, © Springer-Verlag London 2015

2.1.3 Meniscal Tears Classification

Most meniscal tears appear due to degenerative causes, only few of them deriving from traumatic actions. Degenerative tears occur in older patients and are usually the result of normal tissue ageing, whereas traumatic injuries occur in younger people due to shear forces that the tibio-femoral joint creates during sport activities and trauma. These two pathogenic paths also divide the meniscal tears in acute (first 2–3 weeks) and old (older than 3 weeks) lesions.

Meniscal tears can also be classified by their shape, location and extent. Most traumatic tears are "bucket-handle" and flap lesions. Horizontal tears are usually created by a degenerative background (Figs. 2.1, 2.2, 2.3, 2.4, 2.5, 2.6, 2.7, 2.8, 2.9 and 2.10).

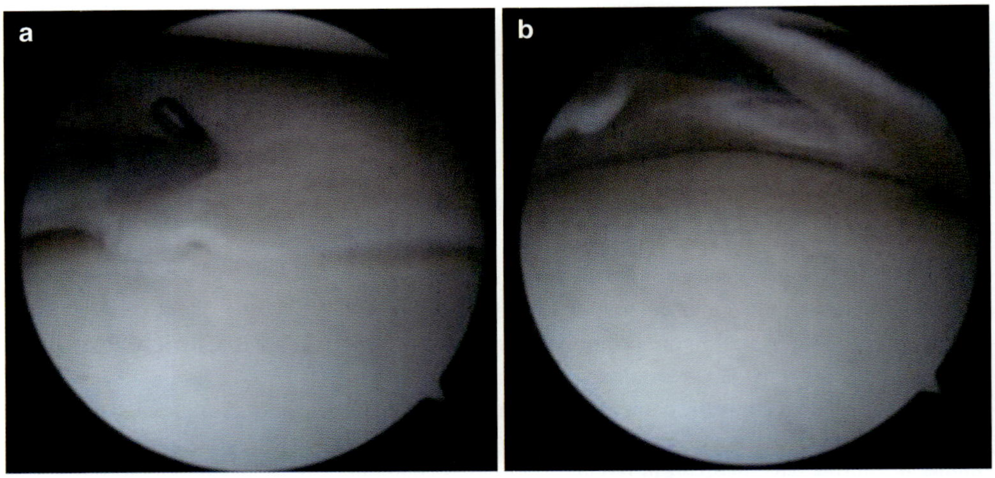

Fig. 2.1 Occult lesion of the medial meniscus. The femoral surface can be viewed with no lesions (**a**). Longitudinal meniscal rupture on the tibial aspect (**b**)

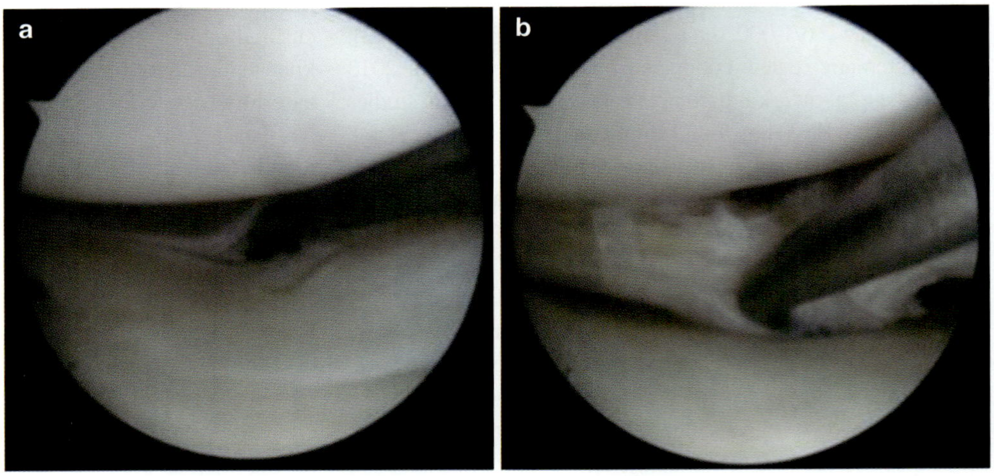

Fig. 2.2 Apparently an incomplete longitudinal rupture of the medial meniscus (**a**). Upon further inspection the full extent of the rupture can be seen expanding further (**b**)

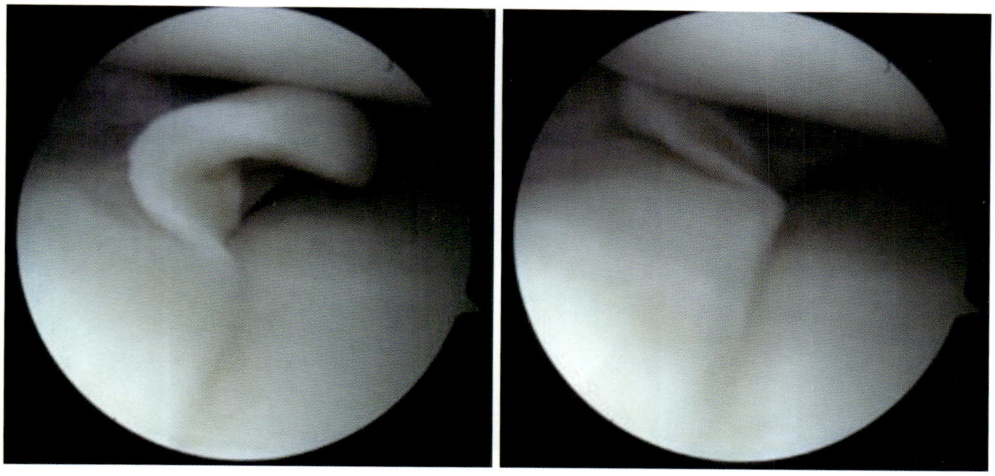

Fig. 2.3 "Parrot-beak" medial meniscal rupture

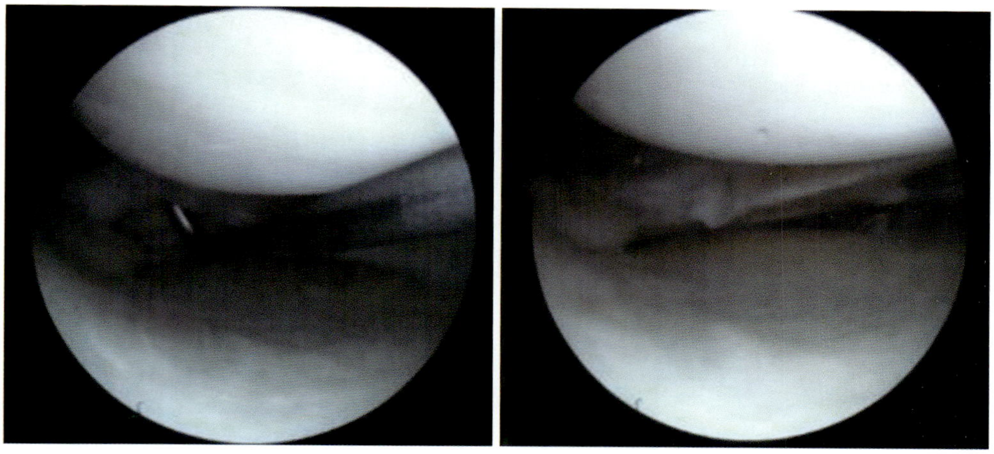

Fig. 2.4 Posterior horn rupture of the medial meniscus associated with an Outerbridge II condral pathology. The lesion extends towards the capsular portion and the insertion of the posterior part of the meniscus

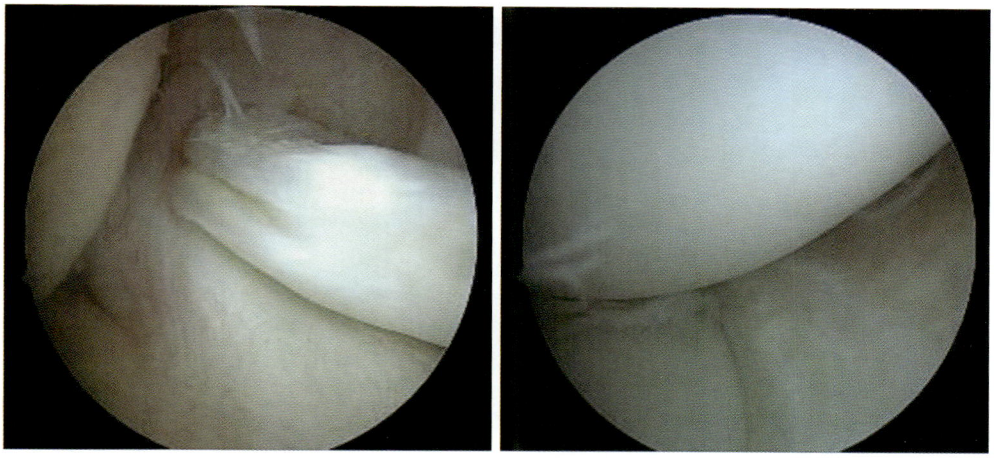

Fig. 2.5 "Bucket-handle" lesion of the medial meniscus associated with an intercondylar dislocation of the torn piece

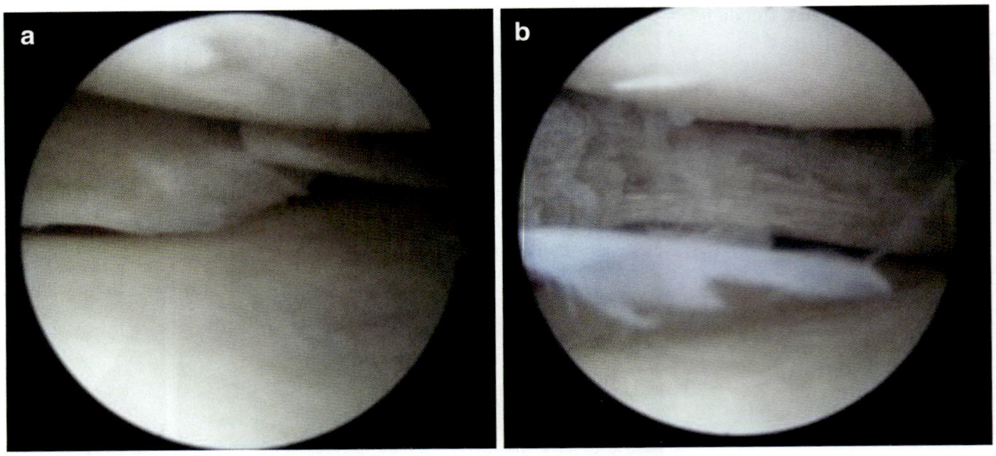

Fig. 2.6 Rupture of the medial meniscus (**a**), which underwent partial meniscectomy (**b**)

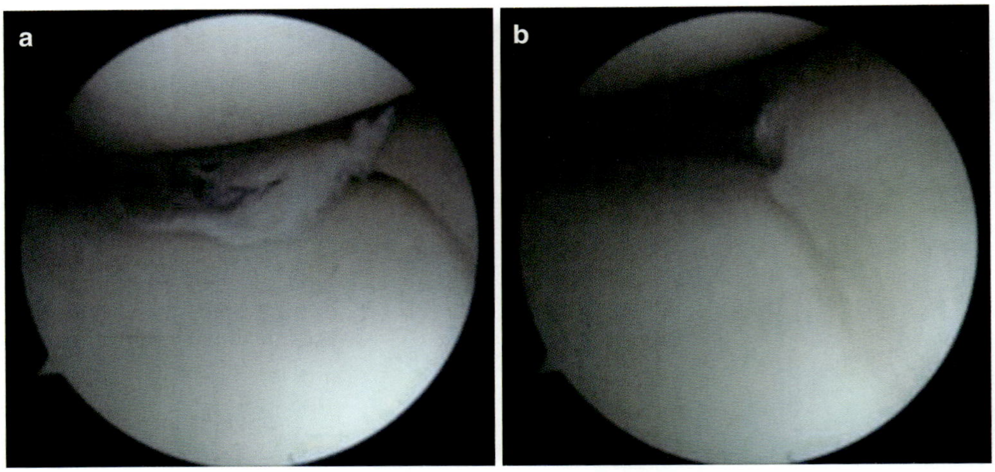

Fig. 2.7 Degenerative lesion located on the posterior portion of the medial meniscus, before (**a**) and after (**b**) the partial meniscectomy

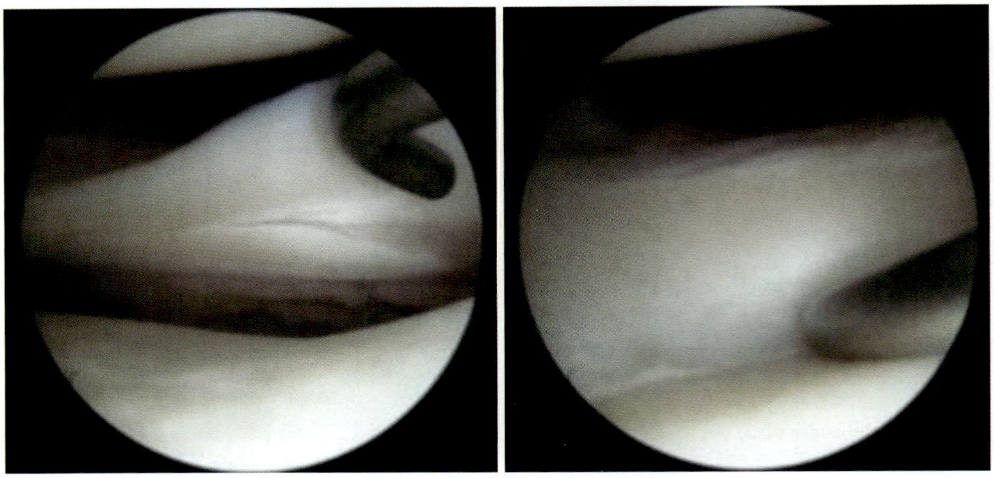

Fig. 2.8 Stable longitudinal tear of the lateral meniscus

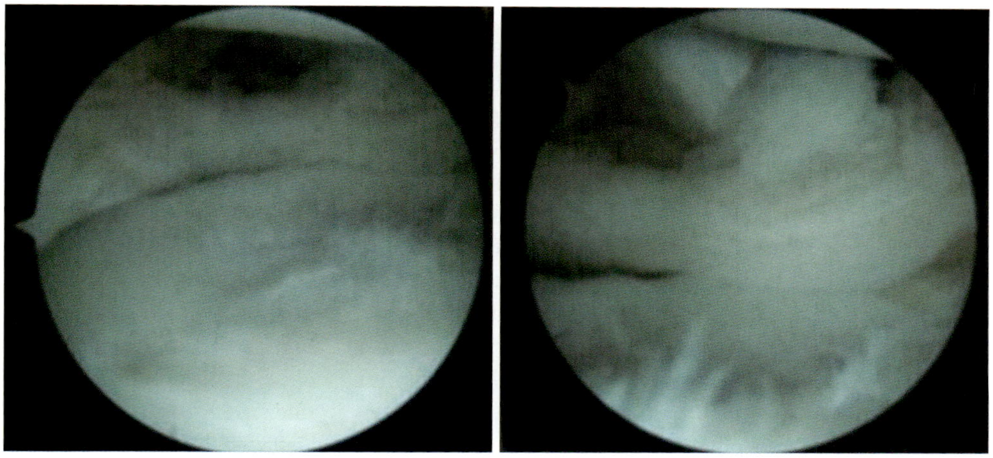

Fig. 2.9 Complete horizontal tear of the external meniscus

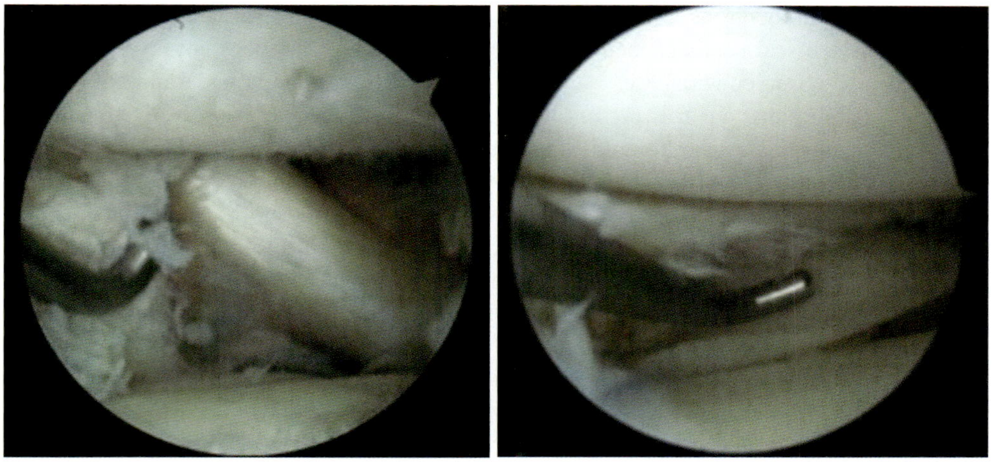

Fig. 2.10 A complex degenerative tear of the external meniscus. Secondary condral pathology Outerbridge II. The popliteal tendon can be seen in the posterior aspect

2.1.4 Imaging

Magnetic resonance Imaging is considered the "gold standard" and is the most frequently used imaging technique in the diagnosis of internal knee injuries. Even though it is a highly sensitive investigation when it comes to finding meniscal injuries, it may often yield false-positive or false-negative results. Thus, it is very important to be able to correlate the imagistic findings with the symptoms of the patient. In a study conducted by Crues et al. in the late 80's, it was showed that at surgery, 89 % of the patients diagnosed on MRI with grade 1 and 2 ruptures, were found to be normal during arthroscopy.

Meniscal tears are defined as an intrasubstance hyperdensity that reaches the surface of the meniscus [8]. The most often depicted meniscal tear is located in the posterior portion of the medial meniscus. This is due to the fact that it is the thickest meniscal segment, and hyperintensity intrasubstance can be observed with ease.

The probability that a tear is present increases if the specific signal changes are seen in more consecutive slices and in both sagittal and coronal planes. The sensitivity decreases to 55 and 30 % if the signal changes are only seen on one slice for the medial meniscus and lateral meniscus respectively [8]. Complete meniscal tears reach both the superior and inferior surfaces, while the partial tears only affect one of the two [9].

Von Engelhardt et al. studied the correlation between a 3-T MRI and arthroscopy meniscal tear diagnosis. They revealed that the MRI showed an increased accuracy in diagnosing medial meniscal tears (complex and horizontal tears were prevalent) than lateral meniscal tears. Regarding the grade III medial meniscal tears, the MRI had a 86 % sensitivity and a 100 % specificity. These two values decreased to 79 and 95 % respectively for the lateral meniscus. Grade II tears had a rate of 24 % missed diagnosis, while grade I lesions were not associated with an arthroscopic tear [10]. This changes dramatically regarding grade 3 lesions which showed a rate of confirmation during surgery of 91.3 % [11]. In 2009 Khanna et al. stated that false MRI results can be avoided by having a better understanding of several misconceptions. Thus, by being able to recognize the "magic angle" phenomenon, knowing the physics of an MRI, the anatomy and the pathophysiology of certain diseases, many of these errors can be avoided [12].

MRI-artrography has proven to be an efficient way of diagnosing meniscal tears, proving high rates of sensitivity and specificity. Mathieu et al. have shown that MR-artrography exceeds MRI regarding these two aspects, reaching values of 100 % sensitivity and 89.6 % specificity, while the MRI's rates were 92.3 and 82.8 % respectively. The study was carried out on 21 patients (15 males) with a mean age of 35.7 years. MR-artrography is indicated in the detection of foreign bodies within the knee joint, detection on secondary tears on operated menisci and assessment before chondral lesion repairs. The lack of lesion depth resolution though, advantages the classic MRI [13].

The ultrasonography is inexpensive and easily accessible. It has been recently put to use in the case of acute internal knee injury. The advantages it has over classic MRI are the cost efficiency, portability of the equipment and duration of assessment. Compared to the MRI, the diagnosis made with ultrasonography has proven to have higher specificity rates (84.2 %/66.7 %), higher correct classification rates (89.5 %/81.5 %) and similar sensitivity rates (91.2 %/91.7 %) [14].

Typically, the patient's lifestyle, size, localization and shape of the tear indicate a certain type of treatment. Conservative treatment is usually an indication in small tears that can be found in patients with a rather sedentary lifestyle that does not involve sport activities, resulting in little to no symptoms. Rathleff et al. conducted a clinical trial that evaluated conservative treatment in patients with MRI-confirmed meniscal lesions. Their success rate for this type of treatment was 58 %, and it was determined using the KOOS and Lysholm score [15]. Large and complex tears require arthroscopic surgery, be it by resection or meniscal suture. Resection is usually an indication when tears involve the free edge of the meniscus which has less chance of healing (due to the lack of vascularization) than the tears in the more vascularized area of the meniscus (near the tibial insertion point).

2.1.5 Incomplete Meniscal Tears During ACL Reconstruction

One of the topics that are still debated is defining the management of incomplete meniscal tears found during anterior cruciate ligament reconstructions. One of the first studies to approach this subject found that stable vertical longitudinal tears, in the periphery of the menisci, have good healing whereas radial tears, in the avascular third of the meniscus, do not have the same favorable healing potential. They recommend for stable longitudinal tears to be left in situ but cannot find a solution for the vertical lesions [16]. Further research has also found that peripheral meniscal lesions associated with surgery for chronic anterior instability do not always require suture if they are limited to the posterior segment [17].

The debate has then focused on laterality and length of the lesions. Shelbourne et al. have shown favorable long term follow-up for lateral meniscal tears left in situ or stimulated by abrasion or trephination that are posterior horn, stable radial flap, or peripheral/posterior third tears which extend less than 10 mm in front of the popliteus tendon [18].

In a previous study, the same authors also found that posterior horn avulsions, vertical tears posterior to the popliteus tendon and other stable tears at the time of index anterior cruciate ligament reconstruction can be left in situ without becoming clinically symptomatic [19].

With regard to the medial meniscus, Shelbourne et al. observed most traumatic stable peripheral vertical medial meniscus tears treated with abrasion/ trephination to be asymptomatic without stabilization [20]. Other studies also found limited stable medial lesions and most lateral tears to have good outcomes when left untreated during ACL reconstruction [21–23]. Furthermore, meniscal rasping is feasible for repairing longitudinal tears in the avascular region of the meniscus, but the healing potential is influenced by the distance to the capsule, length and stability of the tear [24].

Detection of incomplete or subtle meniscal tears is highly dependent on the quality of the MRI as well as the examiners proficiency. A correlation between arthroscopic findings of incomplete meniscal tears and preoperative MRIs performed in different locations found the initial radiologist interpretation failed to identify most medial and all lateral incomplete lesions of either meniscus when the acquisition was performed on a 0.2 T open MRI. Even with the 1.5 T MRI the findings were missed in 47 % of the cases for the lateral meniscus [25]. There were considerable more missed lesions when compared to the literature [26] with all machines but we can conclude that 0.2 T MRIs cannot be used to successfully identify incomplete meniscal tears in the setting of anterior cruciate ligament rupture.

Pujol et al. performed a literature review concerning the healing results of meniscal tears left in situ during anterior cruciate ligament reconstruction and recommend fixation for medial meniscus tears [27]. These findings are supported by other authors that found meniscal repairs at the time of anterior cruciate ligament reconstruction had a lower failure rate than isolated repairs and better long-term outcomes than partial meniscectomy [28]. One explanation might be that longitudinal tears of the medial meniscus in an ACL-deficient knee alter kinematics; particularly the anterior-posterior tibial translation comparable to a partial meniscectomy and that stability can be improved by repair [29].

A more recent review performed by Noyes et al. found that meniscectomy is performed two to three times more frequently than meniscus repair during anterior cruciate ligament reconstruction [30]. This raises concern since meniscectomy significantly alters long term outcomes and favors arthritic changes, especially in the lateral compartment [31]. To a certain degree, this can be attenuated by the fact that lateral meniscus tears are better tolerated and can be excised more parsimoniously hoping they will continue to provide support [32].

Vermesan et al. concluded that incomplete medial meniscal tears left in situ at the time of anterior cruciate ligament can yield favorable outcomes as long as decisions are carefully weighed with regard to length of the lesion. Also, at least in this perspective, anatomic single bundle has proved a sufficient stabilizer for anterior translation of the tibia [33].

2.2 Meniscectomy

Meniscal pathology remains a commonly encountered clinical entity for the practicing orthopedic surgeon. In Clayton and Court-Brown's recent prospective study of musculoskeletal injuries, meniscal injury to the knee was the most common, occurring at a rate of 23.8/100,000 per year. According to the American Academy of Orthopaedic Surgeons, the incidence in the United States is 61/100,000 [34].

The first description of a meniscectomy was provided by Broadhurst, in 1866 in London. Annandale was the first to describe meniscal repair in 1885. Despite the reports of King and Fairbanks, who described the harmful effects of total meniscectomy and the secondary radiographic changes, until the seventies, menisci were considered as functionless evolutionary remnants of leg muscle that could be excised without further relevant consequences for the knee joint [35]. In 1948, Ghormley recommended total excision of any torn meniscus, stating that partial meniscectomy carried a higher risk of joint surface damage [36]. In the fifties, Trillat and Dejour highlighted the role of the meniscal rim. Trillat described intramural medial meniscectomy through a short anteromedial arthrotomy, preserving the medial collateral ligament and the meniscal rim [37]. However, the first arthroscopic partial meniscectomy is generally attributed to Watanabe (disciple of Takagi) in 1962. He designed the first practical arthroscope: the Watanabe number-21 arthroscope, which was produced in series and allowed effective intraarticular exploration [38].

Arthroscopic partial meniscectomy is the most common orthopedic procedure performed in the United States. The aim of the procedure is to relieve symptoms attributed to a meniscal tear by removing torn meniscal fragments and trimming the meniscus back to a stable rim. Most treated meniscal tears are associated with degenerative knee disease, which can range from mild chondral changes not visible on a radiograph to established knee osteoarthritis. Objectives of meniscus surgery are return to previous activity level, relieve symptoms associated with tears, not increase risk of late osteoarthritis, not add further problems [39]. Approximately 700,000 arthroscopic partial meniscectomies are performed annually in the United States alone [40]. Metcalf et al. concluded that partial meniscectomy is better than total meniscectomy because less operative time, enhanced recovery rate, improved long term stability. They also concluded than arthroscopic is better than open meniscectomy with less operative time and quicker recovery post-op [41].

Arthroscopic medial meniscectomy is performed with the patient under spinal or general anesthesia. A tourniquet is applied to the thigh and it can be or not inflated [42]. A thigh holder or lateral post is used to allow for controlled varus and valgus stress. The leg is positioned in a leg holder, which allows valgus stress to be exerted across the joint to open up the medial compartment for adequate visualization [43]. The patient may be positioned so that the leg can be draped off the side of the bed if using a lateral post or the end of the bed can be lowered when using a thigh holder [44].

The antero-medial and antero-lateral portals are sufficient to achieve the majority of medial meniscectomies. First, the antero-lateral portal will be performed to introduce the arthro-trocar sleeve and the arthroscope [45]. The anterolateral portal is the primary viewing portal for knee arthroscopy. With the knee flexed to 90°, the inferior pole of the patella, the lateral border of the patella and the lateral joint line are palpated [46]. An incision is made with a no. 11 blade approximately 1 cm above the joint line and in line with the lateral border of the patella. A vertical incision angled toward the intercondylar notch is used unless a horizontal portal is preferred. In either case, great care is taken to protect the meniscus and intraarticular structures [47]. The trocar sleeve will be introduced after cutting the skin and the patella with a scalpel and then it will be directed to the intercondylar notch, the knee being flexed at 30° or 45°. Then, the arthroscope will be directed towards the femoral-patellar joint, with the knee in extension, to start the exploration [48].

The anteromedial portal is created with the knee at 30° of flexion. The 30° scope needs to be rotated to obtain an unobstructed view of the anterior aspect of the medial meniscus and anterior capsule [49]. The anteromedial portal will be performed by trans-illumination in the dihedral anteromedial angle above the anterior segment of the medial meniscus. Then the probe will be introduced to palpate both menisci on their two sides by lifting them and the two cruciate ligaments. The anteromedial portal will be more or less high and medial according to the lesion localization [50].

The lateral meniscus shows anatomic particularities different from those of the medial meniscus. The accessibility of the anterior segment is often difficult. The standard arthroscopic meniscectomy portals are used and in case an accessory portal may be use, through the patelar tendon. For arthroscopic lateral meniscectomy, the lateral skin incision should be superior to the joint line and for arthroscopic lateral meniscectomy, the lateral skin incision should be superior to the joint line [51].

Arthroscopic partial meniscectomy is a 10–20 min procedure where torn or mobile areas are removed and edges contoured to prevent further tears. It has the advantage that immediate partial weight bearing is allowed. Partial meniscectomy is indicated in complex tears, flap tears, radial tears, rupture in the white-white zone, degenerative tears and degenerative horizontal cleavage [52].

Metcalf described basic principles to adhere to when performing partial meniscectomy procedure. This includes: remove all mobile fragments, do not leave sudden changes in rim contour, do not try to obtain a perfectly smooth rim as some remodeling may occur, use the probe often to reevaluate the tear, protect the meniscus-capsular junction to avoid the loss of hoop stresses, use both manual and motorized instruments to maximize efficiency when uncertain if an area should be resected, we should opt for leaving more meniscus intact rather than compromising biomechanical properties [53].

Meniscus resection – basic steps: instrumental meniscal resection (punch), removal of residual tissue (avoiding thus irritation and hidarthrosis, shaving, coagulation of bleeding vessels. In a "bucket handle tear" first reduction of the displaced meniscus then identification/resection of the posterior basis, identification/resection oft the anterior bases, removal of the meniscal tissue, smoothening of the structure [54]. In a meniscal flap the steps are reduction of the flap, resection, removal of the flap, smoothening. In degenerative meniscla lesion resection is performed along with removal of lost fragments and smoothening. Adequate instruments are use to perform the procedure such as punches, scizors, hook, shaver, radiofrequency, cautery [33].

The arthroscopy ends up with a thorough cleaning of the knee. Any meniscus fragments must be removed without leaving any remnants in the portals which will become a source of chronic pain. The closure of the portals is carried out by several ways: non resorbable sutures, staples or even adhesive tape [55].

In a longer-term study, Burks and colleagues reported 88 % good and excellent results after 15 years follow-up. They also reported that results were not significantly different for medial versus lateral tears. Patients with valgus as opposed to varus alignment had better results after partial medial meniscectomy. Radiographic examinations demonstrated a 0.24 % mean decline in osteoarthritis grade. Of note, their study population consisted of low-demand patients [56].

Full weightbearing ambulation is possible immediately after surgery. In the context of degenerative lesions, sports activity will depend above all on the degree of coexistent cartilage lesions. Physical therapy can be used for residual pain [57]. Patients are allowed to return to full athletic activities when their quadriceps muscle tone returns and they have full painless range of motion. This varies but usually averages 4–6 weeks postoperatively and slightly longer in the setting of degenerative changes [58].

Vermesan et al. compared arthroscopic debridement with intra-articular steroids in degenerative medial meniscal tears. They concluded that arthroscopic debridement has marginal better outcomes. They identified several negative prognostic factors such as obesity, meniscal extrusion and bone marrow edema [33].

Complications are rarely seen. The risk of infection is about 0.1 %. Hydrarthrosis is more common after a lateral than a medial meniscectomy. This can be explained by the congruence of the lateral tibial plateau, which is more convex than the medial one. This incongruence increases the mechanical conflict. Contrary to meniscal repair techniques, arthroscopic meniscectomy is very rarely fraught with vascular or nervous complications [59].

Small reported on the complications of 21 experienced arthroscopists over a 19-month period. The complication rates for arthroscopic partial medial and lateral meniscectomies were 1.78 and 1.48 %, respectively. Partial meniscectomy can be complicated by instrument failure, knee ligament injury, neurovascular injury, iatrogenic damage to articular cartilage through aggressive instrumental manipulation, also can generate further damage to cartilage and can lead to arthritis. Inadequate resection with persistence of meniscal lesion can happen by lack of arthroscopic knowledge, inexperienced surgeon or re-arthroscopy [60].

Knee ligament injury during partial meniscectomy usually involves the medial collateral ligament. This infrequent injury may occur when excessive valgus force is placed on the knee in an attempt to gain better access to the medial compartment [61]. This can make a prolonged recovery but it always heal. Persistent pain after partial meniscectomy may occur because of incomplete resection of the tear or from coexistent knee pathology. When resecting a tear, in an attempt to preserve the maximal amount of menisci, it is possible that torn remnants may be left behind [62] (Figs. 2.11, 2.12, 2.13, 2.14, 2.15, 2.16, 2.17 and 2.18).

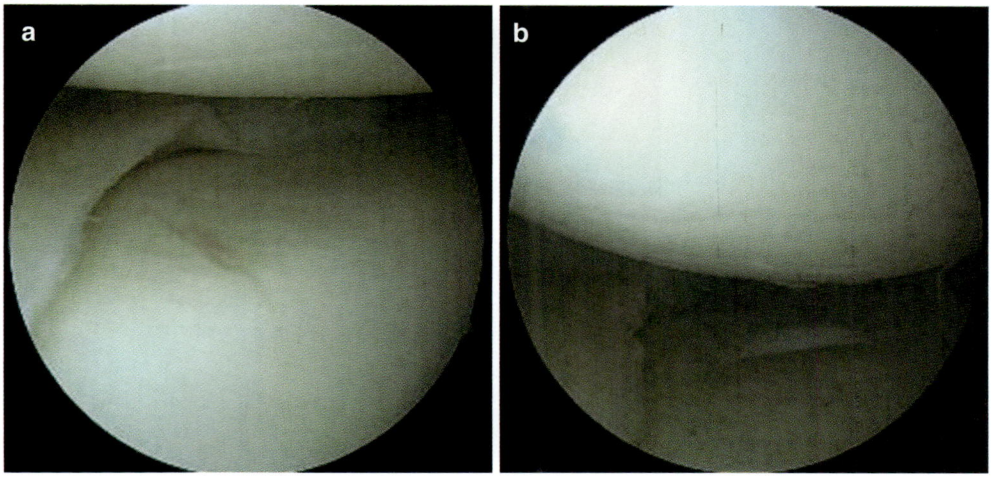

Fig. 2.11 Tear of the medial meniscus' posterior horn. Before (**a**) and after (**b**) the punch meniscectomy

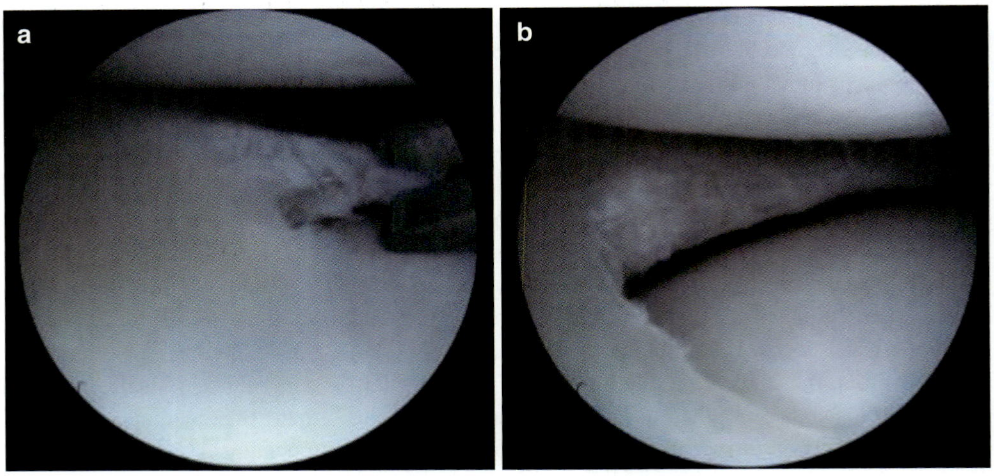

Fig. 2.12 Radial rupture of the medial meniscus before (**a**) and after (**b**) punch meniscectomy

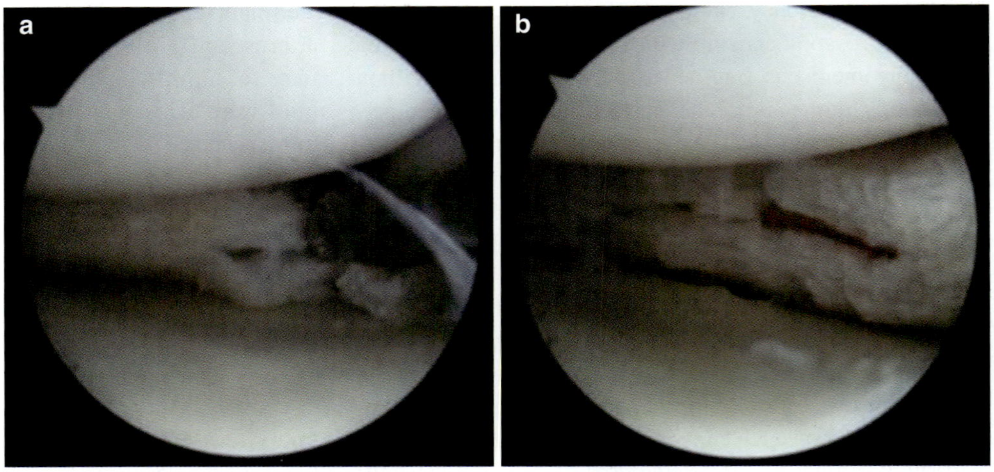

Fig. 2.13 Complex lesion of the medial meniscus – punch meniscectomy (**a**). The post-meniscectomy appearance reveals the lesion extending near the capsular portion of the meniscus (**b**)

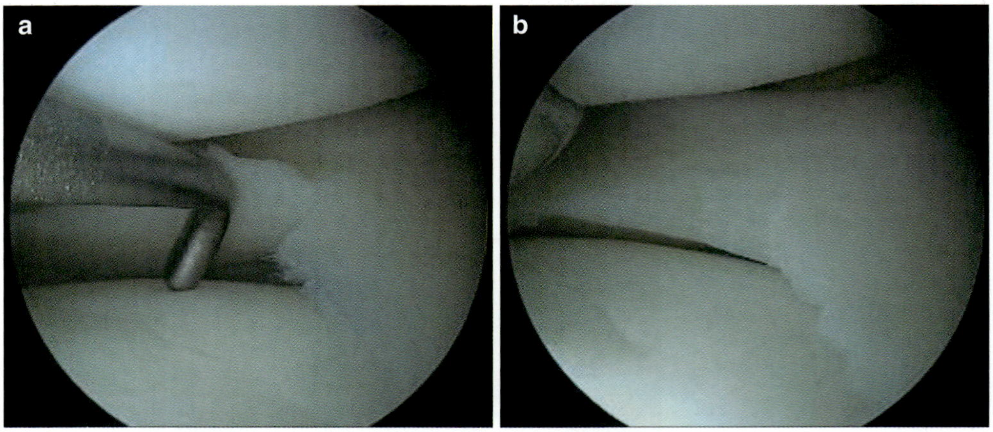

Fig. 2.14 A small tear of the lateral meniscus body showed to us by the help of a probe, before (**a**) and after (**b**) smoothening of the articular border was performed

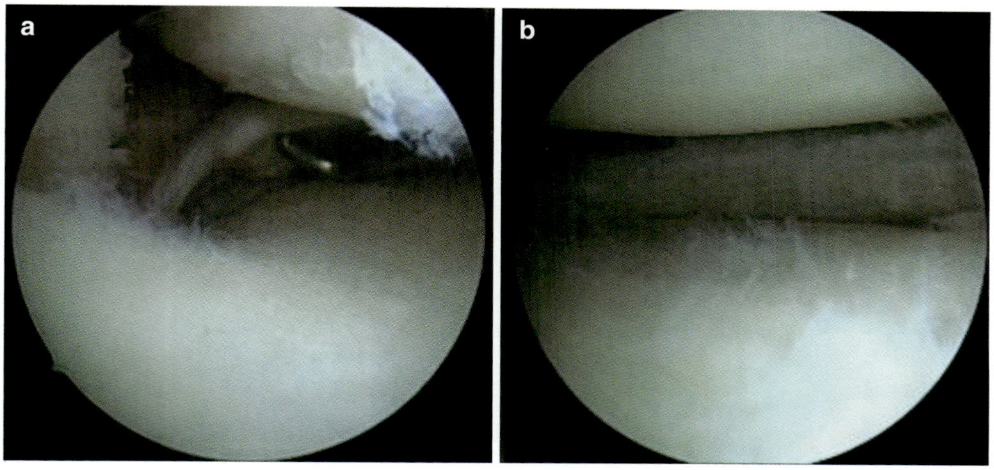

Fig. 2.15 Posterior horn avulsion tear of the medial meniscus and chondral damage (**a**). This particular type is frequently missed on preoperative MRI examination. Punch meniscectomy is performed and the final result can be observed in the second picture (**b**)

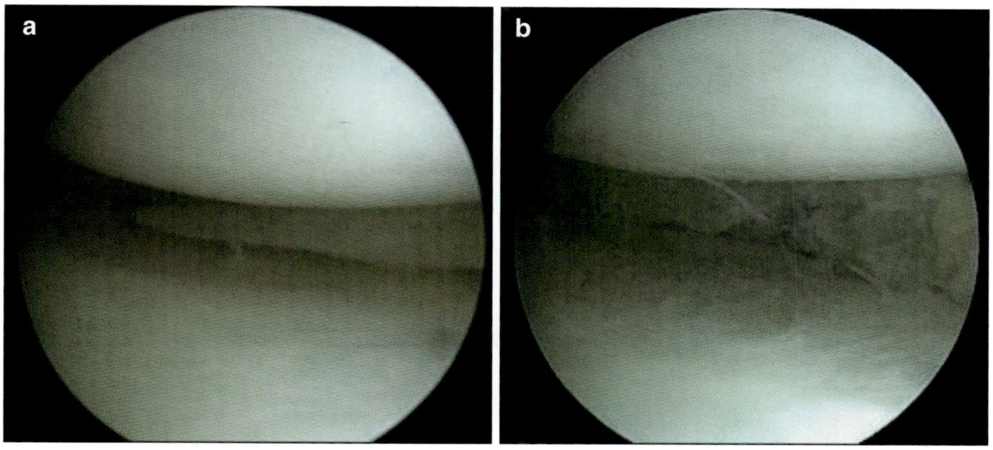

Fig. 2.16 Longitudinal tear of the lateral meniscus posterior horn and body. Subsequent early cartilage damage can be observed (**a**). Meniscus aspect after the meniscectomy has been performed (**b**)

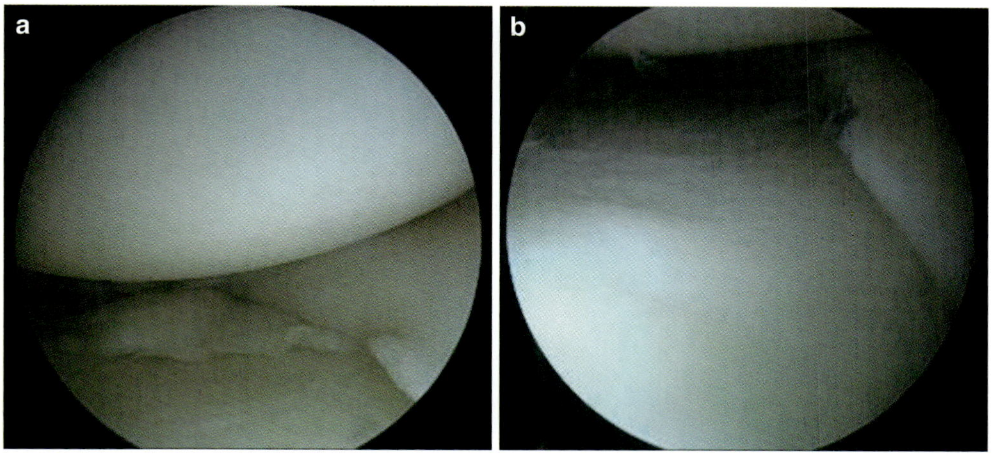

Fig. 2.17 Old tear located on the posterior horn of the lateral meniscus. Cartilage damage can also be observed (**a**). The torn piece is removed and the edges of the meniscus are evened out (**b**)

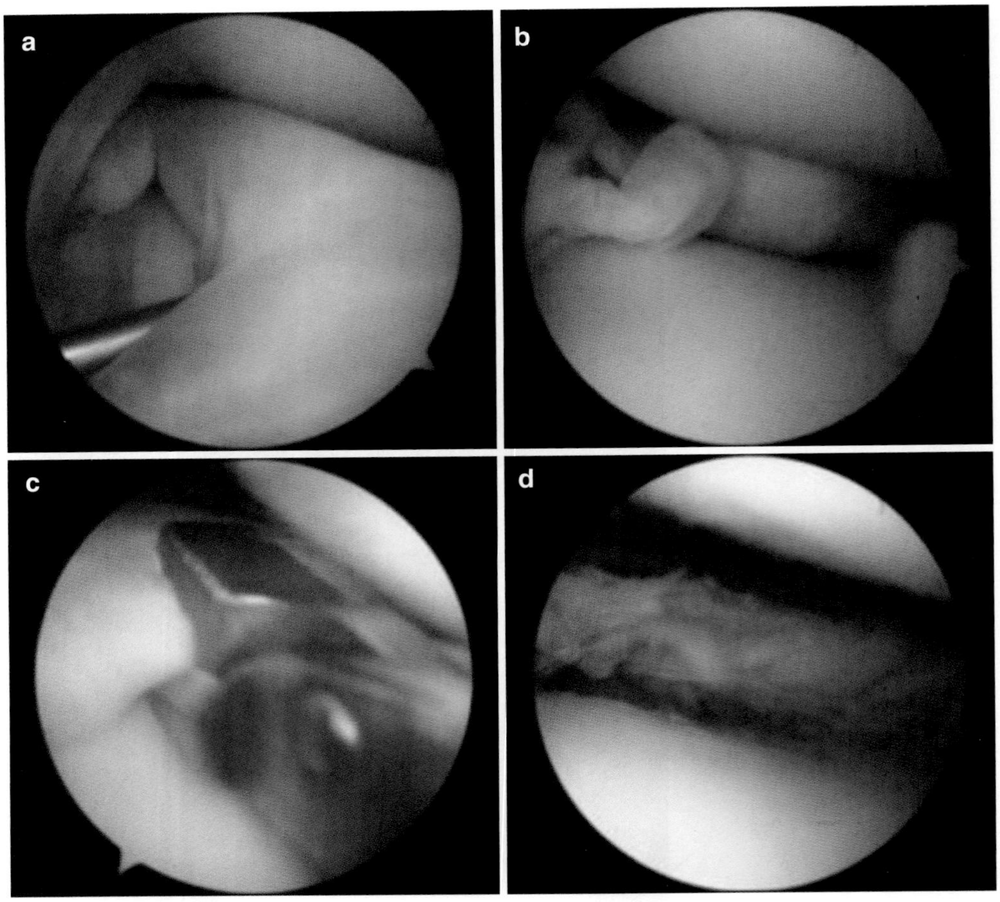

Fig. 2.18 A "bucket-handle" lesion of the external meniscus before (**a**) and after the intercondylar luxation reduction (**b**). Pictures taken during the meniscectomy (**c**), and after the torn piece was removed (**d**)

2.3 Meniscal Preservation

2.3.1 Meniscal Repair

In the eighties, biomechanical studies stated the importance of menisci to load transfer. Kurosawa et al. showed that total meniscectomy reduced the total contact area by a third to a half in a fully extended knee [63]. Menisci transmit up to 50 % of weightbearing forces in extension and about 85 % in flexion. In vitro trials reported about 70 and 50 % of load transmission through the corresponding menisci in the lateral and medial compartment, respectively. This combined knowledge stressed the relevance of meniscal preservation, and partial meniscectomy gained ground over total excision [64].

The development of arthroscopic surgical instruments and techniques facilitated a movement toward meniscus preserving surgery. Rather than resection of the entire meniscus, partial meniscectomy became a mainstay of treatment for symptomatic tears. Short-term results of partial meniscectomy are excellent. Jarequito and associates reported 90 % good and excellent outcomes at 2-years follow-up, with 85 % of patients returning to their desired activity level. At 8 years, though, these results had declined to only 62 % good or excellent outcomes, and only 48 % of patients maintained their desired activity level [65].

Due to the long-term complications that meniscectomy induces, such as joint space narrowing followed by degenerative changes [64, 65], more and more arthroscopists have initiated the trend of meniscal repair. Annandale [66] was the first to perform and report meniscal repairs, but his idea was not received with open arms and it was very soon put aside. With the advances made in arthroscopy, the meniscal repair techniques have evolved and are now used worldwide. The first arthroscopic meniscal repair was performed in 1969 by Ikeuchi [67]. With the development of new implants, all of the repair techniques including inside-out, outside-in and all-inside have become less demanding and now cause less postoperative complications.

2.3.1.1 Basic Principles

In order to easily asses the healing potential of a meniscal tear and to be able to treat it correctly, these injuries were classified according to their location on the meniscus and the grade of vascularization it has. Thus, Arnoczky and Warren have named zone 0 the peripheral meniscosynovial junction, zone 1 the red-red zone, zone 2 the red-white zone and zone 3 the white-white zone [66]. Depending on the zone, the rupture is less likely to heal [68], or not, after a meniscal repair. A tear in the red-red zone is likely to heal, whereas a tear in the white-white zone has little to none healing chances.

Once the type of meniscal tear has been assessed, before doing the repair, the surgeon has to perform arthroscopic debridement if necessary. Pujol et al. proposed that using a posterior portal may improve the precision of the debridement [69]. Bucked-handle tears have to be reduced back to their anatomic position, and needling can be performed for meniscal healing stimulation (Fig. 2.19).

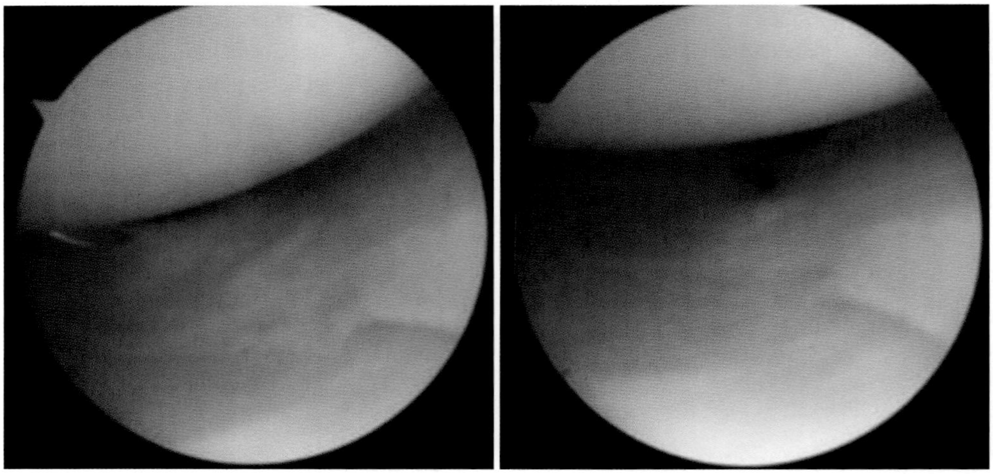

Fig. 2.19 Incomplete rupture of the meniscus located in the red-red zone. Needling is performed

2.3.1.2 Arthroscopically Assisted Repairs

The development of the less invasive techniques aimed at reducing the disadvantages that came along with the open repair. It was meant to allow for a faster recovery, lower the rate of morbidity and grant a good option when dealing with lesions found in the red-white zone. The inside-out and outside-in can be used as complementary repairs in different meniscal tears or long longitudinal tears. Posterior and middle segment ruptures benefit from the inside-out repair, while anterior horn sutures benefit from the outside-in technique better.

Outside-in repairs were first performed by Warren in 1985 [70]. A variation to this technique has been described. A cannulated needle is passed through the tear from the outside, into the knee joint. When the tip has reached the surface of the meniscus, the suture (2 nonabsorbable) is passed through. A second needle is passed on the other side of the rupture and a thin looped nonabsorbable monofilament (2/0) suture is passed. With the help of the probe and an arthroscopic grasp the suture is passed through the loop under arthroscopic visualization. The loop, the suture and the needle are all pulled back out of the joint and tied to one another on the exterior portion of the capsule through a small incision (Figs. 2.20 and 2.21).

The inside-out technique. Most systems mainly consist of long curved single or double-barrel canulas. The stitches can be horizontal or vertical and they usually consist of absorbable or nonabsorbable 2-0 sutures. The sutures are then retrieved through a posterior extraarticular incision (medially or laterally), with the knots being tied outside the joint, over the knee capsule. The disadvantages of this technique are the neurovascular complications that may arise. The posteromedial or posterolateral incision must be positioned carefully as to not harm the saphenous vein and/or nerve and the peroneal nerve respectively.

2.3.1.3 Implant Assisted Repairs

The need for managing meniscal repairs in an all-inside fashion, without the use of any other accessory incisions, has led to the production of various implants that were deemed suited for this task. They are made out of bioabsorbable materials, mostly composed of rigid poly-L-lactic acid (PLLA), and come in many shapes such as screws, anchors, staples, etc.

This type of technique can be performed easily and very fast. It also has a low risk of neurovascular injury and it requires no accessory incision. Some disadvantages have been proven in time. Their strength is lower when compared to vertical sutures [71, 72], and they have a risk of presenting loose bodies, developing synovitis and meniscal cysts, as well as cartilage abrasion [73–76].

2.3.1.4 All-Inside Meniscal Repairs

These types of techniques are the latest developed treatments in the field of meniscal sutures. All of them are achieved with specially designed devices that allow for easy and secure repair using only arthroscopic portals. The principle that they are designed around is positioning one or two anchors behind the capsule while a compressing suture holds the torn parts of the meniscus together. This suture is locked in place with a sliding knot.

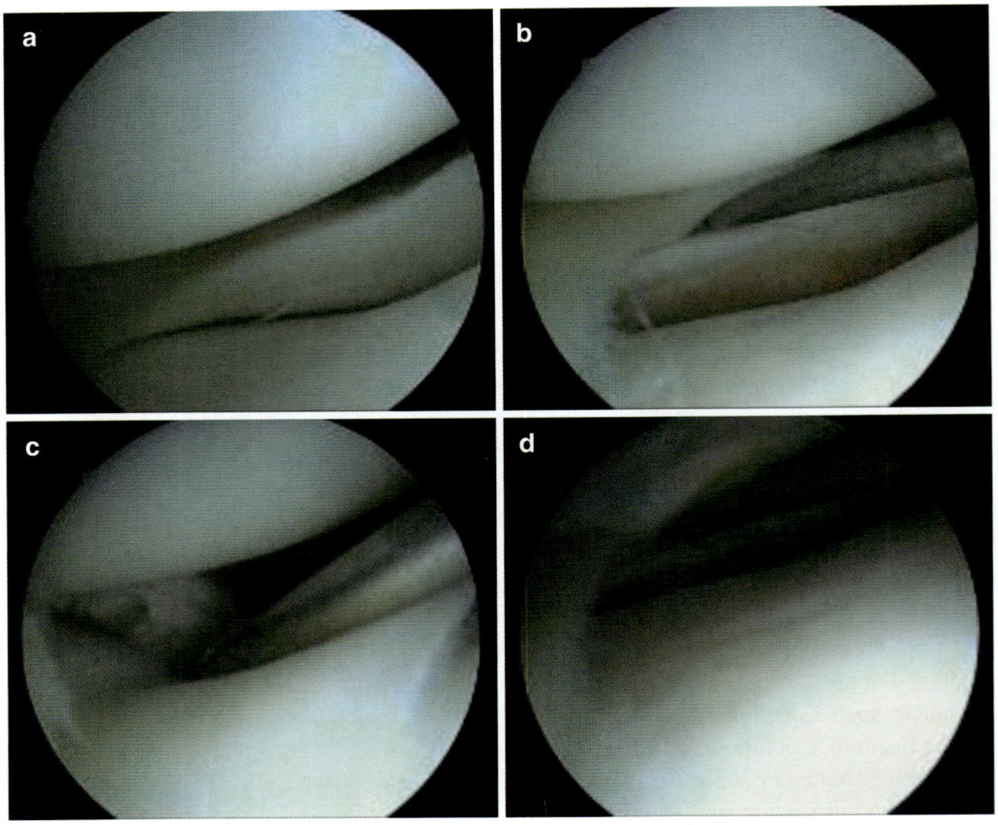

Fig. 2.20 Arthroscopic view of an external meniscal longitudinal rupture (**a**–**d**), indicated with the probe

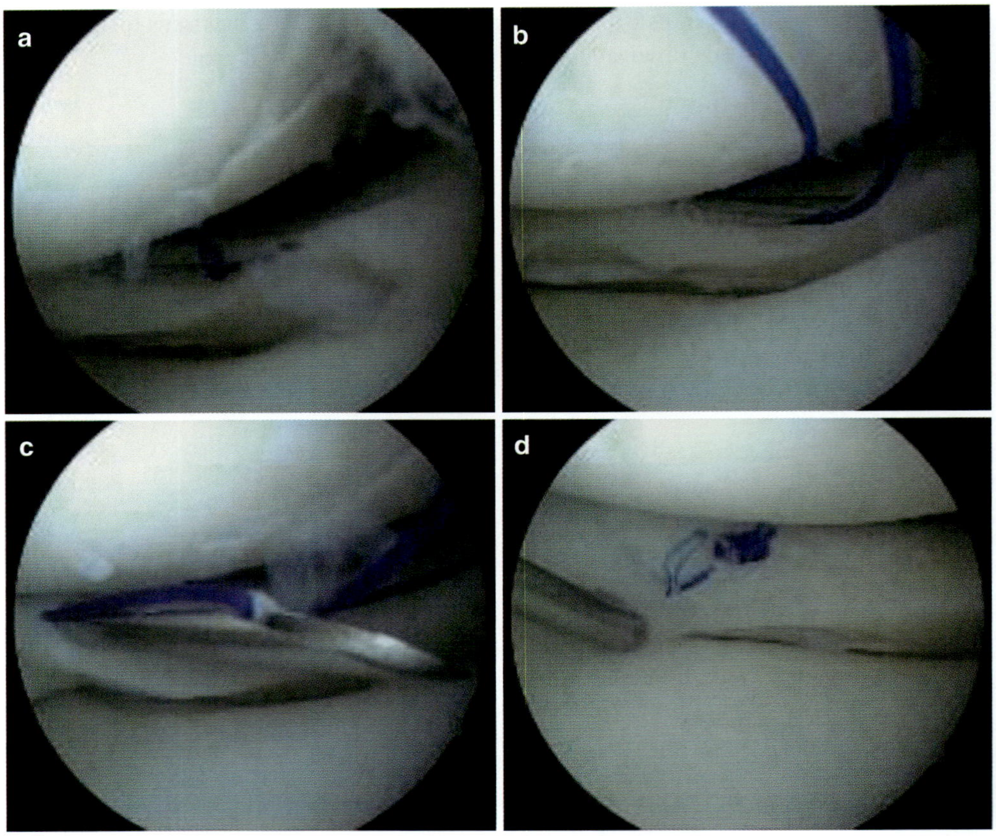

Fig. 2.21 Meniscal suture of the same case above, performed through an inside out technique (**a**–**c**). The final aspect of the tied knot can be viewed in the last picture (**d**)

2.3.1.5 FasT-Fix

Is a successful device manufactured by Smith and Nephew. It consists of two 5 mm polymer anchors with a pre-tied self-sliding knot made up from 2 to 0 non-absorbable ultra high molecular weight polyethylene suture. This system is integrated alongside in an ergonomic "screwdriver-like" handle with anchor-release buttons, a knot-pusher, an adjustable length limiter and a delivery needle which can be curve-shaped or straight. The device allows placing vertical mattress sutures on the femoral as well as on the tibial surface (using the inversed curve-shaped needle) of the meniscus.

It is recommended that we use the anterolateral portal for repairing lateral meniscal tear, and middle-zone medial meniscal tears and the anteromedial portal for the other medial meniscal tears. A proper measurement of the needle depth limit is very important as it reduces neurovascular lesions to the minimum and it allows for a correct positioning of the anchors. A slotted cannula can be used for knee guidance inside the knee in order to avoid unwanted chondral damage and support the needle during the positioning process.

Vertical mattress sutures are made by placing the first implant (anchor) in the capsular side of the meniscus, pulling the suture back out of the meniscus and then re-inserting it in the inner meniscal fragment. The suture is then tensioned and the knot is slid into place and then cut. Several sutures can be placed at a recommended gap of 5 mm from one another. For horizontal mattress sutures the same steps apply, but the first anchor is placed in the posterior side of the meniscus and the second one is deployed anterior to the rupture (Figs. 2.22 and 2.23).

2.3.1.6 Meniscal Cinch

The Meniscal Cinch is developed by Arthrex and even though it is not as compact as the FasT-Fix, it brings some novelties that allow for better device manipulation. The Meniscal Cinch has the shape of a vertical handle with two push pins on top of it that trigger the two anchors. The repair is made with a 2-0 FiberWire suture, which can be placed vertically or horizontally.

When dealing with tears that occurred on the body of the meniscus, the contralateral portal is used for repair, whereas posterior horn repairs can sometimes be obtained using the ipsilateral portal. The implants are deployed by pushing the trocars through the cannula. The Meniscal Cinch also has a depth stop for the needle which needs to be set before starting the trocar insertion, once the measurements have been done. In the same fashion as with the FasT-Fix, the first needle is inserted until it stops on to the depth stop. Pulling back on the needle triggers the implant and removes the trocar from the cannula. After first implant insertion, its trocar can be completely removed from the device in order to not interfere with the second implant. The second trocar is then pushed down from the holding position, the tip of the cannula is moved to the other side of the tear and the process is then repeated to trigger the second anchor. By removing the second trocar and the entire device from the joint and applying tension on the external suture, we make the knot advance to the surface of the meniscus. Then the suture is placed into the suture threader that acts as a knot pusher and a suture cutter at the same time, thus finishing the repair.

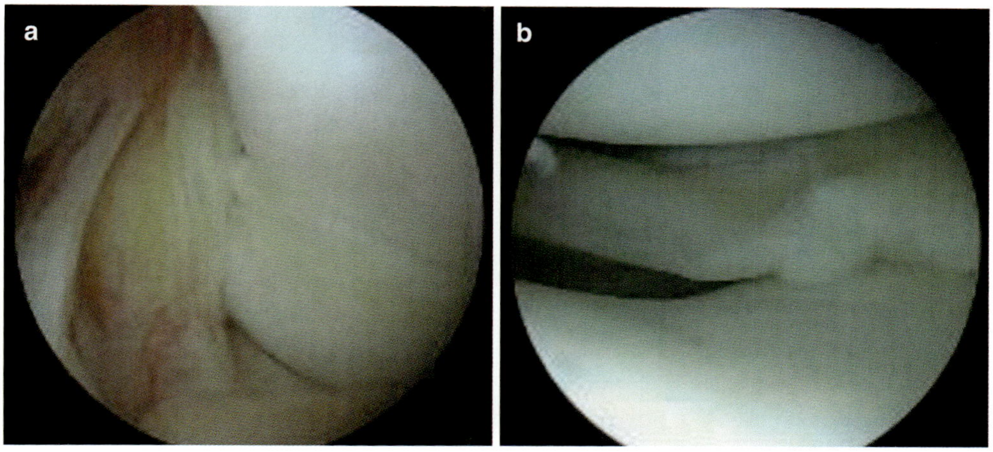

Fig. 2.22 Locked knee that presents a bucket-handle external meniscus tear. Arhtroscopic views before (**a**) and after (**b**) the relocation of the torn meniscus

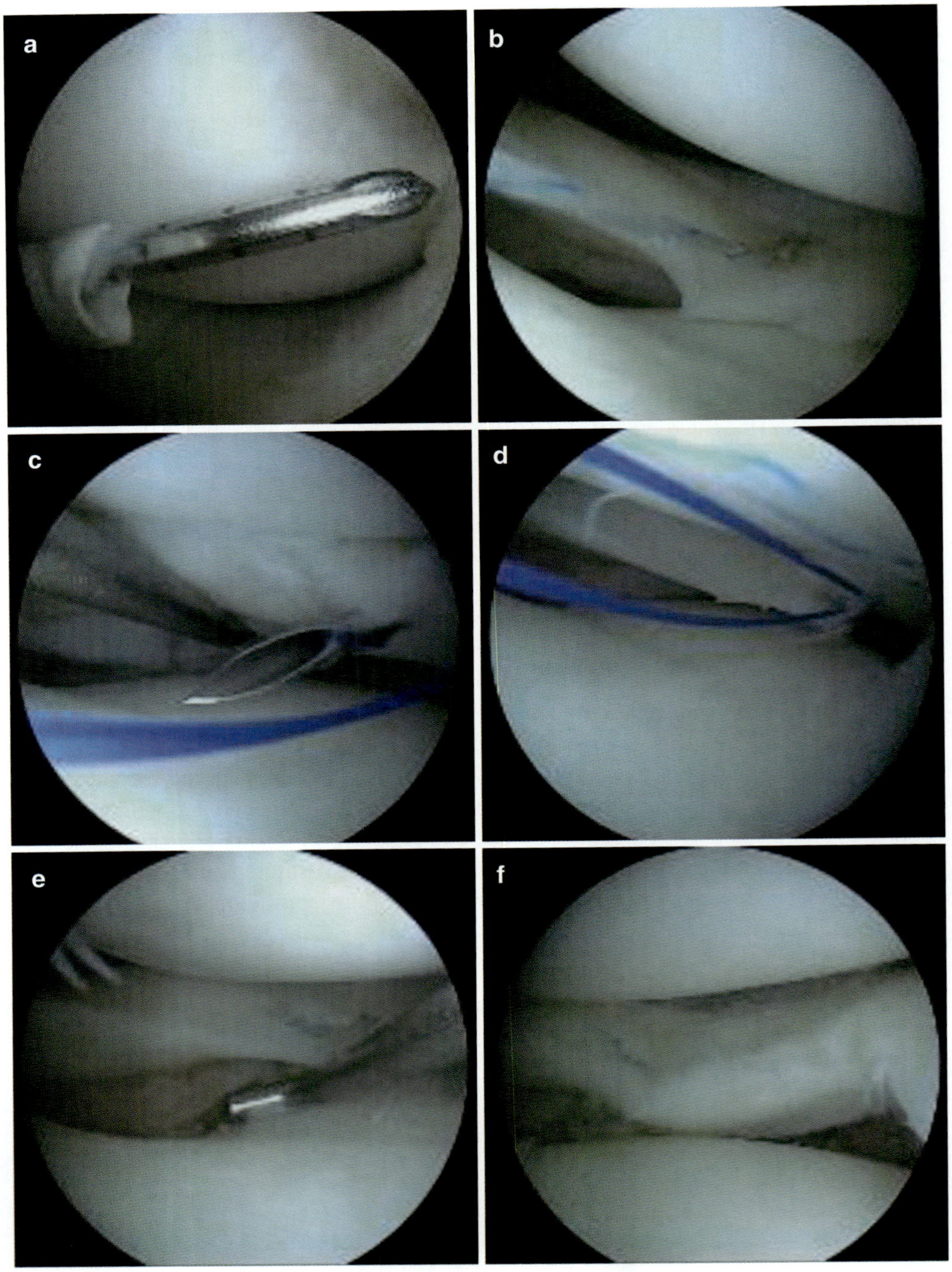

Fig. 2.23 The meniscal rupture shown above is sutured with a combination of outside-in and all inside (FasT-Fix) techniques. Ultra Fast-Fix, Smith & Nephew, Inc. Andover, MA, USA

2.3.2 Meniscal Transplant

The beginnings of meniscal allograft transplants date back to the early twentieth century, when fat tissue arthroplasty [77] and tibial plateau parts transplants [78] were performed. The first free meniscal allograft transplant was reported by Milachowski et al. in 1984, when 23 patients underwent medial meniscal transplantation using allografts which were deep-frozen and lyophilized [79]. However, the developing trend did not follow so successfully, as none of the future solutions such as meniscal scaffolds and xenografts were to obtain satisfactory results [79–82].

Osteoarthritis following complete meniscus removal is a known fact and has been thoroughly documented [83–87]. By removing the meniscus, the contact surface between the femoral condyle and the tibial plateau is decreased, resulting in an increase of contact pressure. The meniscus also allows for joint lubrication, pressure distribution, joint stability and shock absorption. Depriving the knee of all these beneficial factor leads to imminent and irreparable cartilage damage [61, 88–90].

Meniscal transplantation is recommended in three types of clinical patterns:

1. Young patients that had meniscectomy performed in the past and present symptoms in that specific knee compartment, but have low osteoarthritic modifications (<3 based on the ICRS scale) and a stable knee joint. Lateral compartment, symptomatic, meniscus deficiencies are also a common indication [91].
2. Patients with ACL deficiency, which underwent ACL reconstruction and medial meniscectomy and might benefit from a healthy and functional medial meniscus. Thus, knee joint stability is improved and the reconstructed ACL is protected.
3. A rather relative indication can be found in young athletes which have had a total meniscectomy in the past and are yet to encounter any osteoarthritic symptoms [92].

Meniscal allograft transplantation is not recommended to be performed if:

1. High chondral degeneration (3 > according to ICRS) has been suggested to be a contraindication, although its effect on eventual graft failure was not proven to be of great significance [93].
2. Radiograph evidenced osteophytes have been known to favor bad outcomes due to the structural modifications they create on the normal bone surface [94].
3. Varus and valgus deformities exert abnormal pressure on the graft and induce a high rate of failure [94]. Correction osteothomies must be performed prior to the transplant in order to correct the axial misalignment.
4. Joint instability, obesity, synovial disease, inflammatory or infectious arthritis and skeletal immaturity.

2.3.2.1 Research

Animal model transplantation served as a reliable source of research in the field of meniscal transplantation. The best match of an animal model with human meniscal anatomy and biomechanics was discovered in the sheep model by Joshi et al. [95]. Milachowski et al. found that healing was achieved in a sheep model at approximately 6 weeks after transplantation using both lyophilized and deep-frozen allografts. Arnoczky et al. performed meniscal allograft transplantation in dogs. The result was a grossly normal and healed menisci [96]. Posterior horn disruption was signaled in three cases. This was later confirmed by Elliot et al. who reported meniscal healing and capsule attachment at 12 weeks after transplantation [95]. Later cartilage assessment revealed insignificant differences between allograft transplantation and meniscectomy on most of the animal models [96–101]. All in all, meniscal healing and capsular attachment was found in most models, the downside being the degeneration found in the meniscus itself. Also, we can state that restoring cartilage quality is hard to achieve through allograft transplantation.

2.3.2.2 Graft Selection, Harvesting and Preservation

Of course, human meniscal allograft transplantation is a risk involving procedure. As with all transplants, the first risk is disease spreading. Choosing a right donor must be done according to Health Organization directives, and it must respect specific standards. Screening tests are ran for HIV-1 and HIV-2, hepB, hepC, syphilis and HTLV-1. The harvested probe is placed in a thioglycate broth culture medium to ensure that bacteriological contamination does not exist [102, 103]. They are also cultured for aerobic end anaerobic fungi and bacteria for at least a week.

The perfect menisci donor should preferably be under 45 years old, have no history of knee osteoarthritis (inflammatory or post-traumatic) and no meniscal damage. Usually a 1 cm slice of the entire tibial plateau is cut, containing the two menisci, followed by another mid-section sagittal cut of the specimen, without damaging the insertion of the two menisci.

Due to the lack of proven advantages compared to preserved grafts and need for a high amount of logistics, we will not be covering the fresh, viable meniscal allograft transplantation. Cryopreserved meniscal allografts are gradually frozen and stored at a temperature of −196 °C, after being treated with an antiseptic agent and culture medium. The information on the amount of viable cells remaining after this process has been scarce, thus the method is still under question [104].

Freshly frozen allografts are packaged and stored in a freezer at −80 °C after being treated with an antibiotic saline solution. They can be kept like this for as long as 5 years and do not present mechanical properties alteration. Freeze-dried allografts are frozen under a vacuumed and dried environment. Cellular viability can be obtained through this method only if cryoprotective solutions are applied, otherwise the graft would be a dry nonviable tissue [105, 106]. Furthermore, due to the difficulty of the sterilizing procedure, irradiation at 25 kGy must be applied. From a clinical point of view, these types of grafts are not suitable for transplantation [97, 107, 108].

2.3.2.3 Surgical Technique

The meniscal allograft transplantation procedure can be done either via open technique or arthroscopic. Fixation-wise, there are two main options in meniscal transplantation. The graft can either be sutured to the soft tissue, or attached to the tibia alongside with bone blocks in specially drilled tunnels. From what has been studied, no clinical or radiological difference has been found between these two fixation options.

Graft preparation is an important step of this procedure, as it ensures most of the outcomes. The meniscus is fixed on a cork board with three needles, and its upper side is marked with a skin marker. Horizontal sutures are placed every 4–5 mm from one another, starting from the posterior horn and moving towards the anterior horn. The number of required sutures averages between 6 and 8. These sutures are also fixed to the board, in sequence. Depending on the transplanted meniscus, a medial or lateral 8 cm parapatellar incision is made with the knee flexed at 90°. The capsule is opened and the medial collateral ligament or the lateral collateral ligament, popliteus tendon and iliotibial band must be cut loose. This is achieved by performing a small osteotomy at their insertion points with a curved osteotome. Once this process is done, we can easily open the required knee compartment to obtain a gap of 2 cm by applying a valgus force or placing the leg in the figure-four position.

The remnant meniscus must be trimmed so that its outer rim stays intact, as it will serve as a support for the future graft. The meniscus' insertions can also be trimmed to fit the implant. Next, the allograft is introduced inside the knee and the sutures are passed through the meniscal rim from inferior to superior and then transferred to another suture holder from posterior to anterior. Now the allograft can be fixed by gently pulling on each suture and tying it with a knot. This is also done progressively from posterior to anterior in order to perform a secure and optimal fit to the meniscal rim.

Once this is done, the knee can be flexed in a normal 90° flexed position without any varus or valgus applied, and the bony insertions of the tendons are fixed with screws. The last step is securing the anterior horn of the graft to the tibia with an anchor.

2.3.2.4 Arthroscopic Technique

The knee is positioned as for a normal arthroscopic procedure and a standard 30° knee arthroscope can be used. Before initiating the transplant procedure itself, the surgeon must remove all fibrous/scar tissue that is present near the implantation zone. This improves the chances of graft re-vascularization and facilitates its integration. The only preparation the graft needs, are two sutures, one at each implantation area (posterior and anterior horn extensions).

The bone tunnels are drilled using an ACL guide aimed at the insertion points of the posterior and anterior horn. A semi-rigid wire is inserted through each of the tunnels, and both are extracted through the portal that coincides with the meniscus that is about to be implanted. In order to allow the graft to be inserted into the joint, the portal must be enlarged so that it fits a fingertip and that no other soft parts are interposed.

The semi-rigid wires are attached to the sutures on the menisci and we start inserting the graft by pulling on the posterior wire until the posterior horn is firmly positioned. The same action is repeated for the anterior guiding wire. Afterwards, the meniscus can be sutured to the peripheral rim through a combination of inside-out and outside-in techniques. Now the two sutures can be tied together on the anterior surface of the tibia. A rigid hinge orthosis is recommended for 6 weeks with the knee flexed at 20°.

2.3.3 Meniscal Reconstruction with Artificial Substitutes

2.3.3.1 Collagen Meniscus Implant (CMI)

The idea of creating such an implant started from one main hypothesis – that the meniscus possesses the ability to regenerate itself, if provided with the proper biologic environment, and that it can be supported by a bioengineered matrix scaffold [109–112]. It already is known that type I collagen has the appropriate properties that makes it suitable for tissue and organ repair [113]. This makes it viable for it to develop on a properly engineered matrix scaffold.

The scaffold must have the right biomechanical properties in order to maintain survivability inside the knee and function like a normal meniscus when the collagen has developed on it [114, 115]. Growth factors and other similar biologic factors can be implemented in the matrix in order to allow the regeneration and remodeling process to occur [109–111, 113].

This was tested on immature pigs knees and the results were promising. After each evaluation period (1, 3, 6 weeks) since the implantation of a CMI on 80 % meniscus resected knees, results were observed. There was no sign of cartilage wear, tissue destruction or joint degeneration. Furthermore, they observed signs of tissue regeneration – granulation tissue and vascular proliferation [111].

As more and more improvements were added to the CMI, the human clinical trials that followed these upgrades, had good results. A large prospective study on more than 300 patients was conducted in the US in 16 different investigation sites. Positive results were obtained, especially for patients which underwent previous partial meniscectomy, and it was concluded that CMI can support growth of collagenous tissue that can serve the role of the menisci with improved clinical outcomes [112].

2.3.4 Conclusion

The number of meniscal repair techniques has grown over the past years, as a need to develop an alternative technique to meniscectomy. It is known that loss of joint stability and loss of tissue requires its replacement. As ACL reconstruction became the golden standard in ACL tears and the instability that it produces, it is not improbable that meniscal sutures or transplantation may just be the future standard treatment, given the right patients and their daily needs.

Meniscus allograft implantation offered satisfactory results in 70 % of the patients, when compared to total meniscectomy, regardless of the preservation technique that was used. However, considering the larger number of patients that receive only a partial meniscectomy, the field of CMI and different innovative matrix scaffold technique seems to have a better prediction, given the possibility of carving the implant to fit the remnant meniscus. It seems that in the field of meniscal repair, the knowledge obtained so far is only the tip of the iceberg, leaving room for more innovative research and the development of new techniques.

2.4 The Osteoarthritic Knee

Degenerative meniscal tears can represent an initiation factor for the onset of knee osteoarthritis. Virtually all such cases will have degenerative medial meniscus lesions accompanying the chondral defects. Nevertheless, these meniscal lesions have been shown to appear in high number also in asymptomatic knees. These findings are common in the general population and increase with age [40]. In addition, the prevalence of articular cartilage damage in patients undergoing arthroscopic surgery for meniscal lesions increases with age, weight, medial compartment and knee contractures [116].

Controversy surrounds whether the pain is caused by the unstable meniscus or by osteoarthritis, since the degenerative rupture of the meniscus can merely be an effect of knee osteoarthritis and incidental finding on an MRI performed for painful osteoarthritis (Fig. 2.24). In addition, there is no consensus in the literature about the preoperative factors predictive for the relief of pain following arthroscopic meniscectomy in the presence of early stage knee osteoarthritis. The treatment options for such cases include physiotherapy, intraarticular injections of hyaluronic acid and steroids and arthroscopic debridement, as conservative methods to alleviate symptoms until progression of disease and age will deem suitable for joint replacement procedure.

The popularity of arthroscopy in osteoarthritic knees has increased due to its short surgery time, low costs, fast recovery and immediate benefit output. Besides the clear pain relief it offers to patients, arthroscopy also allows them to continue with their daily activities, without disabling them for a long recovery period.

Burman in 1934 [117] reported the benefits of arthroscopic mechanical washout of the knee in osteoarthritis. Haggart introduced in 1940 [118], mini-open arthrotomy procedures such as resecting hypertrophic synovial, osteophytes and extracting loose bodies from the joint. In 1941, Magnuson reported complete recovery in 60 out of 62 patients knee osteoarthritis treated by arthroscopic debridement [119]. In 1981, Sprague reported his results on a large series of patients who had undergone arthroscopic treatment for degenerative osteoarthritis. His results were satisfying as he achieved good results in 74 % of the patients at a mean of 14 months after surgery. He found a rate of failure of 16 %, while 10 % of the patients presented with fair results [120].

The role of arthroscopy in patients with knee osteoarthritis is still debated. There are studies that show the lack of improvement after treatment, and studies that demonstrate that it can be marginally better than other types of treatment. The multitude of techniques, performed by many investigators associated with many individual variables that the patients have, may turn out to produce uneven results between similar studies.

In 2002, Moseley et al. presented the results of a Level I investigation, concerning the arthroscopic treatment of knee osteoarthritis. He evaluated the pain in the operated knee, 24 months after surgery using a 12-item knee pain scale. The result was somehow disappointing. They concluded that the outcomes following arthroscopic lavage or debridement is no better than placebo in patients with knee osteoarthritis. Some faults did exist in this trial though. The results were not stratified by grade of OA and also by OA localization (the results were combined for all three compartments) [121].

Kirkley et al. realized another randomized trial study in 2008. They compared medical and physical therapy with medical, physical and arthroscopic treatment in patients with knee OA. The arthroscopy associated lavage (at least 1 l of saline solution) with one or more of the following: debridement, synovectomy, meniscectomy, excision of loose bodies or osteophyte resection. The SF-36 score after 2 years – 37.0/37.2 – was similar, showing basically no differences between outcomes [122].

Another recent multicenter, randomized, controlled trial involving symptomatic patients with meniscal tears and mild-to-moderate osteoarthritis (METEOR) performed by Katz et al. also found little difference between arthroscopic meniscectomy and physical therapy in this population [Katz]. However, they also had an important number of patients from the physical therapy group eventually undergo arthroscopic surgery [123].

A recent study by Vermesan et al. compared the use of intraarticular steroids with arthroscopic debridement in patients with knee osteoarthritis. They found that the arthroscopic group performed better in terms of symptom improvement at 4 weeks after surgery. After 1 year, 4.2 % of the patients were converted to a total knee replacement [33]. They also concluded that bone marrow edema, extrusion of the meniscus, obesity and the duration of the clinical symptoms were negative prognostic factors.

In 1997, Steadman et al. presented the results of a clinical trial involving microfractures in patients with knee OA. After a mean follow-up of 7 years, 75 % out of the total of 298 patients presented with good results, 20 % had unchanged symptoms and 5 % had poor results. Second look arthroscopy revealed that 77 patients presented hyaline cartilage cell proliferation on the treated area [124] (Figs. 2.25, 2.26 and 2.27).

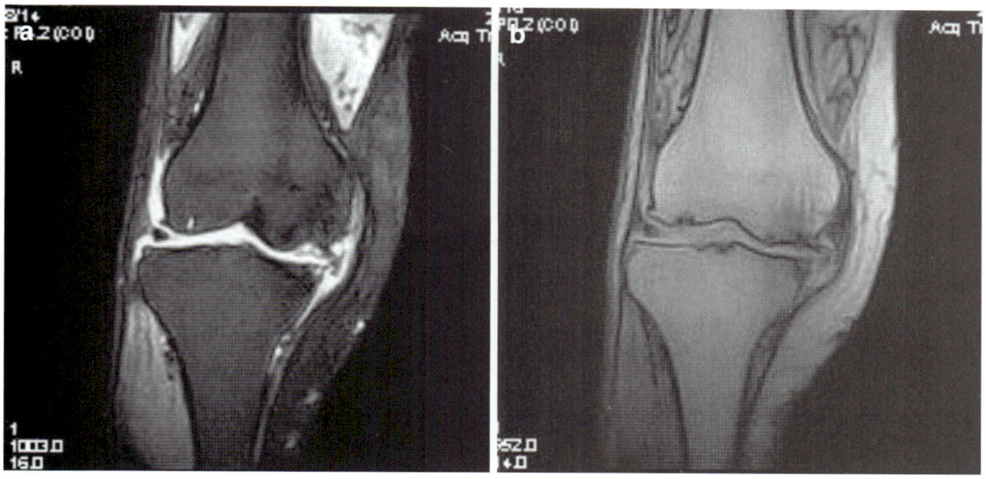

Fig. 2.24 Coronal STIR (**a**) and T2 (**b**) MRI scans of a 69 year-old woman with advanced osteoarthritis

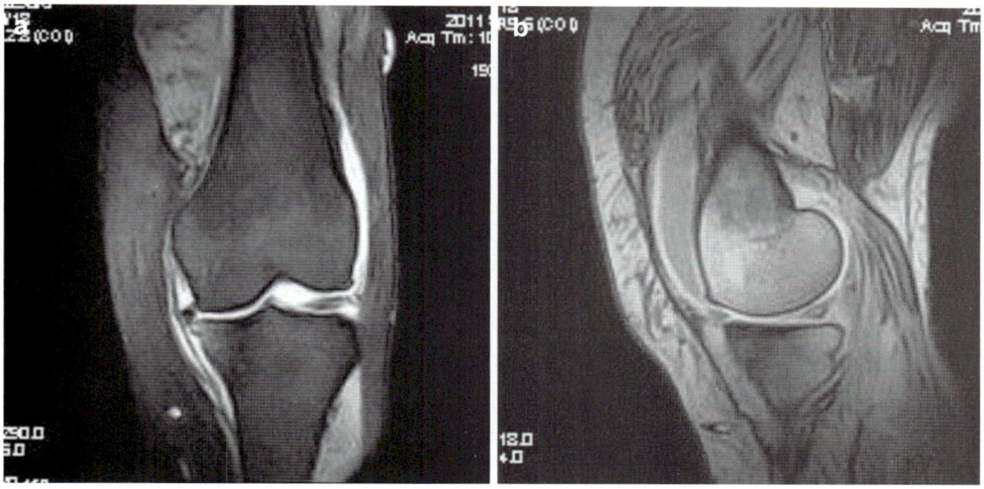

Fig. 2.25 A 60 year old woman MRI scans showing clear signs of knee osteoarthritis. We can notice the asymmetry between the two tibio-femoral compartments, the tight medial compartment and the varus deviation of the knee (**a**). Meniscal extrusion and osteophytes can also be observed (**b**)

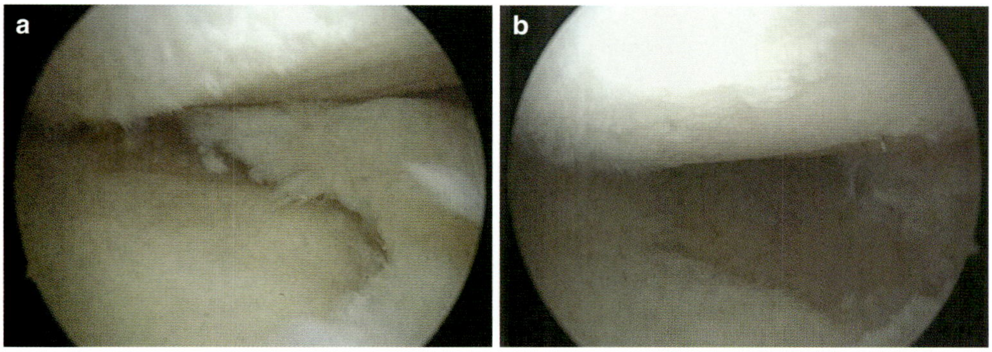

Fig. 2.26 Outerbridge IV condropathy of the internal compartment with mirrored chondral lesions and meniscal degeneration (**a**, **b**)

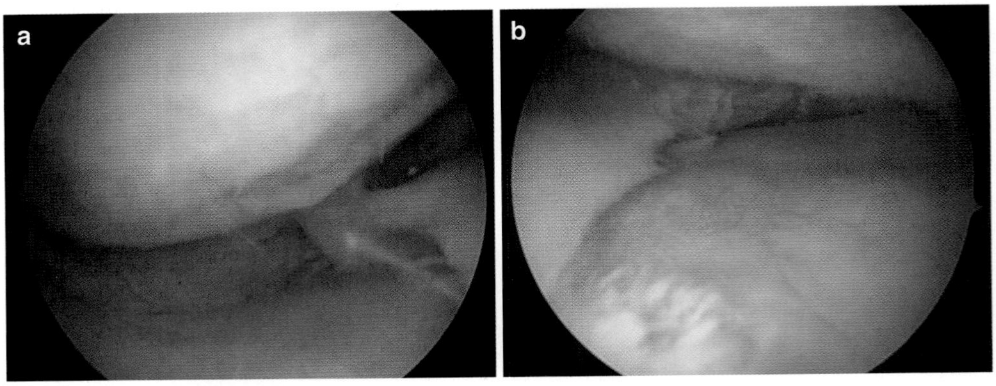

Fig. 2.27 Medial meniscus posterior horn meniscectomy performed on a patient with advanced knee osteoarthritis (**a**, **b**)

References

1. Praemer A, Furner S, Rice DP. Musculoskeletal conditions in the United States. Rosemont: American Academy of Orthopedic Surgeons; 1999.
2. Renstrom P, Johnson PJ. Anatomy and biomechanics of the menisci. Clin Sports Med. 1990;9:523–38.
3. Shiraev T, Anderson SE, Hope N. Meniscal tear – presentation, diagnosis and management. Aust Fam Physician. 2012;41(4):182–7.
4. Snoeker BA, Bakker EW, Kegel CA, Lucas C. Risk factors for meniscal tears: a systematic review including meta-analysis. J Orthop Sports Phys Ther. 2013;43(6):352–67. doi:10.2519/jospt.2013.4295.
5. Sri-Ram K, Salmon LJ, Pinczewski LA, Roe JP. The incidence of secondary pathology after anterior cruciate ligament rupture in 5086 patients requiring ligament reconstruction. Bone Joint J. 2013;95-B(1):59–64. doi:10.1302/0301-620X.95B1.29636.
6. Belzer J, Cannon Jr WD. Meniscus tears: treatment in the stable and unstable knee. J Am Acad Orthop Surg. 1993;1:41–7.
7. Ercin E, Kaya I, Sungur I, Demirbas E, Ugras AA, Cetinus EM. History, clinical findings, magnetic resonance imaging, and arthroscopic correlation in meniscal lesions. Knee Surg Sports Traumatol Arthrosc. 2012;20(5):851–6.
8. Niitsu M. Magnetic resonance imaging of the knee. Berlin/New York: Springer; 2012.
9. De Smet AA, Mukherjee R. Clinical, MRI, and arthroscopic findings associated with failure to diagnose a lateral meniscaltear on knee MRI. AJR Am J Roentgenol. 2008;190(1):22–6.
10. von Engelhardt LV, Schmitz A, Pennekamp PH, Schild HH, Wirtz DC, von Falkenhausen F. Diagnostics of degenerative meniscal tears at 3-Tesla MRI compared to arthroscopy as reference standard. Arch Orthop Trauma Surg. 2008;128(5):451–6. Epub 2007 Oct 30.
11. Crues 3rd JV, Mink J, Levy TL, Lotysch M, Stoller DW. Meniscal tears of the knee: accuracy of MR imaging. Radiology. 1987;164(2):445–8.
12. Khanna S, Crues 3rd JV. Complexities of MRI and false positive findings. Ann N Y Acad Sci. 2009;1154:239–58. doi:10.1111/j.1749-6632.2009.04393.x.
13. Mathieu L, Bouchard A, Marchaland JP, Potet J, Fraboulet B, Danguy-des-Deserts M, Versier G. Knee MR-arthrography in assessment of meniscal and chondral lesions. Orthop Traumatol Surg Res. 2009;95(1):40–7.
14. Cook JL, Cook CR, Stannard JP, Vaughn G, Wilson N, Roller BL, Stoker AM, Jayabalan P, Hdeib M, Kuroki K. MRI versus ultrasonography to assess meniscal abnormalities in acute knees. J Knee Surg. 2014;27:319–24.
15. Rathleff CR, Cavallius C, Jensen HP, Simonsen OH, Rasmussen S, Kaalund S, Ostgaard SE. Successful conservative treatment of patients with MRI-verified meniscal lesions. Knee Surg Sports Traumatol Arthrosc. 2013:1–6 [Epub ahead of print].
16. Weiss CB, Lundberg M, Hamberg P, DeHaven KE, Gillquist J. Non-operative treatment of meniscal tears. J Bone Joint Surg Am. 1989;71(6):811–22.
17. Beaufils P, Bastos R, Wakim E, Cho SH, Petit-Jouvet C. Meniscal injury in the plastic reconstruction of the anterior cruciate ligament. Meniscal suture or abstention. Rev Chir Orthop Reparatrice Appar Mot. 1992;78:285–91.
18. Shelbourne KD, Heinrich J. The long-term evaluation of lateral meniscus tears left in situ at the time of anterior cruciate ligament reconstruction. Arthroscopy. 2004;20(4):346–51.
19. Fitzgibbons RE, Shelbourne KD. "Aggressive" nontreatment of lateral meniscal tears seen during anterior cruciate ligament reconstruction. Am J Sports Med. 1995;23:156–9.
20. Shelbourne KD, Rask BP. The sequelae of salvaged nondegenerative peripheral vertical medial meniscus tears with anterior cruciate ligament reconstruction. Arthroscopy. 2001;17:270–4.
21. Pierre A, Hulet C, Locker B, Schiltz D, Delbarre JC, Vielpeau C. Outcome of 95 stable meniscal tears left in place after reconstruction of the anterior cruciate ligament. Rev Chir Orthop Reparatrice Appar Mot. 2001;87:661–8.
22. Zemanovic JR, McAllister DR, Hame SL. Nonoperative treatment of partial-thickness meniscal tears identified during anterior cruciate ligament reconstruction. Orthopedics. 2004;27(7):755–8.
23. Yagishita K, Muneta T, Ogiuchi T, Sekiya I, Shinomiya K. Healing potential of meniscal tears without repair in knees with anterior cruciate ligament reconstruction. Am J Sports Med. 2004;32(8):1953–61.
24. Uchio Y, Ochi M, Adachi N, Kawasaki K, Iwasa J. Results of rasping of meniscal tears with and without anterior cruciate ligament injury as evaluated by second-look arthroscopy. Arthroscopy. 2003;19(5):463–9.
25. Vermesan D, Prejbeanu R, Laitin S, Georgianu V, Haragus H, Nitescu S, Tatullo M, Tattoli M, Caprio M, Cagiano R. Meniscal tears left in situ during anatomic single bundle anterior cruciate ligament reconstruction. Eur Rev Med Pharmacol Sci. 2014;18(2):252–6.
26. De Smet AA, Norris MA, Yandow DR, et al. MR diagnosis of meniscal tears of the knee: importance of high signal in the meniscus that extends to the surfact. AJR Am J Roentgenol. 1993;161:101–7.
27. Pujol N, Beaufils P. Healing results of meniscal tears left in situ during anterior cruciate ligament reconstruction: a review of clinical studies. Knee Surg Sports Traumatol Arthrosc. 2009;17:396–401.
28. Paxton ES, Stock MV, Brophy RH. Meniscal repair versus partial meniscectomy: a systematic review comparing reoperation rates and clinical outcomes. Arthroscopy. 2011;27(9):1275–88.
29. Ahn JH, Bae TS, Kang KS, Kang SY, Lee SH. Longitudinal tear of the medial meniscus posterior horn in the anterior cruciate ligament-deficient knee significantly influences anterior stability. Am J Sports Med. 2011;39(10):2187–93.
30. Noyes FR, Barber-Westin SD. Treatment of meniscus tears during anterior cruciate ligament reconstruction. Arthroscopy. 2012;28(1):123–30. Epub 2011 Nov 9.
31. Salata MJ, Gibbs AE, Sekiya JK. A systematic review of clinical outcomes in patients undergoing meniscectomy. Am J Sports Med. 2010;38(9):1907–16.
32. Shelbourne KD, Roberson TA, Gray T. Long-term evaluation of posterior lateral meniscus root tears left in situ at the time of anterior cruciate ligament reconstruction. Am J Sports Med. 2011;39(7):1439–43.
33. Vermesan D, Prejbeanu R, Laitin S, Damian G, Deleanu B, Abbinante A, Flace P, Cagiano R. Arthroscopic debridement compared to intra-articular steroids in treating degenerative medial meniscal tears. Eur Rev Med Pharmacol Sci. 2013;17(23):3192–6.
34. Clayton RA, Court-Brown CM. The epidemiology of muculoskeletal tendinous and ligamentous injuries. Injury. 2008;39:1338–44.
35. Fairbank TJ. Knee changes after menisectomy. J Bone Joint Surg Br. 1948;30:664–70.
36. Ghormley RK. Late joint changes as a result of internal derangements of the knee. Am J Surg. 1948;76:496–501.
37. Neyret PH, Walch G, Dejour H. La meniscectomie interne intramurale selon la technique de A. Trillat. Résultats à long terme de 258 interventions. Rev Chir Ortho. 1988;74:637–46.
38. Watanabe M, Takeda S, Ikeuchi H. Atlas of arthroscopy. 3rd ed. Tokyo: Igaku Shoin; 1979. p. 87–91.
39. Cullen KA, Hall MJ, Golosinskiy A. Ambulatory surgery in the United States, 2006. Natl Health Stat Rep. 2009;11:1–25.
40. Englund M, Guermazi A, Gale D, Hunter DJ, Aliabadi P, Clancy M, Felson DT. Incidental meniscal findings on knee MRI in middle-aged and elderly persons. N Engl J Med. 2008;359(11):1108–15.
41. Metcalf MH, Barrett GR. Prospective evaluation of 1485 meniscal tear patterns in patients with stable knees. Am J Sports Med. 2004;32:675–80.

42. Andersson-Molina H, Karlsson H, Rockborn P. Arthroscopic partial and total meniscectomy: a long term follow-up study with matched controls. Arthroscopy. 2002;18:183–9.
43. Becker R, Schroder M, Starke C, Urbach D, Nebelung W. Biomechanical investigations of different meniscal repair implants in comparison with horizontal sutures on human meniscus. Arthroscopy. 2001;17(5):439–44.
44. Hede A, Larsen E, Sandberg H. Partial versus total meniscectomy a prospective, randomised study with long-term follow-up. J Bone Joint Surg Br. 1992;74:118–21.
45. Barber FA, Herbert MA. Meniscal repair devices. Arthroscopy. 2000;16(7):754–6.
46. Asik M, Sener N, Akpinar S, Durmaz H, Göksan A. Strength of different meniscus suturing techniques. Knee Surg Sports Traumatol Arthrosc. 1997;5:80–3.
47. Johnson DS, Stewart H, Hirst P, Harper NJ. Is tourniquet use necessary for knee arthroscopy. Arthroscopy. 2000;16:648–51.
48. Orengo P, Zahlaoui J. Chirurgiedesménisques. Encycl Med Chir, Paris, Techniques chirurgicales, Orthopédie trauma- tologie, 44785, 4.10.06, 18 p.
49. Neyret P, Walch G, Dejour H. La méniscectomie interne intra-murale selon la technique de A. Trillat: résul- tats à long terme de 258 interventions. Rev Chir Orthop. 1988;74:637–46.
50. Trillat A. Les lésions méniscales internes. Les lésions méniscales externes. Chirurgie du genou. Journées Lyonnaises de chirurgie du genou. 1973. 04/1971. Simep, ed., Villeurbanne.
51. Gillquist J, Oretorp N. Arthroscopic partial meniscectomy. Clin Orthop Relat Res. 1982;167:29–33.
52. Northmore-Ball MD, Dandy DJ. Long-term results of arthroscopic partial meniscectomy. Clin Orthop Relat Res. 1982;167:34–42.
53. Metcalf RW. Arthroscopic meniscal surgery. In: McGinty JB, editor. Operative arthroscopy. New York: Raven Press; 1991. p. 203–36.
54. Escalas F, Quadras J, Caceres E, et al. T-Fix anchor sutures for arthroscopic meniscal repair. Knee Surg Sports Traumatol Arthrosc. 1997;5:72–6.
55. Vandermeer RD, Cunnigham FK. Arthroscopic treatment of the discoid lateral meniscus: results of long term follow-up. Arhroscopy. 1989;5:101–9.
56. Burks RT, Metcalf MH, Metcalf RW. Fifteen-year follow-up of arthroscopic partial meniscectomy. Arthroscopy. 1997;13:673–9.
57. Panisset JC, Neyret P. Méniscectomie sous arthroscopie. Encycl Med Chir. Techniques chirurgicales- Orthopédie-traumatologie. 2002; 12:44–765.
58. Chatain F, Robinson AHN, Adeleine P, Chambat P, Neyret P. The natural history of the knee following arthroscopic medial meniscectomy. Knee Surg Sports Traumatol Arthrosc. 2001;9:15–8.
59. Smillie IS. Injuries of the knee joint. London: Churchill Livingstone; 1978.
60. Small N. Complications in arthroscopic surgery performed by experienced arthroscopists. Arthroscopy. 1988;4:215–21.
61. Tapper EM, Hoover NW. Late results after meniscectomy. J Bone Joint Surg Am. 1969;51:517–26.
62. Matsusue Y, Thomson NL. Arthroscopic partial medial meniscectomy in patients over 40 years old: a 5- to 11-year follow-up study. Arthroscopy. 1996;12:39–44.
63. Markolf KL, Mensch JS, Amstutz HC. Stiffness and laxity of the knee-the contributions of the supporting structures. A quantitative in vitro study. J Bone Joint Surg Am. 1976;58:583–94.
64. Kurosawa H, Fukubayashi T, Nakajima H. Load- bearing mode of the knee joint: physical behavior of the knee joint with or without menisci. Clin Orthop Relat Res. 1980;149:283–90.
65. Jareguito JW, Elliot JS, Leitner T, et al. The effects of partial lateral meniscectomy in an otherwise normal knee: a retrospective review of functional, clinical, and radiographic results. Arthroscopy. 1995;11:29–36.
66. Annandale T. An operation for displaced semilunar cartilage. Br Med J. 1885;1:779.
67. Ikeuchi H. Surgery under arthroscopic control. In: Proceeding of the Societe Internationale d'Arthroscopie. Rheumatology. 1975;14:57–62.
68. Arnoczky SP, Warren RF. Microvasculature of the human meniscus. Am J Sports Med. 1982;10:90–5.
69. Pujol N, Panarella L, Selmi TAS, Neyret P, Fithian D, Beaufils P. Meniscal healing after meniscus repair. A CT arthrography assessment. Am J Sports Med. 2008;36:1489–95.
70. Rodeo SA, Warren RF. Meniscal repair using the outside-to-inside technique. Clin Sports Med. 1996;15(3):469–81.
71. DeHaven KE, Black K, Griffiths HJ. Open meniscus repair. Technique and two to nine year results. Am J Sports Med. 1989;17:788–95.
72. Warren RF. Arthroscopic meniscus repair. Arthroscopy. 1985;1:170–2.
73. Arnoczky SP, Lavagnino M. Tensile fixation strengths of absorbable meniscal repairs as a function of hydrolysis time. Am J Sports Med. 2001;29:118–23.
74. McDermott ID, Richards SW, Hallam P, Tavares S, Lavelle JR, Amis AA. A biomechanical study of four different meniscal repair systems, comparing pull-out strengths and gapping under cyclic loading. Knee Surg Sports Traumatol Arthrosc. 2003;11:23–9.
75. Anderson K, Marx RG, Hannafin J, Warren RF. Chondral injury following meniscal repair with a biodegradable implant. Arthroscopy. 2000;16:749–53.
76. Calder S, Myers PT. Broken arrow: a complication of meniscal repair. Arthroscopy. 1999;15:651–2.
77. Cole BJ, Carter TR, Rodeo SA. Allograft meniscal transplantation: background, techniques, and results. Instr Course Lect. 2003;52:383–96.
78. Rijk PC. Meniscal allograft transplantation – part I: background, results, graft selection and preservation, and surgical considerations. Arthroscopy. 2004;20:728–43.
79. Milachowski KA, Weismeier K, Wirth CJ. Homologous meniscus transplantation. Experimental and clinical results. Int Orthop. 1989;13:1–11.
80. Locht R, Gross A, Langer F. Late osteochondral resurfacing for tibial plateau fractures. J Bone Joint Surg Am. 1984;66:328–35.
81. de Groot J, de Vrijer R, Pennings A, et al. Use of porous polyurethanes for meniscal reconstruction and meniscal prosthesis. Biomaterials. 1996;17:163–73.
82. Kohn D, Rudert M, Wirth C, et al. Medial meniscus replacement by a fat pad autograft. Int Orthop. 1997;21:232–8.
83. Menche DS, Phillips GI, Pitman MI, Steiner GC. Inflammatory foreign-body reaction to an arthroscopic bioabsorbable meniscal arrow repair. Arthroscopy. 1999;15:770–2.
84. Ross G, Grabill J, McDevitt E. Chondral injury after meniscal repair with bioabsorbable arrows. Arthroscopy. 2000;16:754–6.
85. Allen PR, Denham RA, Swan AV. Late degenerative changes after meniscectomy. Factors affecting the knee after operation. J Bone Joint Surg Br. 1984;66:666–71.
86. Fairbank TJ. Knee joint changes after meniscectomy. J Bone Joint Surg Br. 1948;30-B:664–70.
87. Johnson RJ, Kettelkamp DB, Clark W, et al. Factors effecting late results after meniscectomy. J Bone Joint Surg Am. 1974;56:719–29.
88. McNicholas MJ, Rowley DI, McGurty D, et al. Total meniscectomy in adolescence: a thirty-year follow-up. J Bone Joint Surg Br. 2000;82-B:217–21.
89. Bourne RB, Finlay JB, Papadopoulos P, et al. The effect of medial meniscectomy on strain distribution in the proximal part of the tibia. J Bone Joint Surg Am. 1984;66:1431–7.
90. Krause WR, Pope MH, Johnson RJ, et al. Mechanical changes in the knee after meniscectomy. J Bone Joint Surg Am. 1976;58:599–604.
91. Levy IM, Torzilli PA, Warren RF. The effect of medial meniscectomy on anterior-posterior motion of the knee. J Bone Joint Surg Am. 1982;64:883–8.

92. Shoemaker SC, Markolf KL. The role of the meniscus in the anterior-posterior stability of the loaded anterior cruciate- deficient knee. Effects of partial versus total excision. J Bone Joint Surg Am. 1986;68:71–9.
93. Walker PS, Erkman MJ. The role of the menisci in force transmission across the knee. Clin Orthop. 1975;109:184–92.
94. Johnson DL, Bealle D. Meniscal allograft transplantation. Clin Sports Med. 1999;18:93–108.
95. Joshi M, Suh J, Marui T, et al. Interspecies variation of compressive biomechanical properties of the meniscus. J Biomed Mater Res. 1995;29:823–8.
96. Messner K, Gillquist J. Prosthetic replacement of the rabbit medial meniscus. J Biomed Mater Res. 1993;27:1165–73.
97. Arnoczky S, Warren S, McDevitt C. Meniscal replacement using a cryopreserved allograft. Clin Orthop. 1990;252:121–8.
98. Elliot D, Jones III R, Setton L, et al. Joint degeneration following meniscal allograft transplantation in a canine model: mechanical properties and semiquantitative histology of articular cartilage. Knee Surg Sports Traumatol Arthrosc. 2002;10:109–18.
99. Aagaard H, Jörgensen U, Bojsen-Möller F. Reduced degenerative articular changes after meniscal allograft transplantation in sheep. Knee Surg Sports Traumatol Arthrosc. 1999;7:184–91.
100. Jackson D, McDevitt C, Simon T, et al. Meniscal transplantation using fresh and cryopreserved allografts. Am J Sports Med. 1992;20:644–56.
101. Stone K, Rodkey W, McKinney L, et al. Autogenous replacement of the meniscus cartilage: analysis of results and mechanisms of failure. Arthroscopy. 1995;11:395–400.
102. Szomor Z, Martin T, Bonar F, et al. The protective effects of meniscal transplantation on cartilage. J Bone Joint Surg Am. 2000;82A:80–8.
103. von Lewinski G, Pressel T, Hurschler C, et al. The influence of intraoperative pre-tensioning on the chondroprotective effect of meniscal transplants. Am J Sports Med. 2006;34:397–408.
104. Tomford WW, Doppelt SH, Mankin HJ, et al. 1983 bone bank procedures. Clin Orthop Relat Res. 1983;174:15–21.
105. Tomford WW, Thongphasuk J, Mankin HJ, et al. Frozen musculoskeletal allografts. A study of the clinical incidence and causes of infection associated with their use. J Bone Joint Surg Am. 1990;72:1137–43.
106. Fabbriciani C, Lucania L, Milano G, et al. Meniscal allografts: cryopreservation vs deep-frozen technique. An experimental study in goats. Knee Surg Sports Traumatol Arthrosc. 1997;5:124–34.
107. Delloye C, De Halleux J, Cornu O, et al. Organizational and investigational aspects of bone banking in Belgium. Acta Orthop Belg. 1991;57 suppl 2:27–34.
108. Delloye C, Naets B, Cnockaert N, et al. Harvest, storage and microbiological safety of bone allografts. In: Delloye C, Bannister G, editors. Impaction bone grafting in revision arthroplasty. New York: Marcel Dekker; 2004.
109. Yahia LH, Drouin G, Zukor D. The irradiation effect on the initial mechanical properties of meniscal grafts. Biomed Mater Eng. 1993;3:211–21.
110. Yahia L, Zukor D. Irradiated meniscal allotransplants of rabbits: study of the mechanical properties at six months postoperation. Acta Orthop Belg. 1994;60:210–5.
111. Rodkey WG. A look beyond the horizon. In: Feagin Jr JA, Steadman JR, editors. The crucial principles in care of the knee. Philadelphia: Lippincott Williams & Wilkins; 2008.
112. Rodkey WG, Stone KR, Steadman JR. Prosthetic meniscal replacement. In: Finerman GAM, Noyes FR, editors. Biology and biomechanics of the traumatized synovial joint. The knee as a model. Rosemont: American Academy of Orthopaedic Surgeons; 1992.
113. Stone KR, Rodkey WG, Webber RJ, et al. Future directions: collagen-based prosthesis for meniscal regeneration. Clin Orthop Relat Res. 1990;252:129–35.
114. Stone KR, Rodkey WG, Webber RJ, et al. Meniscal regeneration with copolymeric collagen scaffolds: in vitro and in vivo studies evaluated clinically, histologically, biochemically. Am J Sports Med. 1992;20:104–11.
115. Rodkey WG, DeHaven KE, Montgomery WH, et al. Comparison of the collagen meniscus implant to partial meniscectomy: a prospective randomized trial. J Bone Joint Surg Am. 2008;90:1413–26.
116. Ciccotti MC, Kraeutler MJ, Austin LS, Rangavajjula A, Zmistowski B, Cohen SB, Ciccotti MG. The prevalence of articular cartilage changes in the knee joint in patients undergoing arthroscopy for meniscal pathology. Arthroscopy. 2012;28(10): 1437–44.
117. Burman MS, Finkelstein H, Mayer L. Arthroscopy of the knee joint. J Bone Joint Surg Am. 1934;16:255–68.
118. Haggart GE. Surgical treatment of degenerative arthritis of the knee joint. J Bone Joint Surg Br. 1940;22:717–29.
119. Magnuson PB. Joint debridement: surgical treatment of degenerative arthritis. Surg Gynecol Obstet. 1941;73:1–9.
120. Sprague 3rd NF. Arthroscopic debridement for degenerative knee joint disease. Clin Orthop. 1981;160:118–23.
121. Moseley JB, O'Malley K, Petersen N, et al. A controlled trial of arthroscopic surgery for osteoarthritis of the knee. N Engl J Med. 2002;347:81–8.
122. Kirkley A, Birmingham TB, Litchfifield RB, et al. A randomized trial of arthroscopic surgery for osteoarthritis of the knee. N Engl J Med. 2008;359:1097–107.
123. Katz JN, Brophy RH, Chaisson CE, de Chaves L, Cole BJ, Dahm DL, Donnell-Fink LA, Guermazi A, Haas AK, et al. Surgery versus physical therapy for a meniscal tear and osteoarthritis. N Engl J Med. 2013;369(7):677–8.
124. Steadman JR, Briggs KK, Rodrigo JJ, et al. Outcomes of microfracture for traumatic chondral defects of the knee: average 11-year follow-up. Arthroscopy. 2003;19:477–84.

3 The Anterior Cruciate Ligament

Radu Prejbeanu, Horia Haragus, and Florin Ramadani

3.1 Injury Patterns

3.1.1 Epidemiology

The anterior cruciate ligament of the knee (ACL) is the most reconstructed ligament in the human body. Granan et al. gathered data from Denmark, Norway and Sweden as part of the Scandinavian registry. The overall annual incidence of primary ACL reconstructions ranged between 32 and 38 per 100,000 inhabitants. This rose to 71–91 for the target population (15–39). There was a slight predominance of males (57–60 %). The median age at injury was 23–27 and at surgery 25–30, with a median time from injury to surgery of 7–10 months. Soccer, handball and skiing were the top injuring sporting activities (13–50 %). The reconstruction averaged approximately 1 hour and was predominantly performed as outpatient surgery (38–79 %). Simultaneous meniscal (35–55 %) and cartilage (17–27 %) lesions were common and led to less favorable outcomes. Meniscectomy was the most frequent procedure for meniscal injuries (69–80 %). Autologus hamstrings were the most used grafts (61–86 %), followed by bone – patellar tendon – bone (14–38 %). All knee injury and osteoarthritis outcome (KOOS) subscales improved up to 2 years postoperatively, with no difference between single and double bundle procedures. The highest increase was seen in function and sports, pledging for an injury of the young and physically active population [1–3].

There can be certain epidemiological differences between particular study cohorts and Nordic ligament registries. In the Multicenter Orthopedic Outcomes Network (MOON) the patients were younger (23), the time from injury to surgery was shorter (2.4 months) and the common injuring sports were basketball, soccer and American football. In addition, chondral defects were also more common (42 %) and allografts were more frequently used (13 %) in primary reconstructions compared to the Norwegian ligament registry [4]. These differences were much smaller when an American community based registry was compared to the Norwegian and soccer was the most frequent sport that led to ACL reconstruction in both registries [5]. A meta-analysis has found higher ACL tear incidences in sports for women compared to males. The same study found the highest variation in incidence related to training level in downhill skiing (0.63 for recreational skiers and 0.03 for professional respectively) [6].

3.1.2 Anatomy, Bundles, Function

Descriptive and functional data on the cruciate ligaments of the knee begun to emerge in the mainstream literature at the beginning of the last century. It has since been recognized that the ACL is the main restrain for anterior tibial translation as well as internal tibial rotation. Numerous attempts for repair and reconstruction have been proposed with limited success. The development of the arthroscopic techniques has boosted the applicability of ligamentous reconstruction, in favor of repair, due to the limited healing capacity of the torn ACL [7].

The anterior cruciate ligament has been described as a multifascicular structure originating on the antero-medial aspect of the tibia, with a sagittal and coronal oblique course towards the posterior aspect of the medial side of the lateral femoral condyle. The multiple collagen bundles are mainly

R. Prejbeanu, MD, PhD • H. Haragus, MD, PhD (✉)
Department of Orthopedics and Trauma,
University of Medicine and Pharmacy 'Victor Babes' Timisoara,
2 Eftimie Murgu Square, 300041 Timisoara, Romania

I-st Clinic of Orthopedics and Trauma,
Emergency Clinical County Hospital Timisoara,
10 Iosif Bulbuca Blvd, 300736 Timisoara, Romania
e-mail: raduprejbeanu@gmail.com; horia.haragus@yahoo.com

F. Ramadani, MD, PhD
Unfallchirurgie, Klinikum Wels-Grieskirchen,
42 Grieskirchner St, Wels A-4600, Austria

University of Medicine and Pharmacy 'Victor Babes' Timisoara,
Timisoara, Romania
e-mail: florin.ramadani@liwest.at

R. Prejbeanu (ed.), *Atlas of Knee Arthroscopy*,
DOI 10.1007/978-1-4471-6593-4_3, © Springer-Verlag London 2015

grouped into two fascicles, named after their tibial insertion the anteromedial (AM) and posterolateral (PL) bundles. This aspect is already evident from the fetal stage and is maintained in the adult form [8].

With the knee in extension, the two bundles are parallel, with the AM in front of the PL. Most ACL reconstruction is done with the knee flexed, and therefore the femoral insertion of the ACL bundles is important to be understood in a rotatory fashion depending on the flexion angle. Therefore, as the knee is flexed, the PL insertion moves forward and becomes more shallow and low compared to the AM and the two bundles become crossed. This pattern makes the fibers tension differently during the knee range of motion: the AM bundle is tauter in flexion (60°) and the PL in extension respectively with direct implications for stability [9, 10].

The AM bundle is the main restrain to anterior tibial translation and the PL stabilizes the knee near full extension and against tibial rotation [10] and they both work in a synergistic manner. This pattern has important implications in clinical diagnosis of ruptures as well as reconstruction. A study by Zantop et al. showed that sectioning of the AM bundle increased anterior tibial translation at 60° and 90° of flexion and the isolated section of the PL bundle increased anterior tibial translation at 30° respectively. Furthermore, PL insufficiency resulted in a significant increase in combined rotation at 0° and 30° [11]. Extraarticular structures might also play an important role in rotational stability. The antero-lateral ligament has been recently brought back to attention as an important extraarticular stabilizer in extension and early flexion. Additional repair or reconstruction of this structure resists internal tibial rotation and might improve postoperative pivot shift [12].

The femoral attachment of the ACL has been described to have relatively constant bony landmarks compared to the tibial footprint. It is located on the medial aspect of the lateral femoral condyle, posterior to the lateral intercondylar ridge (also named the 'resident's ridge' since it can be confused with the posterior margin of the condyle). It has been determined to have an average area of 196.8 mm^2, with the AM bundle having a larger footprint compared to the PL. The lateral bifurcate ridge sometimes divides the insertion of the two bundles on the femur [13]. In vivo measurement of the femoral footprint of the ACL found a mean length of approximately 16.5 mm. The diameter of the PL was approximately 2 mm smaller than the PL [14]. The AM inserts posterior to the PL with some degree of variability. When the knee is flexed to 90°, the AM bundle is attached between the 9.30 and 11.30 o'clock positions and the PL bundle between the 8.30 and 10 o'clock. When the posterior condyle was used as reference, Edwards et al. found the center of the AM bundle was at an average of 68 % in a shallow-deep direction and 55 in a high-low direction and the PL at 56 and 62 % respectively [15].

For the tibial insertion, the attachments of the PL and AM bundles were positioned on average at 10 and 17 mm anterior to the over-the-back tibial interspinous ridge and 4 and 5 mm lateral to the medial tibial spine border [16]. Together they form a broad insertion with relatively high variability compared to the femoral footprint. In vivo measurements found high individual variability of the size of the ACL insertions, which correlate with the patient's height and weight. The tibial footprint has a mean length of 17 mm with the AM bundle having a diameter approximately 2 mm larger than the PL [14].

The ACL is narrower in the middle portion and much thicker at the insertions, especially on the tibia. In a cadaver study, the average length of the ACL was determined to be 31 mm with an isometric behavior during motion. The same study determined the average inclination to the long axis of the femur with the knee in 90° of flexion of 28° [17]. The isometry of the bundles has been challenged by later studies such as that of Amis et al. [9]. The AM bundle is close to isometric when the knee is flexed while the PL slackens. When the whole ACL is stretched, the shorter PL fibers are subjected to higher tensile strains [18].

The ACL main blood supply is derived from branches of the middle genicular artery. These form a network in the synovial membrane that surrounds the ligament, with secondary contributions from the medial and lateral geniculates at the tibial insertion. The bony attachments are of less nutritive importance. The dense connective tissue of the ACL is composed mainly of type I collagen fibers with sporadic fibroblasts. In the anterior middle portion there is an avascular zone with fibrocartilaginous tissue. The ACL is innervated from branches of the tibial nerve. Especially around the insertions, these fibers have proprioceptive function [19, 20] (Fig. 3.1).

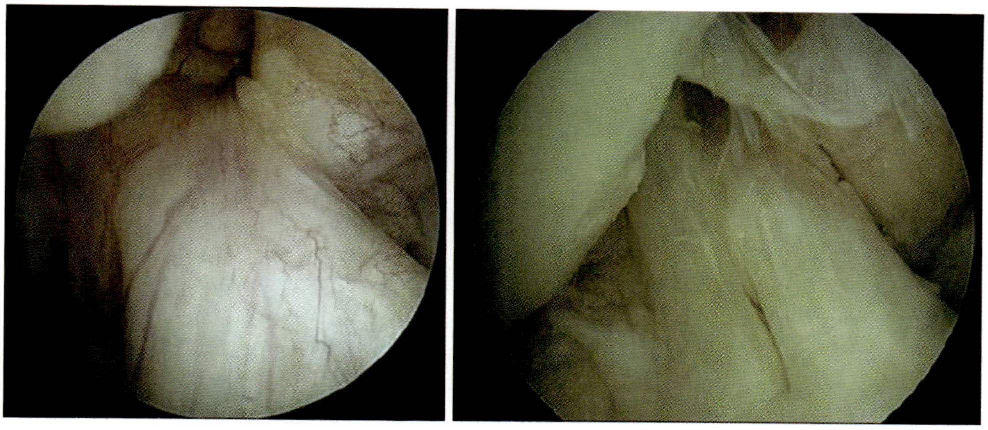

Fig. 3.1 Normal aspect of the ACL through the anterolateral and anteromedial portals and the knee close to 90° of flexion. The synovial vasculature is visible, as well as the large tibial insertion and the twisted narrower body. The bundle structure can sometimes be apparent. The femoral insertion is more difficult to visualize when the ACL is not ruptured (Kundnan)

3.1.3 Injury Mechanism and Patterns

A large number of ACL ruptures are isolated and occur through non-contact injuries. Understanding the causative mechanism might help determine methods for prevention. Anterior tibial shear forces with the knee close to full extension during landing are considered to be the main cause for noncontact ACL injuries. These forces are mainly determined by quadriceps contracture, as demonstrated by both experimental and in vivo studies [21, 22].

When the knee is at less than 30° of flexion, the hamstrings pull no longer exhibits a protective effect on anterior tibial translation. As the knee is flexed, the ACL is unloaded. Internal tibial rotation acts synergistic and increases the combined knee loading, whereas valgus or valgus stress does not significantly increase the loading of the ACL [23].

Although the ACL is also a restraint to forced valgus, this function was considered to be mostly exhibited after the medial collateral ligament (MCL) is torn. Recent cadaveric studies have shown that the ACL strain levels that can be reached during landings are lower than those needed to produce injury to the MCL [24]. It is therefore likely that valgus stress plays a role in the injuring pattern in combined triad injuries such as MCL, ACL and medial meniscus. Nevertheless, internal tibial torque combined with knee valgus during pivot landings loads the ACL and especially the AM bundle even before the MCL is torn [25].

In addition, compression and posterior directed ground reaction forces during landing further contribute to increase the ACL loading [26]. One compression and internal torsion cadaver study showed that the ACL failed when these motions were exaggerated. However, after the ligament was torn, the models exhibited abnormal movement characterized by external tibial rotation and knee valgus [27]. This might explain the descriptive findings associated with noncontact injuries. Video analysis of ACL injuries in team handball confirmed these experimental determinations and observed two prevalent mechanisms. The most common was described as a plant and cut movement with the knee extended and supplemental valgus and tibial rotation. The second was forced valgus and external rotation while landing on a single limb, also with the knee close to full extension [28].

Women are at higher risk for ACL tears from noncontact injuries but the contributing factors are ill defined. Females have been shown to have increased tibial rotation and decreased hamstrings activity, which might contribute to this gender difference [29]. They have smaller ACL cross-sectional dimensions and increased lateral tibial slope, which produce greater strains on the AM bundle during pivot landings [30]. There is also an increased tibial plateau slope in ACL injured knees but imaging studies are inconsistent to determine a cut-off value [31].

Associated meniscal, chondral and bone bruises are common in patients with ACL tears. Abduction and multiplanar loading seem to be directly related to bone lesions of the tibial plateau [32]. Most ACL ruptures are complete, including both bundles. However, an observation by Zantop et al. has found up to one-quarter of the tears to be of a single fascicle. The rupture pattern of the ACL predominates at the femoral insertion, although in 44 % of cases the AM and PL bundles did not rupture at the same location. The remnant stump is thus mainly attached to the tibial insertion and can have various shapes and sizes. The longer the time from injury to reconstruction, the more absent and faded the tibial remnant is found (Figs. 3.2 and 3.3). Furthermore, reconstructed ACLs tear differently depending on the surgical procedure [33].

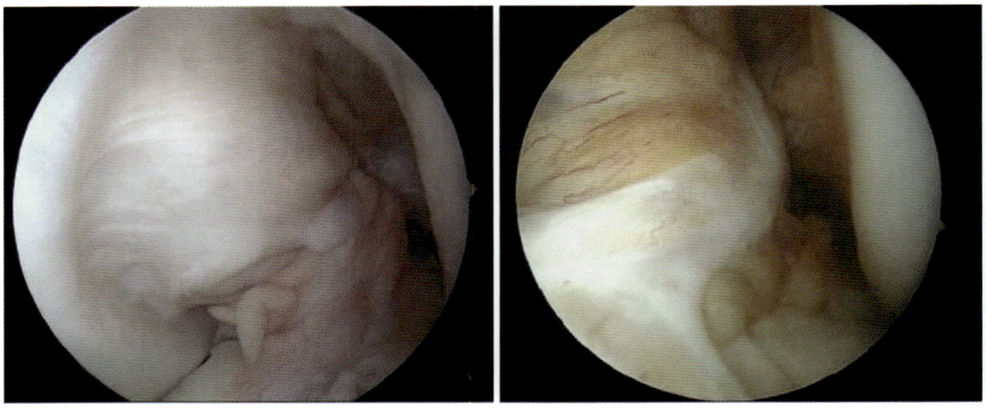

Fig. 3.2 Different shapes and sizes of the ACL remnants: from totally absent to ganglia shaped, adhered to the posterior cruciate ligament (PCL) and covered in synovia and ligaments with scar continuity

Fig. 3.2 (continued)

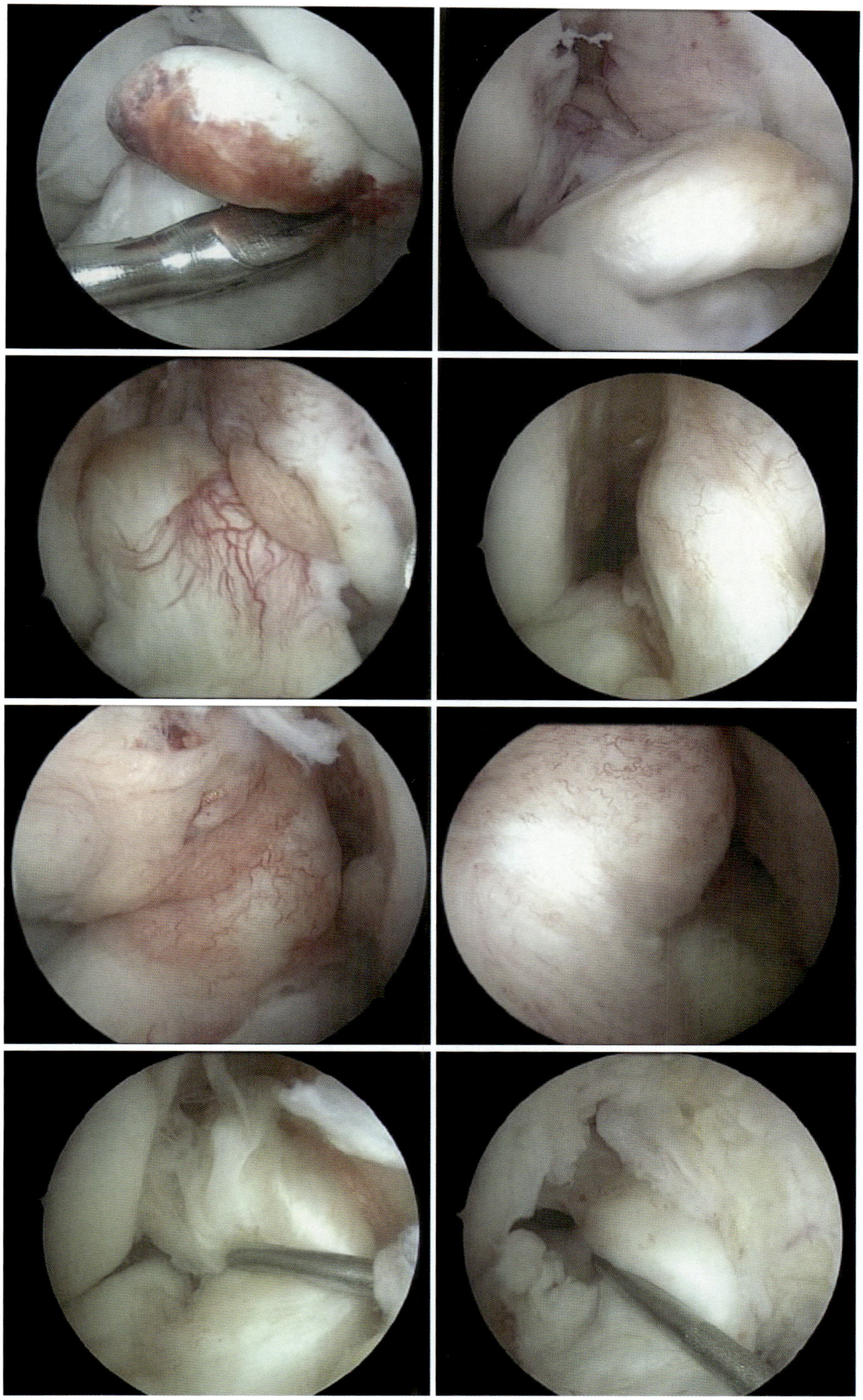

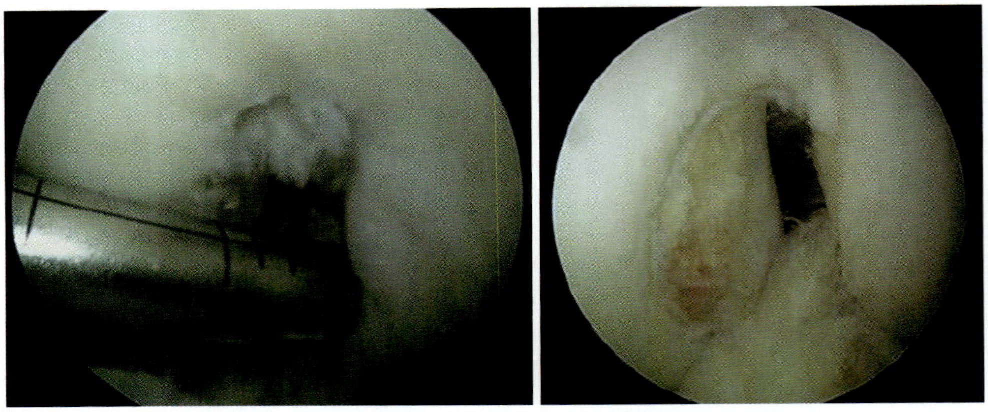

Fig. 3.3 A narrow notch can predispose to ACL ruptures but it is unclear whether this is caused by impingement or by association with smaller ACL sizes [34]

3.2 Diagnosis and Indication for Surgery

The ACL tear should be diagnosed by a thorough medical history, clinical examination and imaging studies. However, the clinical proof of anterior-posterior instability is the most common and important finding. The majority of ruptures are complete, although partial (single bundle) are also encountered but are more difficult to identify.

Acute presentations follow a recent traumatic event, most commonly during sports and, as shown earlier, as a non-contact injury. When this is the case, the knee is usually painful and difficult to examine. The patients can sometimes accurately describe the femur abnormally moving away from the tibia with spontaneous reduction. A 'pop' can also be heard. Swelling most commonly accompanies acute presentations and is caused by hemarthrosis. This is not mandatory and can also occur with osteochondral fractures. The overall acute clinical picture is determined by associated meniscal and chondral lesions [35]. The presence of acute swelling and suspected hemarthrosis no longer has indications for aspiration or diagnostic arthroscopy. Noninvasive imaging studies such as Magnetic Resonance Imaging (MRI) can offer a much better understanding of the lesions and prepare for definitive operative treatment. The emergent standard radiographic examination almost always fails to identify any lesions and stress x-rays are practically never performed routinely.

Isolated ACL tears can be interpreted as simple sprains and further referral to a specialist or MRI examination is not performed. After the initial acute phase the patient returns to daily activities. Subjective giving way is not always encountered during the daily routine but is more prevalent when the patient attempts to return to sports. This way, many months can pass until definitive diagnosis is made. When the ACL tear becomes chronic, the patient usually presents to the orthopedic specialist with due to recurrent instability or secondary chondral and meniscal lesions.

Anterior tibial translation with the knee flexed to 90°, known as the anterior drawer test, is the easiest clinical examination method that can be performed to determine instability. It is very specific but has a relatively high rate of false negative determinations. When this test is performed at only 20° of flexion, the test is known as Lachman and is the most reliable and sensitive clinical examination than can be routinely performed for ACL insufficiency [36]. Probably the most challenging part of performing these tests is being able to have the patient completely relax the hamstrings and quadriceps muscles. It is recommended to have the patient supine and perform gentle but firm maneuvers, especially in the acute setting, when pain can seriously and adversely influence the examination. Compared to the acute presentation, chronic ACL insufficiency usually leads to increased laxity and more pregnant anterior tibial translation [37]. The amount of anterior translation is as important as the firmness of the end point. A complete chronic tear should not have a clearly perceptible stop on anterior drawer or Lachman tests. Based on the absolute and relative (compared to contralateral) amount of translation and the presence of a firm end point, the positive anterior drawer and Lachman tests are evaluated by three severity grades: '+ to +++'.

As easy and useful these tests are, they rely on the examiners clinical abilities, experience and discernment. The KT-1000 (MedMetric, San Diego, USA) and the subsequent KT-2000 are the most widely accepted and used instrumented measures of antero-posterior knee laxity. A determined manual maximal difference of 3–4 mm compared to the contralateral side, especially when the absolute value is over 10 mm is a definitive confirmation of ACL insufficiency [38, 39].

The tibial plateau anterior translation also has a rotational component. The lateral plateau is more mobile as the knee is flexed. When the ACL is insufficient and the knee is flexed from near full extension to 30° of flexion, while simultaneously applying compressive and valgus loads, the anterior tibial subluxation is reduced. This can be clinically evaluated as the pivot shift test and gives a more accurate determination of knee stability during dynamic function. When performed under anesthesia it is both pain free for the patient if positive and much more sensitive. However, these particularities limit its use for diagnostic purposes. Jakob et al. described the three levels grading system currently used in practice mainly to evaluate posterolateral corner integrity and outcomes after ACL reconstruction [40]. Residual pivot shift is related to persistent subjective knee complaints, poor clinical outcomes and progression of osteoarthritis [41, 42]. Quantitative determination of the pivot shift has been recently attempted by determining spatial position and acceleration of electromagnetic sensors with promising results [43].

The MRI is the imaging modality of choice in patients with ACL injuries. It can identify tears with up to 95 % accuracy. In addition, it gives details on menisci, bone bruising, possible cartilage lesions, size and orientation of the native ACL and its insertions, thickness of the patellar and quadricipital tendons. High magnetic field machines produce better resolution, which is especially helpful for partial tears. Complete tears are seen as total discontinuity of the fibers. Incomplete tears are focal hemorrhage, non-homogenous hyperintense interruptions which appear to still have some fibers in continuity. Sagittal T2 acquisitions are the most important series to be examined. However, the coronal plane obliquity of the ligament gives a distorted and incomplete aspect of all ACL fibers on orthogonal series. This is why the standard knee protocols have a dedicated sagittal oblique acquisition. To clarify even further the state of the entire ACL fibers, a coronal oblique series can be added, parallel to the ACL in the sagittal plane. Partial tears can sometimes be misleading to identify on MRIs performed in the acute phase (Figs. 3.4 and 3.5).

In our clinic we treat both professional and recreational athletes whom had injured their ACL during sports activity. The ACL repair is usually done at 4–8 weeks after the injury. A subsidence of the acute posttraumatic inflammation is recommended, and this period will vary between cases. An absolute connection between early surgery and postoperative arthrofibrosis has not been demonstrated. Some studies found patients operated in the first 3 weeks had an increased incidence of arthrofibrosis [45] while others showed that early reconstruction (during the first 2 weeks) led to sooner return to sports and better clinical and laxity testing results [46]. Additional factors such as patient's predisposition to excessive connective tissue formation, associated lesions and the overall magnitude of the injury as well as the postoperative rehabilitation regimen play a considerable role in the surgical outcome. On the other hand, concomitant cartilage damage and delayed reconstruction are major risk factors for inferior outcome after ACL reconstruction [47].

The main indication for ACL reconstruction is symptomatic and clinically evident antero-posterior knee laxity in the absence of advanced joint degeneration. Associated ligamentary laxities need to be excluded or identified prior to planning for reconstruction. PCL tears can also produce anterior tibial translation but with a firm endpoint and sagging. Unaddressed MCL ruptures will give exaggerated anterior movement of the medial tibial plateau that could be confused for ACL insufficiency. Chronic MCL tears will not provide adequate support for valgus loads and will lead to ACL reconstruction failure. Undiagnosed posterolateral corner insufficiency can lead to poor clinical outcomes, persistent positive pivot shift and ACL reconstruction failure.

3.2.1 Outcomes After ACL Reconstruction

ACL reconstruction allows the patients to return to sporting activities and improves the functional outcomes [48]. However, one study found that half of patients operated 10–20 years ago, showed signs of osteoarthritis (OA) with associated pain and functional impairment. The same authors found inconclusive evidence to support the protective role of repair or reconstructive surgery of the ACL or meniscus against osteoarthritis development [49]. A comparison of conservative and reconstructive ACL surgery found similar physical activity levels for both groups at 11 years follow-up. ACL reconstruction led to higher stability but also increased risk for osteoarthritis. Nonetheless, the risk of secondary meniscal tears is reduced after reconstruction, which indirectly reduces the negative effects of OA [50]. The extraarticular augmentation procedure from the Rizzoli Institute of Bologna, Italy only demonstrated progressive joint narrowing for patients having concomitant medial meniscal surgery [51]. A retrospective evaluation performed in Pittsburg identified an almost 40 % incidence of radiographic OA approximately 8 years after ACL surgery. Prior medial meniscectomy, 2 or greater medial chondrosis and obesity were the best predictors for OA development [52]. An analysis of the MOON (Multicenter Orthopaedic Outcomes Network) cohort found patients were able to perform sports function at 6 years, but the activity level continued to decline from baseline evaluation. In addition, lateral meniscus treatment, allograft, smoking and obesity were negative predictors for long-term outcomes [53]. More than a 3-fold increase prevalence of OA was found after ACL reconstructed knees compared with the contralateral. The prevalence of OA was similar between the B-PT-B and hamstrings grafts. A meniscus resection was also a strong predictor of symptomatic degeneration [54]. In the Swedish ACL register, older aged patients (over 40 years) recorded lower preoperative KOOS scores. These patients exhibited the greatest improvement in for all subscales up to 5 years, even though they had more cartilage and meniscus injuries and longer intervals from injury to reconstruction [55]. Fourteen years after operative or nonoperative management of ACL injury, the reconstructed cohorts had less need for subsequent meniscal surgery and less decline of functional scores. The difference in pivot-shift results was not significant, as well as final outcome scores (Tegner – Lysholm, International Knee Documentation Committee – IKDC) or the rate of radiographically evident degeneration [56, 57].

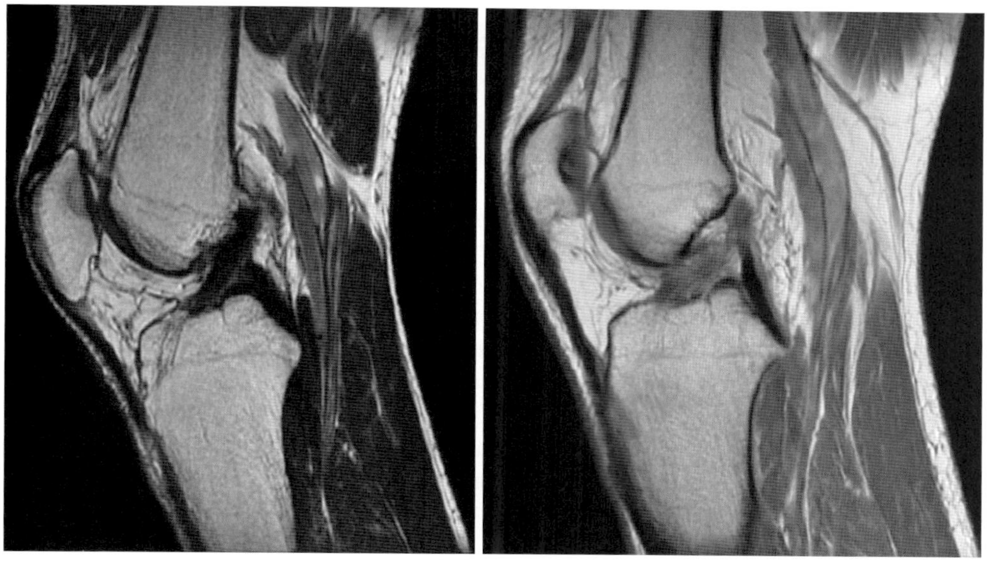

Fig. 3.4 Sagittal oblique images obtained with a 1.5 T machine depicting a normal, continuous, homogenous, hypointense ACL and a torn, hyperintense, discontinued in the proximal part ACL respectively

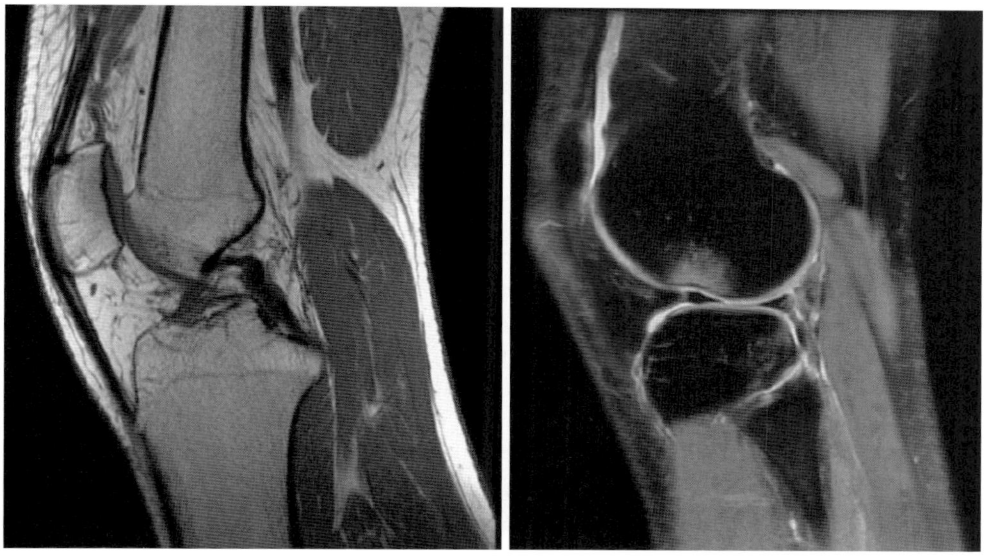

Fig. 3.5 Indirect signs associated with ACL tears: a curled PCL due to anterior tibial translation and lateral femoral condyle and tibial plateau bone bruises [44]

3.3 Skeletal Immaturity

Over the years attitudes have changed towards favoring early surgical treatment as opposed to conservative management. Clear evidence shows that the same correlations from the adult populations exist in the skeletally immature patients regarding increase meniscal and chondral injuries with delayed treatment. This is concerning because studies have shown that, regardless of knee stability obtained after ACL reconstruction, meniscectomy accelerates degenerative joint changes [58]. Lawrence et al. [59] found that out of 70 young patients who underwent surgical reconstruction of an acute ACL tear more than 12 weeks after the injury more were noted to have a significant increase in irreparable medial meniscal tears and lateral compartment chondral injuries (odds ratio 11.3) at the time of reconstruction. When a subjective sense of knee instability was present, this association was even stronger (odds ratio 11.4). Dumont et al. [60] performed a retrospective chart review of 370 pediatric patients undergoing primary arthroscopic ACL reconstruction. They identified that index ACL reconstructions after more than 150 days since injury have a higher rate (odds ratio 1.8) of medial meniscus tears than those treated earlier. Increased age (odds ratio 1.6) and weight (odds ratio 2.2) are independently associated with a higher rate of medial meniscus tears. Patients with ACL tears and a medial or lateral meniscus tear are more likely to have a chondral injury in that particular compartment than those without meniscal ruptures.

Regarding the most appropriate graft choice there is growing support in favor of autologus hamstrings (semitendinosus and gracilis) and concern with bone – patellar tendon – bone since the bone plugs have led to premature physeal ossifications in animal models. Gebhard et al. [61] analyzed 28 patients who underwent ACL reconstruction with hamstrings, 16 patients with bone-patella-bone, 12 patients with quadriceps grafts and 12 patients with facia lata. The mean follow-up was 32 months. Neither leg length discrepancy nor angular deformities were noted. None of the four methods studied showed major differences in outcome compared to the other.

Thus, surgical stabilization should be considered as the first line of treatment for immature patients with ACL tears. The existing literature suggests that transphyseal reconstruction can be safely done in this population if a few rules are considered, and there are physeal-sparing procedures that provide excellent results with less theoretical risk to the growth plate. Conservative or delayed surgical treatment, which carries an increased risk of secondary joint injury, should be reserved only for selected cases [62].

This change of perspective has not been fully agreed upon especially regarding surgical procedure with respect to physeal growth plates. Moksnes et al. [63] performed a recent literature review and found that there is no consensus on the management of anterior cruciate ligament injuries in skeletally immature, and that the methodological quality of published studies is questionable. The transphyseal reconstructions, physeal-sparing reconstructions, and nonoperative treatment algorithms that are advocated have little supportive data.

In the literature the standard bone age evaluation for pediatric ACL reconstructions is the one proposed by Tanner and Whitehouse; this system scores 20 indicators on hand and wrist radiograph, yielding total scores ranging from 0 to 100. Even though we were not able to use this scale in retrospect the probable estimate Tanner stage in our patients was III and IV. Example of MRI appearance can be seen in Figs. 3.6, 3.7, 3.8, and 3.9.

Similar studies have found favorable results for autologus hamstrings grafts using transphyseal techniques [65–67]. Redler et al. [68] showed that transphyseal ACL reconstruction with autogenous quadrupled hamstring graft with metaphyseal fixation in skeletally immatures (14.2 years) yielded excellent functional outcomes in a high percentage of patients without perceived clinical growth disturbance at a mean of 43.4 months.

Drill hole placement during ACL reconstruction produces a zone of physeal injury. The overall volume of injury is relatively low, which reduces the risk of physeal arrest. With careful placement, the region of injury is central on the tibia, and the total volume of injury can be less than 5.0 % of the physeal volume. For the femur, the total volume can be less than 5.0 % as well. However, the region of injury is peripheral, which carries a higher risk of physeal arrest. For the tibia, drill holes that started more medial, distal, and with a steeper angle of inclination reduced the amount of physis and apophysis violated when compared with holes placed more lateral, proximal, and with a shallow angle of inclination [69–71].

Other authors [71] have used MRIs to identify physeal sparring directions of the femoral tunnel using transphyseal techniques and proposed drilling from the center of the ACL femoral footprint to the insertion of the popliteal tendon; this could result in a mean tunnel length of 27–30 mm, and it might allow the safe placement of a femoral tunnel at least 7 mm in diameter in patients 6–17 years old. The center of the ACL femoral footprint and the popliteal insertion are easily identifiable landmarks and will allow safe, reproducible, anatomic ACL reconstruction in the skeletally immature patient.

A retrospective case series of 933 knees with a mean age at the time of surgery of 15 years and an average follow-up from index surgery of 6.3 years evaluated the overall prevalence of arthrofibrosis and found it to be 8.3 %; 77 knees had at least one procedure to treat arthrofibrosis after ACL reconstruction. Arthrofibrosis was defined as a loss of 5° or more of extension or a loss of 15° or more flexion compared with the contralateral knee that required a follow-up procedure. Risk factors for arthrofibrosis were female sex, higher age (16–18 years odds ratio 3.51), patellar tendon autograft (odds ratio 1.7), and concomitant meniscal repair (odds ratio 2.08). Prior knee surgery and ACL reconstruction within 1 month of injury were not significantly associated with arthrofibrosis after ACL reconstruction [72].

Frosch et al. [73] identified a total of 55 articles reporting on 935 patients (median age 13 years) with a median follow-up of 40 months; their review found the weighted rate of leg-length differences or axis deviations was 1.8 % and that of reruptures was 4.8 %. Excellent or good function (International Knee Documentation Committee grade A or B) was achieved in 84.2 % of knees and Lysholm scores averaged 96.3. Transphyseal reconstruction was associated with a significantly lower risk of leg-length differences or axis deviations compared with physeal-sparing techniques (1.9 % versus 5.8 %; relative ratio 0.34) but had a higher risk of rerupture (4.2 % versus 1.4 %; relative ratio 2.91). Sutures did not result in any growth disturbances, with a weighted rerupture rate of 4.6 %. Fixation far from the joint line fared better than close fixation with regard to this endpoint (1.4 % versus 3.2 %; relative ratio 0.42). Bone-patellar tendon-bone grafts, which are also less likely to fail, were associated with higher risks of leg-length differences or axis deviations than were hamstrings (3.6 % versus 2.0 %; relative ratio 1.82). Meta-regression did not show a significant impact of the publication year on event rates.

Kaeding et al. [74] aimed to determine whether any anterior cruciate ligament reconstruction technique is clinically superior in skeletally immature patients having at least one of the following criteria: chronologic or bone age of less than 15 years in boys or less than 14 years in girls, Tanner stage I, II, or III and at least 10 cm of total growth after the reconstruction. Thirteen case series were included. Four studies used physeal-sparing techniques. Six studies used transphyseal techniques. Two studies used a combined technique, and a multicenter study reported results of both techniques. Within the physeal-sparing group, there were two studies that used an entirely extra-epiphyseal technique and two studies that used intra-epiphyseal techniques. Overall clinical outcomes were excellent, with growth complications being very rare in all of these series. The authors concluded that both physeal-sparing and transphyseal reconstructions can produce excellent clinical outcomes with a very low incidence of growth complications in Tanner stage II and III patients. Tanner stage I patients had excellent clinical results with physeal-sparing techniques (both extra- and intra-epiphyseal techniques). Not enough Tanner stage I patients underwent transphyseal techniques to support or discourage their use. This evidence supports considering the expansion of transphyseal reconstruction indications from Tanner stage IV patients to Tanner stage II and III patients.

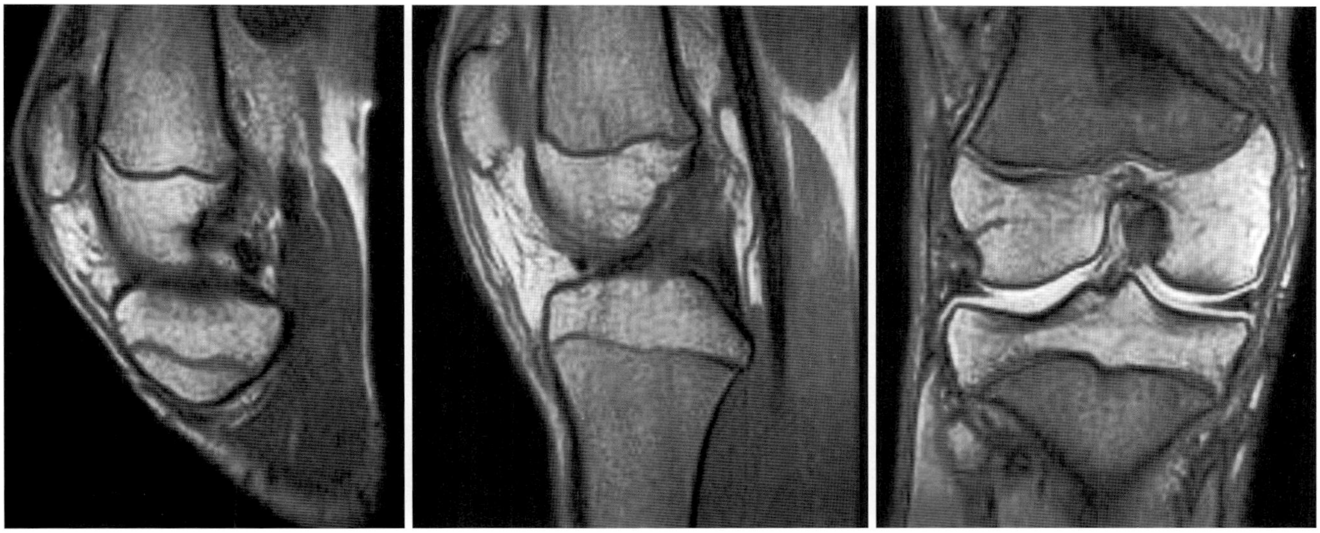

Fig. 3.6 RISE and T1 sagittal and T1 coronal views of 16 years old boy with open physis and torn ACL

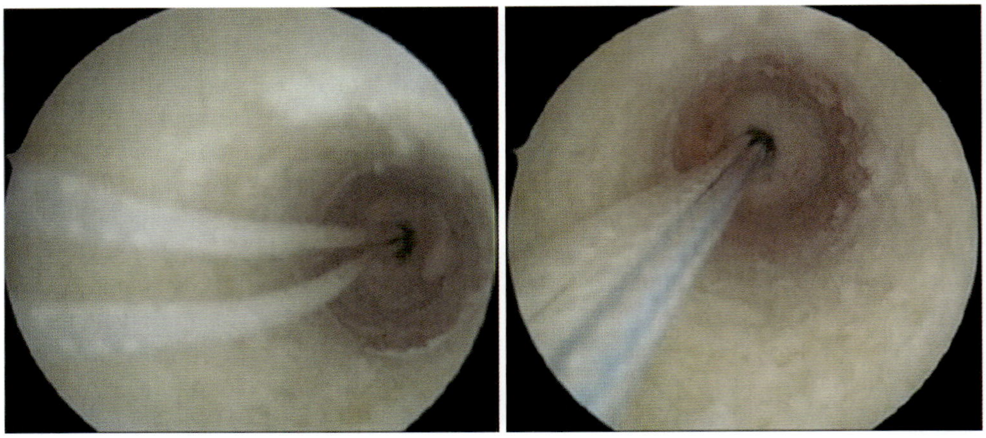

Fig. 3.7 Femoral tunnel of two cases showing the arthroscopic view of the transphyseal ACL reconstruction [64]

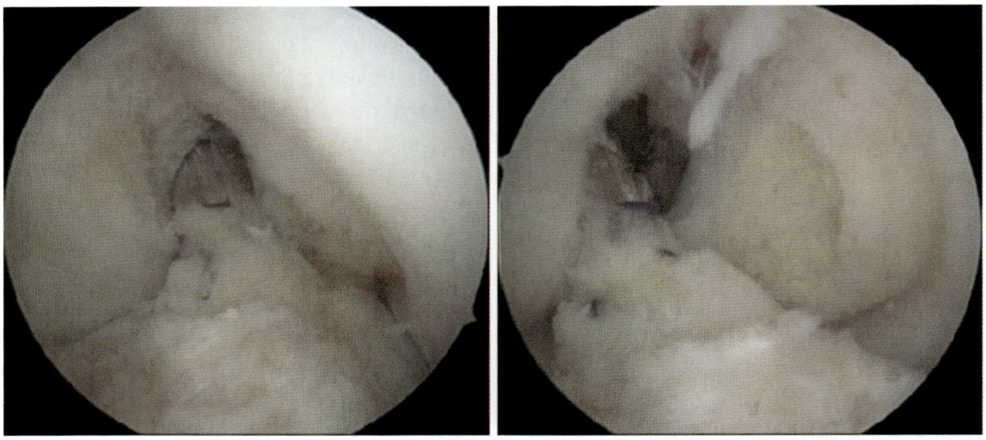

Fig. 3.8 Lateral portal views of the case above of 16 years old boy with anatomic single bundle (transphyseal) ACL reconstruction using ipsilateral hamstrings (semitendinosus and gracilis) autograft (quadruple) [64]

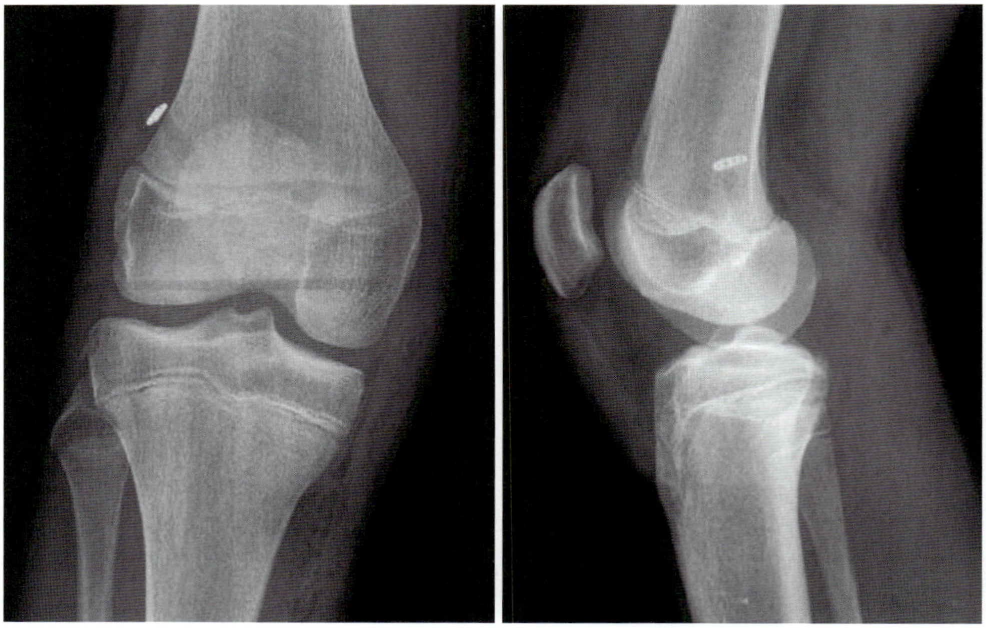

Fig. 3.9 Show AP and lateral radiographs of a 16 years old boy with open physis and ACL reconstruction using transphyseal technique with hamstrings autograft, cortical femoral fixation and absorbable tibial interference screw [64]

3.4 Graft Healing and Stump Preservation

ACL (anterior cruciate ligament) reconstruction is a constantly evolving procedure. The ever-changing trends follow the common goal to restore preinjury anatomy and function as closely as possible [75]. With all the progress that has been made during the last years towards better understanding of the graft healing process and individually tailored surgery and rehabilitation, this target has not yet been fully achieved.

After reconstruction, the neoligament goes through a series of transformations that will lead to graft – tunnel integration and ligamentization of the intraarticular portion; this later process brings the tendinous structure closer to the original ligament. Amiel et al. proposed the term 'ligamentization' to describe the gradual transformation of the autologus B-PT-B graft into a neoligament that resembled the native ACL. The histological and biochemical metamorphosis occurred by 30 weeks and led to ligamentous cell morphology and increased concentration of type III collagen, not normally present in the patellar tendon as well as increased content of glycosaminoglycans [76].

The early phase is characterized by necrosis and hypocellularity. It lasts for the first month, during which the graft depends on synovial fluid nutrition [77]. After 6 weeks, revascularization occurs and the graft goes through intense cell proliferation. This intermediate period lasts until 3 months postoperatively. The final stage of structural remodeling continues over 6 months. In this later period, the graft begins to resemble the native ACL. This process was described for allografts and studied on animal models. During the early stages of revascularization and cell proliferation, allografts show significant delay compared to autografts. These differences start to fade by 1 year even though they continue to exhibit lower mechanical properties and anterior-posterior laxity [78].

It has been long suggested that preservation of the ACL stump and the Hoffa fat pad might be beneficial, especially for the early healing period [79]. However, while the grafts remain viable during this course, complete necrosis and cell replacement in humans does not follow the animal model [80]. Histologically the neoligaments resemble the native ACL but ultrastructural differences of collagen fibers distribution do persist [81]. One of the topics that are still debated is defining the importance of ACL remnants for the final functional outcome. Moreover, restoring proprioception of the ACL reconstructed knee has been hypothesized to be an integral part for successful outcome. The ACL has very poor healing capacity manly due to poor vascularization that is even further damaged after injury.

Denti et al. [82] and Barrack et al. [83] have found mechanoreceptors after ACL reconstruction with tendinous grafts and proposed that a reinnervation of the neoligament had occurred. Georgoulis et al. [84] using gold staining found that Ruffini and Pacini type mechanoreceptors existed in the subsynovial layer and near the femoral and tibial insertions of the ACL in remnant stumps connected to the PCL. Adachi et al. [85] observed a positive correlation between the number of proprioceptors and the accuracy of joint position sense. The authors even found mechanoreceptors in patients having a long interval between injury and the ACL reconstruction and concluded that surgeons should consider preserving ACL remnants to improve clinical outcome.

Gohil et al. [86], in a randomized control trial investigated whether limited debridement of the intercondylar notch and the residual stump of the ruptured ACL leads to earlier revascularization after ACL reconstruction using autologous four-strand hamstring tendon grafts as evaluated by postoperative MRI. Their results indicate that minimal removal of remnants leads to earlier revascularization within the mid-substance of the graft over midterm evaluation.

Lee et al. [87] presented results of the 16 subjects that had undergone ACL reconstruction with the remnant-preserving technique described in a previous article at a mean follow-up of 35.1 months. At the last examination, the patients were evaluated with the IKDC scale and HSS score as subjective tests; stress radiographs, Lachman test, and anterior drawer test by use of the KT-2000 arthrometer as objective tests and single-legged hop test, reproduction of passive positioning, threshold to detection of passive motion, and single-limb standing test as functional tests. On the basis of the extent of ACL remnant, patients were divided into more and less than 20 % respectively. A statistical comparison of the final results revealed that the difference was not significant in terms of mechanical stability, but a significant difference was detected in functional outcome and proprioception regarding the threshold to detection of passive motion at 30° and reproduction of passive positioning at 15° and 30°. In a subsequent study, [88] Ruffii (globular or ovoid corpuscle with thin capsule) and Golgi (fusiform corpuscle with thin capsule) type mechanoreceptors were found predominantly around insertion sites, located in the subsynovial layer and rarely in the interfascicular matrix in the normal (control) ACLs and more uniformly distributed in the remnant stumps collected from injured knees. Immunohistochemical staining method proved to be reliable and relevant in terms of specifically identifying the presence of mechanoreceptors in the normal and tibial remnant of the ruptured ACLs [89]. In the control group 40 % of slices contained mechanoreceptors. However, only one third of the remnant group showed viable mechanoreceptors (one or two per stump) and these were identified in 11 % of the total slices.

Dhillon et al. [85] examined ACL remnants by conventional light microscope. The monoclonal antibody against NFP stained the axons cylinders carrying proprioception. The monoclonal antibodies against S-100 stained free nerve endings and Schwann cells. H&E was used for detailed histological evaluation of synovial lining, sub synovial vascularity, intravascular morphologically normal mechanoreceptors, degenerative changes, and inflammation [90]. Papalia et al. [78] presented a literature review regarding the rationale for preserving the ACL remnants during reconstruction. Seven studies were included. The authors observed that ACL remnants might accelerate the vascularization and the ligamentization of the graft and contribute to faster graft innervation leading to a better proprioception. However, the current assessment methods do not lead to hard evidence that preservation of the remnant confers clinically relevant advantages over its excision.

Our tibial stump preservation technique is comparable to that described by Lee et al. [91] and Locherbach et al. [92] in the sense that ACL remnants are used as a biological sleeve for the graft. We also use ipsilateral quadruple hamstrings autograft and the tibial tunnel was performed inside and through the tibial ACL stump by careful sequential drilling that stopped before completely penetrating the ligamentous remnant.

One concern with tibial remnant preservation is the potential for intraoperative or future roof impingement. We found that accurate placement of tibial tunnel exit point, careful progression of pulling sutures through the middle of the remnant and sizing of the graft diameter prevents overstuffing the intercondylar notch. Nevertheless, occasionally we had to perform minimal adjustments of the ACL remnant after the graft was in final position to prevent progression towards future development of cyclop-like lesions due to stump preservation [93].

The ACL is, as are all key ligaments, important in defining proprioception and body spatial positioning using mechanoreceptors and neural endings. The role of this structures have only recently been credited to their full potential and importance in early recovery, prevention of reinjury and full return to pretrauma body kinematics. Whenever remnants are preserved, bony landmarks remain covered and potential for tunnel misplacement can arise. We consider that preservation of the tibial remnant only does not alter significantly the orientation (Figs. 3.10 and 3.11).

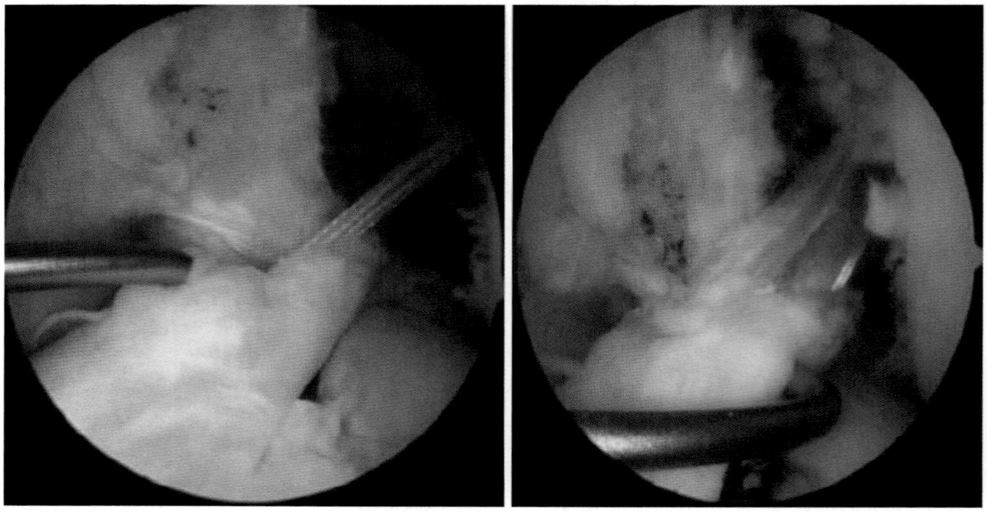

Fig. 3.10 Arthroscopic view of the exit point of the tibial tunnel with the remnant ACL stump preserved and showed with the probe; in the second image, the neoligament passing through the remaining tibial insertion and surrounded by the stump to promote healing whilst preventing impingement

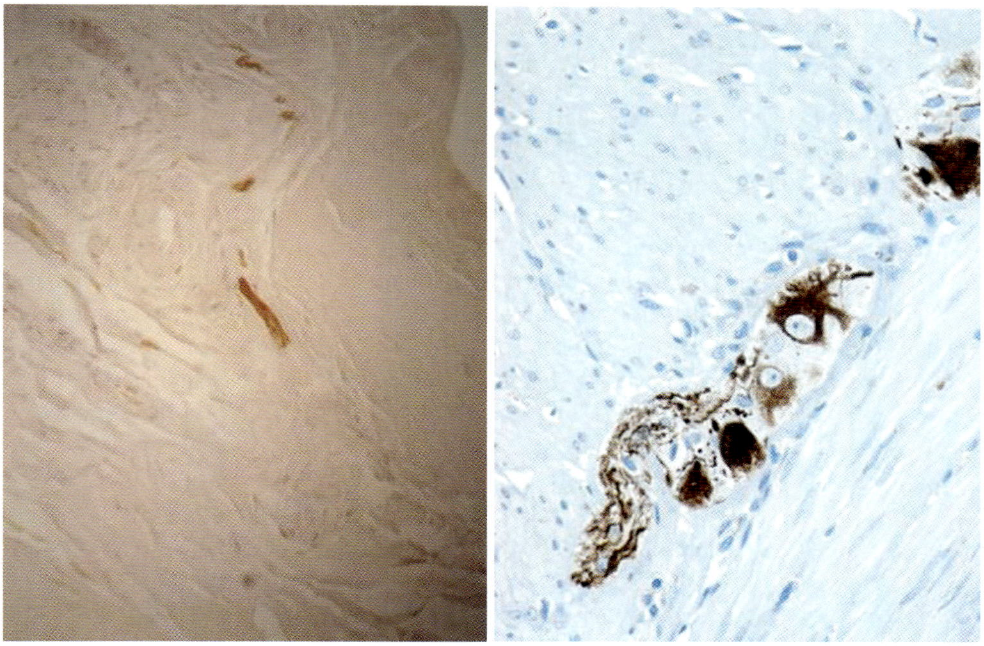

Fig. 3.11 Focal free nerve terminals evidenced by immunohistochemical S-100 staining and mechanoreceptors from the tibial biopsy stained using anti-NF

3.5 Current Anterior Cruciate Ligament Reconstruction

Anterior cruciate ligament (ACL) lesions and their treatment are one of the most debated topics in orthopedics and knee surgery today. While the surgical indication still is a question to some, most orthopedic surgeons agree that reconstruction is the only viable option for a successful management of an ACL deficient knee. This being said, the debate continues as to which graft is most suited for a better outcome, which implants from the wide array that are available on the market have the best results and even which technique is the best.

3.5.1 The Transtibial Technique

The transtibial technique (TT) has been the first widely used arthroscopic reconstruction technique, with favorable outcomes reported in the late '80. In the late '90, the works of Professor Freddie Fu from Pittsburg and others have raised concern regarding the graft placement and function using this surgical procedure. In addition, the clock dial referencing was considered an inappropriate single plane description of a three dimensional position. More research into the biomechanics of the ACL saw the advent of the double bundle technique (DB).

The over-the-top position of the graft on the femur was anterior and medial to the native ACL insertion [9, 17]. In knees with hyperextension and a vertical notch roof, the TT technique required notchplasty and a more posteriorly placed tibial tunnel to prevent impingement [94]. This led to extremely vertical and nonphysiological grafts that were found to have less resistance to anterior translation and especially less rotational stability compared to double bundle anatomic reconstruction [95]. The current switch to anatomic reconstruction has greatly limited the need for notchplasty, mainly to osteophyte removal from the lateral condyle border (Fig. 3.12). Experimental studies have repeatedly showed that the femoral attachment of the native ACL is on the lateral femoral condyle and never on the notch roof. A correctly positioned tibial tunnel will never allow for a correct placement of the femoral aperture in the native insertion [96]. Further research provided additional data to support femoral tunnel drilling through the antero-medial portal. When compared to the TT technique, it offered better function and closer obliquity to the native contralateral ACL [97, 98]. With regard to the tibial tunnel aperture, the results are somewhat inconclusive between the two techniques. It has been shown that trans tibial technique places the tibial tunnel in the same position as the trans antero-medial portal or more posterior in order to achieve better placement of the femoral tunnel [97–99].

It is now universally accepted that ACL reconstruction via transtibial technique fails to accurately position femoral and tibial tunnels within the natural insertion site [100]. In addition, freedom of femoral drilling through the AM portal will also allow for a more anterior placement of the tibial tunnel [99]. This in turn will lead to a more oblique and natural graft placement with improved restoration of anatomy and stability with ACL reconstruction compared with conventional transtibial drilling techniques [101].

The introduction of the anatomic ACL reconstruction technique changed the way surgeons drill the femoral tunnel, by using an antero-medial portal instead of the traditional tibial tunnel. This subsequently changed the positioning of the tunnels and the resulting obliquity of the graft. One of the first materials that evaluated neoligament obliquity in ACL reconstructed patients found a continuous and homogeneous graft similar to the native ACL, but with a more vertical position that does not recreate the normal sagittal obliquity. Nevertheless, these more vertical grafts were still found to control anterior posterior knee displacement [102].

Ahn et al. compared the antero-medial and TT techniques and found a significant vertical angle in the coronal and sagittal plane for the TT reconstructions compared with the native ACL. In addition, the more horizontally the angle of the tibial tunnel can be the closer will be the result compared to the native ACL [103] When the tibial remnant stump was preserved, magnetic resonance imaging showed significantly larger grafts with progressive remodeling and no increase in the incidence of cyclops lesions [104]. MRI proves to be the most useful imaging method in determining outcome after ACL reconstruction. It gives reliable information on graft healing, integrity, length, position, inclination angle, obliquity, impingement syndromes and potential associated lesions. It may even identify ACL impingement against PCL (posterior cruciate ligament) with the knee extended, which cannot be detected by conventional arthroscopy [105].

Three dimensional (3D) volume rendered (VRT) computed tomography (CT) is a useful tool for planning accurate femoral tunnel positioning when aiming for anatomic ACL reconstruction. The direct insertion of the ACL is located in the depression between the resident's ridge and the articular cartilage margin on the lateral femoral condyle [106]. 3D CT reconstructed volumes (VRT) are reliable and can be used to assess the tunnel position regarding stability and outcome [107]. Although not as widely used, 3D MR imaging were proved accurate and can also be used for preoperative templating in anatomic ACL reconstruction (Figs. 3.13 and 3.14) [108].

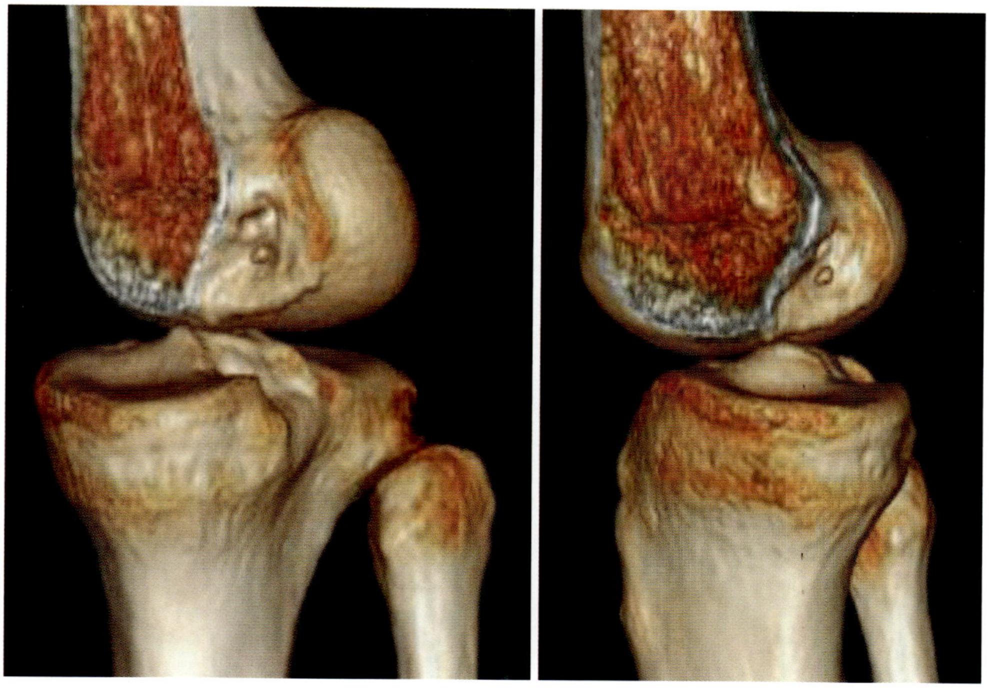

Fig. 3.12 A patient with previous single bundle ACL reconstruction using the transtibial technique (TT) and ipsilateral patellar tendon autograft. 3D CT (three dimensional computed tomography) reconstructions shows the high, non anatomic placement of the femoral tunnel on the roof of the notch

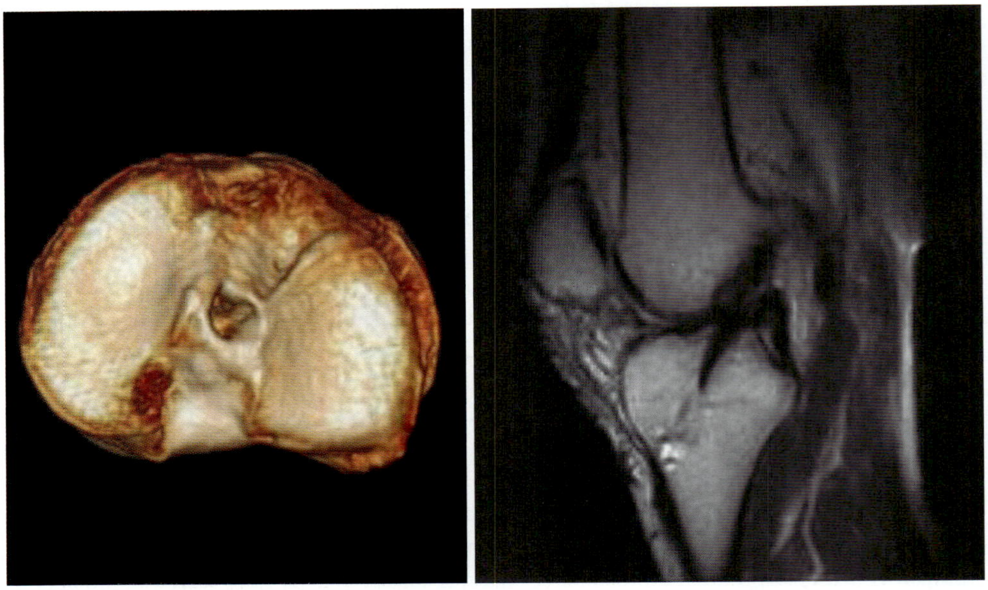

Fig. 3.13 The same case, 3D CT volume rendering showing the non-anatomic, posterior tibial tunnel aperture. The result is a vertical although homogenic hypointense aspect of the neoligament on the sagittal T2 MRI (*right*)

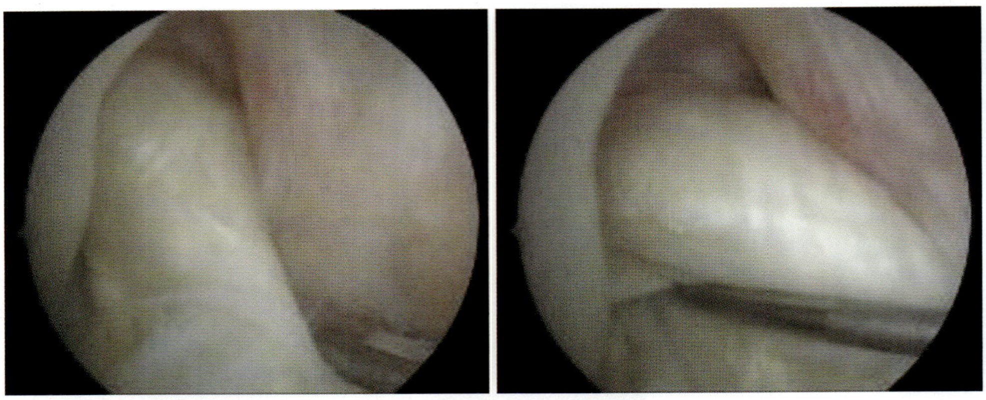

Fig. 3.14 Arthroscopic views of the same case through the anterolateral portal showing a healed and integrated vertical graft; the arthroscopic evaluation was performed in order to perform a partial medial meniscectomy resulting from a recent noncontact sporting injury

3.5.2 The Anatomic Single Bundle Reconstruction

The anatomic single bundle technique appeared initially as a therapeutic alternative in cases where anatomic DB technique could not be performed (small knees, narrow notch) and later gained increased use by surgeons due to easier technique, shorter operating room time and comparable results to the DB technique. The anatomic single bundle (SB) reconstruction technique has been found to more accurately reproduce the femoral footprint and the orientation of the graft. By comparison, with the classical TT technique the tibial tunnel placement resulted in a more vertical graft than native ACL. It has thus been underlined the importance of thorough knowledge of the anatomical landmarks of the ACL [109]. Nonetheless, in many cases normal graft obliquity is not restored with either technique. This may be caused by the single bundle technique itself [110].

The senior authors have been performing ACL reconstructions for more than a decade, with almost 1,000 treated cases each. In the beginning, we used the TT single bundle technique with autologous ipsilateral bone-patellar tendon-bone (B-PT-B) graft fixed with 2 interference screws. Presently, our most versatile and recommended procedure is the anatomic SB reconstruction with autologous ipsilateral quadrupled hamstring graft, cortical button femoral and interference screw tibial fixations. Nonetheless, many types of grafts and fixations can be used equally successful. This technique was applied to both professional and amateur athletes with excellent functional outcomes. A knee MRI is performed on a regular basis to investigate for possible associated ruptures of the menisci, lesions of the cartilage or lesions of the collateral ligaments even though clinical tests (Lachmann, anterior drawer test) are sufficient for the diagnosis of the ACL rupture (Fig. 3.15).

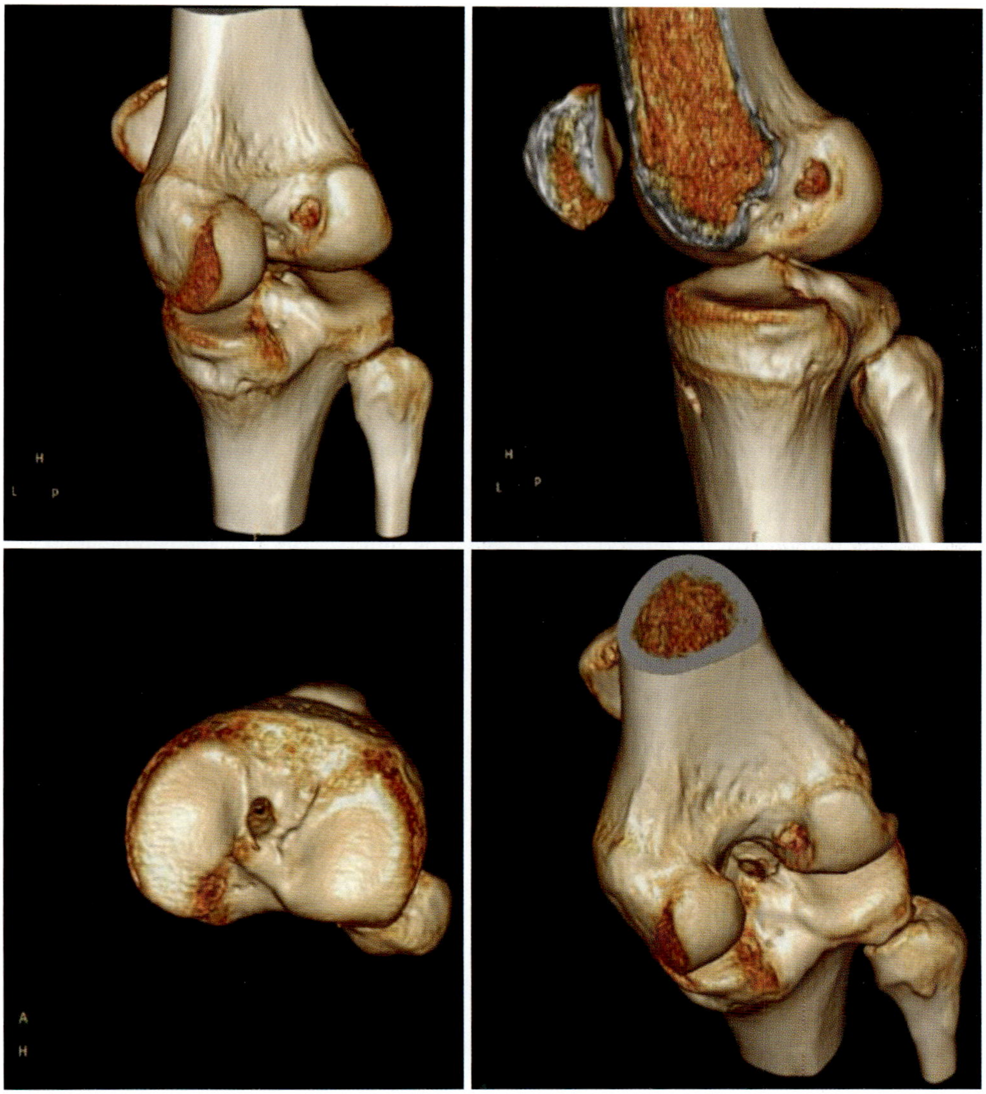

Fig. 3.15 By contrast, the 3D reconstructions of an anatomic single bundle reconstruction shows both tunnel apertures to be centered and sized to the native insertions

3.5.2.1 Surgical Technique

A clinical exam can be repeated after the patient is relaxed from the anesthesia. We do not perform routine exploratory arthroscopy if the preoperative evaluation is conclusive and proceed directly to graft harvesting (see Sect. 3.7). The arthroscopic exploration is performed in a standard fashion (see Sect. 1.2.4). We routinely only use two portals: a slightly higher and centrally placed antero-lateral and a lower and deeper antero-medial, to improve tibial aperture visualization and tunnel direction. Any associated lesions are addressed first; the remnants are parsimoniously debrided and the tunnels prepared while the graft is being handled on the back table. Stable longitudinal meniscal tears are left in situ, large, recent bucket handle tears are sutured and degenerative complex tears are excised. The target is to preserve as much meniscal tissue as possible (see Sect. 2.2) but the most commonly performed procedure in our patients is partial meniscectomy. For cartilage defects we usually perform microfractures (see Sect. 7.1).

What sets this technique apart from the classic single bundle ACL reconstruction technique is that the drilling of the femoral tunnel is done only after clear identification of the anatomical landmarks of the ruptured ACL. Initially we look for the femoral origin and we proceed with careful shaving to help delineate the borders of the ACL. In cases where the proximal remnant in no longer visible we debride the soft tissues until the bone is exposed. If visible, the intercondylar ridge is the superior limit of the ACL footprint with the knee in over 90° of flexion. For a better view of the notch we recommend moving the arthroscope from the antero-lateral to the antero-medial portal. The old "clock" theory that recommends the placement of the tunnel should be disregarded. One hundred and ten degrees flexion of the knee and an inferiorly placed medial portal are essential for the desired femoral tunnel aperture. The entry point should be the limit between the footprints of the AM and PL bundles, but not higher than the intercondylar ridge. The femoral ACL footprint is centered 1.7 mm proximal to the bifurcate ridge and 6.1 mm posterior to the lateral intercondylar ridge [111].

A mark can be made with the Steadman awl (used for microfractures) or with the guide pin freely or using the appropriately sized posterior wall guide (according the size of the graft). The position should always be checked from the central or medial portals. A 4×4 imaginary grid or intraoperative radioscopy can also be used but we do not routinely use them (Fig. 3.16). The appropriate placement of the femoral tunnel is a key point for a favorable outcome, and the leading cause of failure in cases that are revised (see Sect. 4.3).

Once the position is correct, a graded pin is used to measure the distance to the lateral cortex and decide tunnel length. The use of a 9 mm drill at a transverse angle of 40° with the knee in 102° of flexion was shown to produce a femoral tunnel aperture area that best matched the native ACL footprint [112]. A cadaveric study found that when drilling femoral tunnels through the far antero-medial portal both high and low knee flexion angles could have the potential risks of damage to articular cartilage or the common peroneal nerve [113].

The femoral guide pin is entering through the antero-medial portal and exiting the lateral condyle in a correct direction (Fig. 3.17); progressive reaming to the desired size (usually 8) is achieved with special drills that have a thin rounded body and a short reaming tip. This shape is used to protect the medial condyle cartilage (Fig. 3.18). We recommend sizing the femoral reaming in 0.5 mm increments, especially when cortical button fixation is used. A tight fit of the soft tissue graft in the tunnel is highly desired both in diameter and at the end. Variable loop systems or the smallest loop that will 'flip' should be used. The leading sutures are passed through the loop at the end of the guide pin (Figs. 3.19 and 3.20).

The best reference for the tibial tunnel aperture is the remnant ACL of the native ACL (see Sect. 3.1.2). The guide pin should exit in line with the native fibers, in the center of the stump (Fig. 3.21). If this landmark is not clear, as in old ruptures, the tibial insertion should be centered 7.5 mm medial to the anterior horn of the lateral meniscus, 13 mm anterior to the retro-eminence and 10.5 mm posterior to the ACL ridge [111]. The guide is set to 50–55°. The entry point is placed near the anterior border of the superficial MCL insertion with care not to damage the fibers during drilling. We use the same incision used to harvest the hamstrings or a small 1 cm separate incision if a different graft is used. The tibial tunnel should exit as far anterior and medial to prevent impingement in full extension. The tibial stump should also be trimmed to prevent anterior impingement due to cyclops formation. The more oblique the direction of the tibial tunnel is, the larger the intraarticular aperture becomes and the transition of the neoligament smoother.

However, drills larger than 9 mm angled at 45° produce larger tibial footprints than the native ACL and will likely damage the structures surrounding the aperture [114]. We therefore progressively drill the tibial tunnel to the measured size to prevent proximal aperture irregularities. Furthermore, we also use the full tibia drills as opposed to the femoral designs since this also can affect the final shape of the tunnel [115]. The distal aperture is then debrided from fascial soft tissue and the proximal shaved of excessive residual stump to facilitate graft passage. The minimum recommended graft length in the bone tunnels is 15 mm. Several studies failed to obtain improved fixation of soft tissue grafts with higher lengths in animal models [116, 117].

Once the femoral end is stabilized, the knee is put into several flexion-extension motions for better adjustment of the graft tension in the tibial tunnel. With the knee in approximately 30° of flexion and 8 kg force of pulling on the ligament the tibial fixation is completed. The proximal tibia should be pushed backward to counteract the anterior pull of the help during tensioning. There is no clear data on the amount of tension required as well as the reproducibility in real conditions [118]. Applying reduced pulling tension during tibial fixation might leave the ACL graft slack. However, increased tension appears to impede the healing during the ligamentization process and favor the development of stiffness in the immediate postoperative period. Histological analysis of grafts implanted under higher tension forces showed more necrotic areas which led to increased ligamentous laxity compared to grafts with minimal initial tension. Especially tendon grafts, such as the semitendinosus and gracilis have viscoelastic properties and can increase the length by pretensioning (Figs. 3.22, 3.23, and 3.24) (see Sect. 3.7.1).

We no longer use postoperative drains after primary ACL reconstructions, both intraarticular and at the hamstrings donor site. This shift in management was applied several years ago and did not lead to increased rated of effusions, hematomas or infections. All our patients receive pharmaceutical thromboprophylaxis by single subcutaneous injections of low molecular weight heparins up to 1 week. A compressive long leg stockinette is also worn for a minimum of 1 week. Immediate partial weight-bearing is permitted with the aid of 2 crutches for the first 3 weeks. We do not routinely immobilize primary ACL reconstructions but do use orthosis to limit range of motion when concomitant meniscal sutures are performed (see Sect. 2.3.1).

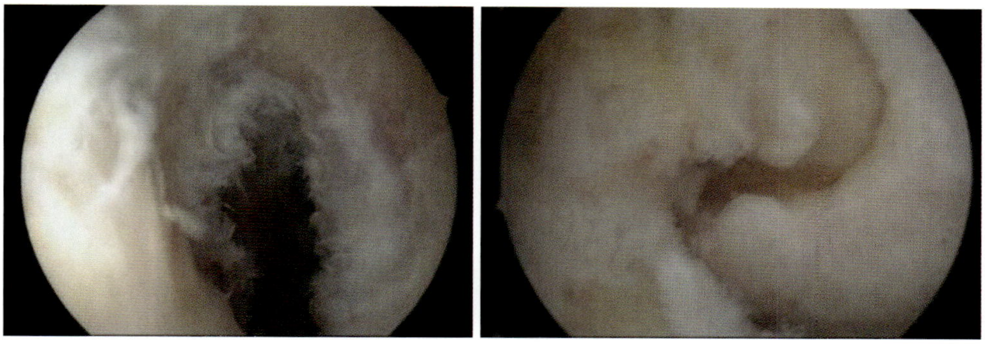

Fig. 3.16 Femoral footprint gently debrided, viewed from the antero-lateral portal with the left knee in high flexion. The only current indication for notchplasty is the presence of large osteophytes on the medial side of the lateral condyle

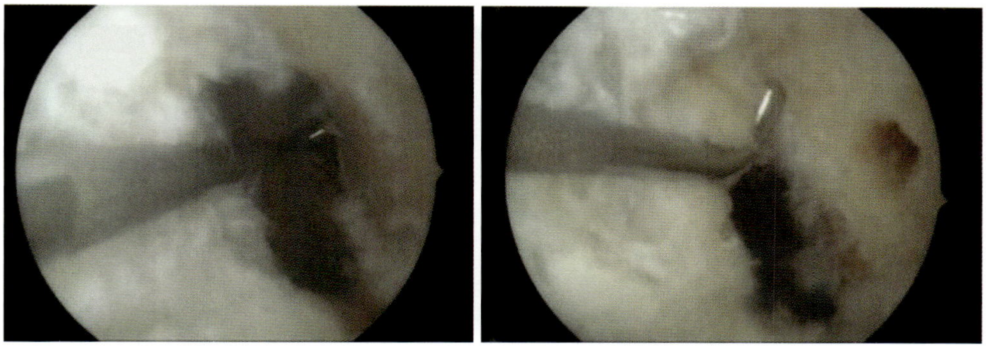

Fig. 3.17 The posterior cortex is referenced and shown in relation to the center of the femoral tunnel (antero-lateral portal view of the left knee)

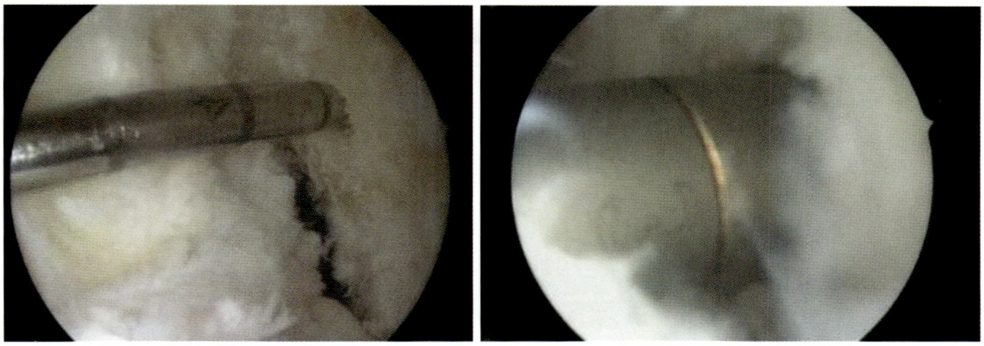

Fig. 3.18 A graded 4 mm pin is used to measure the distance to the lateral cortex (34 mm) and decide tunnel length (25) and loop size (20); progressive drilling to the desired size (usually 8) (antero-lateral portal view of the left knee)

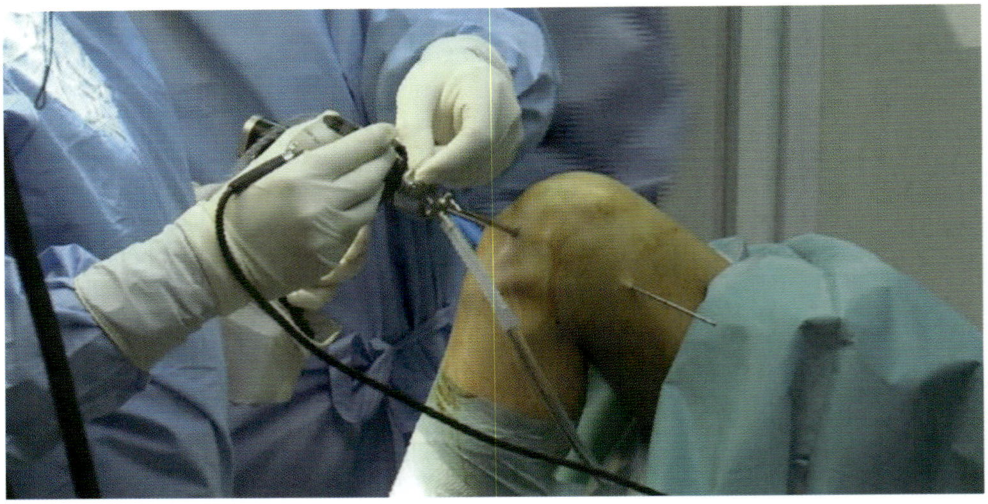

Fig. 3.19 Extra articular view of the left knee flexed to 110°; the patient is supine on a full table and the sterile draping is for general lower extremity use, without a fluid pouch. The arthroscope is through the antero-lateral portal and the femoral guide pin is entering through the antero-medial portal and exiting the lateral condyle in a correct direction

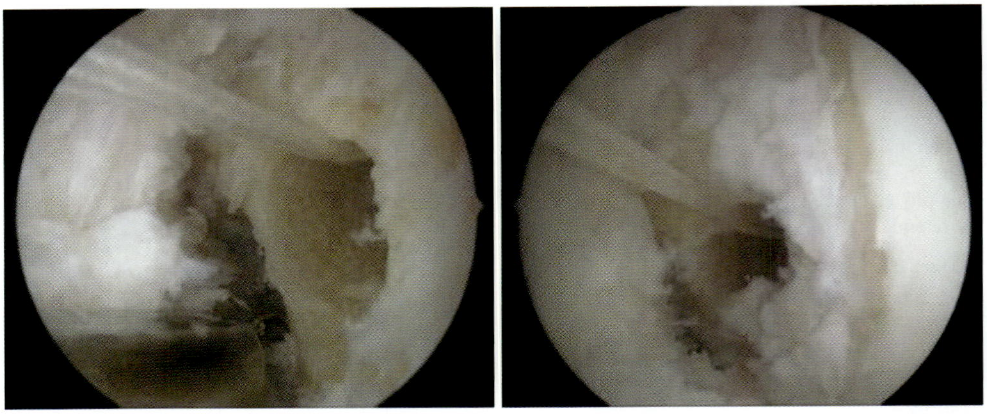

Fig. 3.20 Antero-lateral and antero-medial portal views of the left knee with the femoral aperture in the correct position and the leading sutures running trough

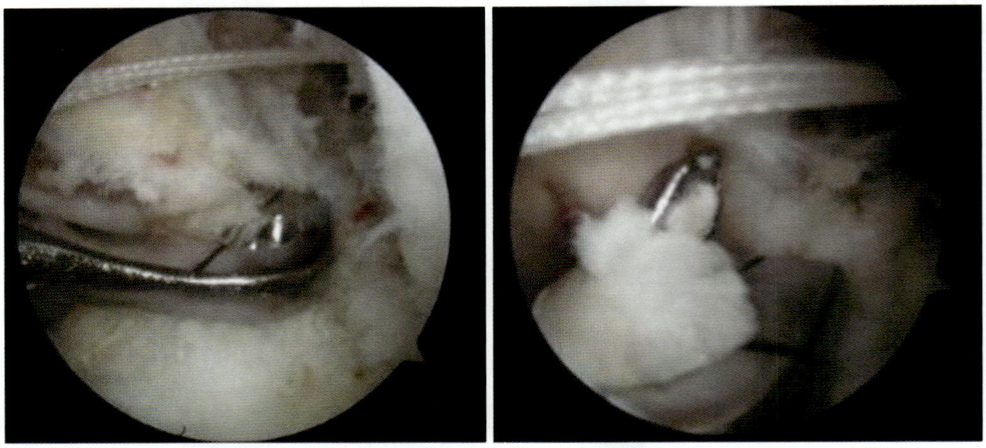

Fig. 3.21 The tibial guide pin is in the middle of the remnant stump (antero-lateral portal view of the left knee)

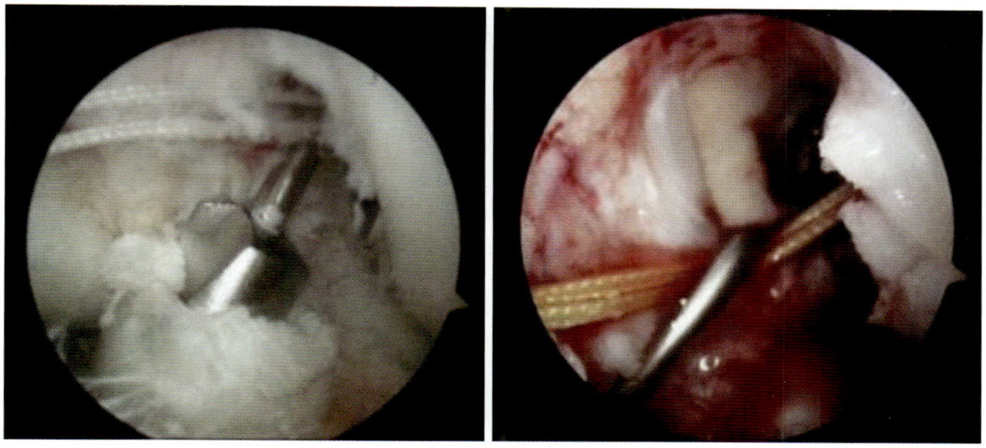

Fig. 3.22 Sequential drilling of the tibial tunnel (antero-lateral portal view of the left knee). "Hooking" the passing suture with the probe to pass it through the tibial tunnel (antero-lateral portal view of the left knee)

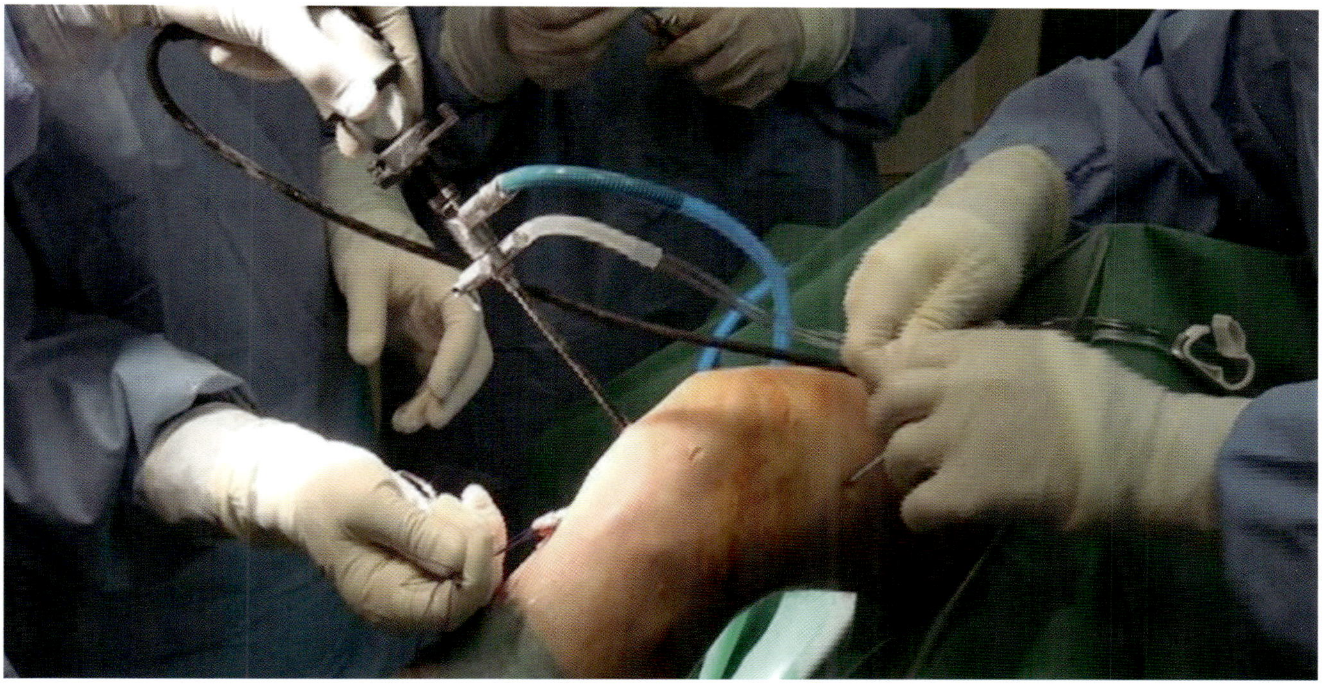

Fig. 3.23 The graft is pulled through the tunnels and the tension is maintained by pulling on the leading sutures; extra articular view of the left knee with the patient supine on the table with the leg segments removed and the feet hanging

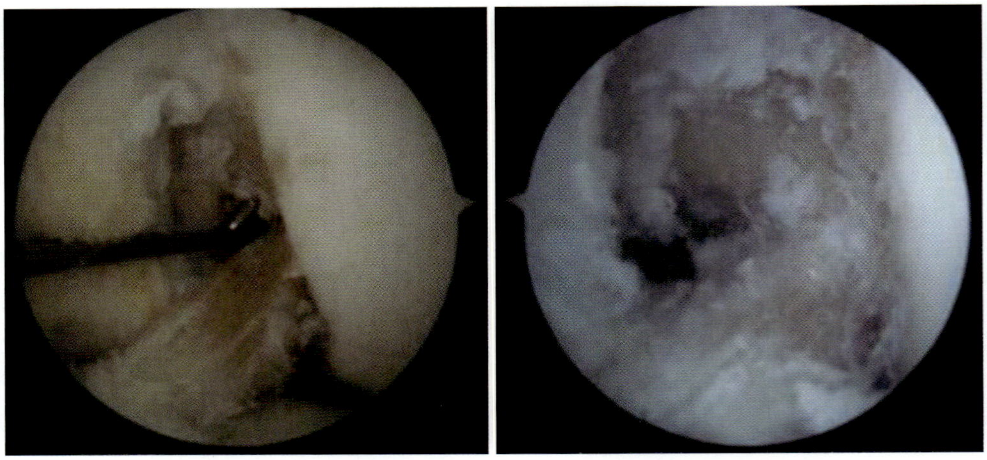

Fig. 3.24 The graft in the final position (antero-lateral and antero-medial portal views of the left knee); the oblique anatomic placement leads to a triangle between the reconstructed ACL and the native PCL

3.5.3 The Double Bundle Technique

The femoral and tibial insertion sites of the native ACL were extensively studied for landmarks, shape and normal variation (see Sect. 3.1.2). This was translated technically in the advent of "anatomic" techniques. The first to emerge was the anatomic double bundle (DB) technique that aimed not only to replicate the number of anatomical bundles of the ACL but also their insertion sites in order to restore knee kinematics to preinjury level [119]. There are several variations in the technique for DB reconstruction. Two standard portals are most commonly used, although some surgeons use a third central or accessory anteromedial to aid visualization. Transtibial DB is possible but the femoral aperture of the PL bundle is very unlikely to be accurately positioned through this approach [120]. A four tunnel approach is therefore recommended and used by the majority of surgeons. The patient is positioned in the same manner as for SB reconstruction. After a brief examination of instability under anesthesia, a standard exploration of the joint is performed (see Sect. 1.2.4).

By far the best graft choices for DB reconstruction are double looped hamstrings or tendon allograft with lateral cortical button fixation. Ideally, the grafts should be larger than 6 mm for the AM and 5 mm for the PL bundle respectively. We harvest the semitendinosus and gracillis tendons through a 3 cm oblique incision centered over their 'pes anserinus insertion'. The semiT is used for the AM bundle which is thicker and longer and the gracilis for the PL (see Sect. 3.1.2).

While the grafts are prepared on the backtable, any associated lesions are addressed. We always try to preserve as much as possible from the menisci. Although we most commonly treat meniscal ruptures by partial meniscectomy, we try to perform limited excisions and whenever possible suture. Outside in techniques are cheaper but require more effort (see Sect. 2.3.1). Small, stable longitudinal ruptures, especially when located on the posterior horn of the lateral meniscus can be successfully left in situ [121]. The ACL remnants and especially the tibial are trimmed just enough to allow for footprint identification and prevent impingement. The medial side of the lateral condyle is gently debrided of soft tissues with a mechanical or radiofrequency shaver.

With the knee flexed at 110–120° the location of the AM and PL bundles are judged and their centers marked with an awl or a small pin (see Sect. 3.5.2.1). If only two portals are used, the position should also be assessed by switching the camera to the anteromedial portal. The AM bundle is placed higher and deeper in the footprint (see Sect. 3.1.2). The tunnel is reamed to the appropriate size and the corresponding guide is placed into the tunnel and rotated so that the PL is located positioned lower and more shallow. By using the guide seen in Fig. 3.25 the two femoral tunnels diverge at 15° and are separated by a 4 mm bonebridge. This is sometimes to wide and will force the tunnels to be located outside the anatomic landmarks. Smaller offset guides are currently available on the market. The tunnel is drilled through the lateral cortex with a 4 or 4.5 guide pin, depending on the fixation system. The AM tunnel is longer and wider and exits more proximal through good cortex. The PL tunnel is shorter and exits more lateral. Care should be taken when reaming because the lateral cortical bone is thin and can easily be reamed through.

The tibial insertion is wider than for SB. The AM bundle aiming device is positioned just medial to the tuberosity, in a more anterior position than for SB and is passed at 55° to the horizontal. It is enlarged to the corresponding size and the appropriate PL drill guide is inserted through the AM tunnel and advanced until it becomes visible on the articular surface. The barrel has a mark on its head that indicates the direction of the PL guide pin. By rotating the guide's handle this line will point toward the native PL bundle attachment (see Sect. 3.1.2). Using this guide, the PL aperture is placed 9 mm posteriorly and laterally to the center of the AM bundle tunnel (Fig. 3.26). The tunnel is then reamed to the graft size. Two different leading sutures are pulled through each femoral tunnel and brought distal from the articular side through the tibial tunnels using a grasp.

The PL bundle graft is pulled first and the AM second, through their corresponding tibial and then femoral tunnels, and the cortical buttons are secured. The small size of the femoral tunnels and their proximity on the lateral condyle makes interference screw fixation more difficult. The knee is then extended and flexed whilst individually manually tensioning the grafts. This assures a comfortable fit of the grafts in the tunnels. The AM bundle should be relatively isometric whereas the PL bundle should exhibit a perceptible amount of variation during the range of motion. The AM bundle is secured first at 50° of flexion. The angle for the PL bundle depends on the length change throughout the knee flexion. If this is less than 3 mm, the bundle should be fixed in 20° of flexion. The more variation is seen, the closer to full extension the fixation is performed. The tibial fixation is made using absorbable interference screws, one size larger than the tunnel diameter. The tension applied to the grafts should be between 5 and 8 kg of force. When in doubt, the tension can be measured using the coil dynamometer from the graft preparation bench. The remainder of the grafts can be cut flush to the cortex or the pulling sutures tight one to another over the bone bridge between the tunnels.

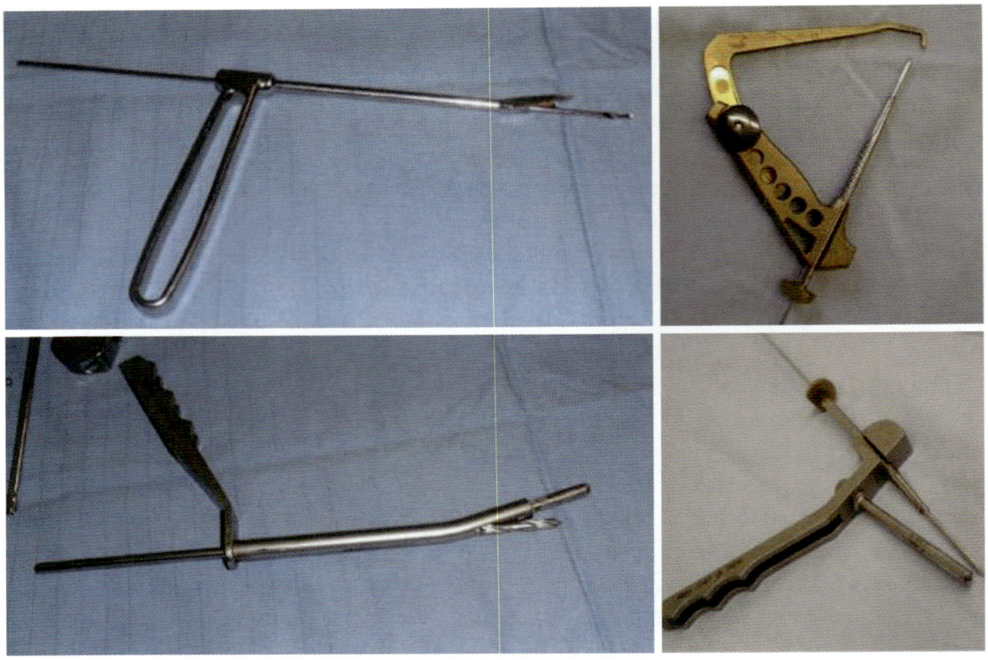

Fig. 3.25 A comparison of the SB and DB tibial and femoral guides, showing how the AM tunnel guides the distance to the PL apertures

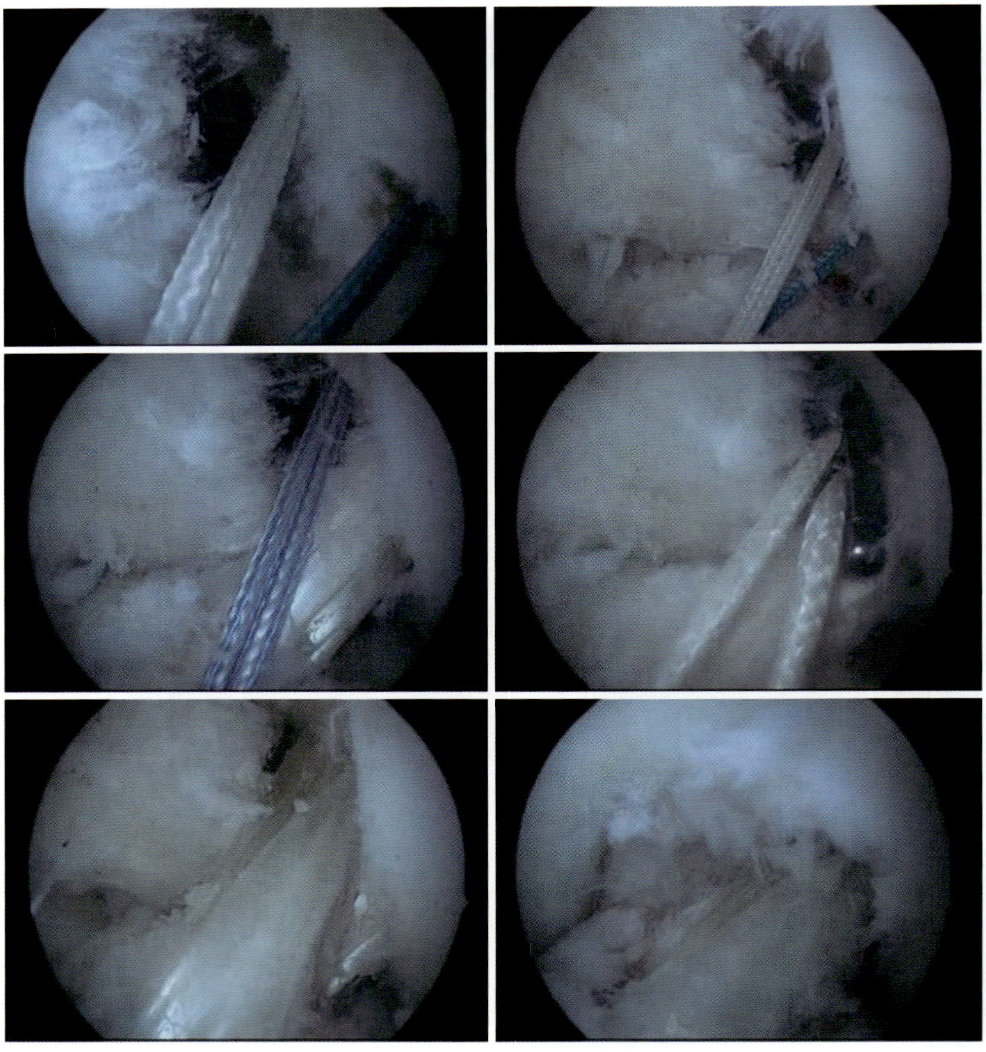

Fig. 3.26 Anterolateral portal views of the left knee. The femoral and tibial apertures of the two bundles are visible. A with leading suture is passes through the AM bundle and a green one through the PL respectively. The PL bundle is pulled through first, followed by the AM. The final aspect with the knee in flexion and extension

3.5.4 The Individualized ACL Reconstruction

The management of a ruptured ACL can differ depending on the patient age, past and future level of activity and the type of injury. For the elderly, sedentary patient conservative treatment and physiotherapy leads to a satisfactory outcome [122]. On the other hand, ACL deficient knees exhibit rotational instability even during activities of daily living. Gait analysis found these patients rotated their tibia internally during the initial swing phase. This abnormal movement might lead to articular degeneration and is attenuated after ACL reconstruction [123].

For the high demand patients such as athletes that wish to return to their previous level of exercise the primary goal is achieving a stable knee, avoiding further damage to the internal structures of the knee (menisci) and early start of rehabilitation and return to sports. Professional athletes are also one of the groups most exposed to the accidental rupture of the ACL. This injury is of the outmost importance to them because the ACL is the primary stabilizer of the knee. Injuries to this ligament can seriously alter an athlete's physical activity level or even end their sporting career. The focus on restoring the native ACL landmarks has led to the popularization of the anatomic double-bundle technique. Recent data however has somewhat failed to show definitive superior outcomes with the double bundle approach. Nonetheless, the anatomic reconstructions, weather single or double bundle have proved superior to the transtibial technique.

The team led by Professor Freddie Fu from Pittsburgh, USA, have devised a flowchart individually tailor ACL surgery. The authors define anatomic reconstructions as the 'functional restoration of the ACL to its native dimensions, fiber orientation, and insertion sites' [73]. This guide requires large footprints to be restored by double bundle procedure in order to provide a closer resemblance to the native architecture. Nevertheless, for smaller knees and footprints the double-bundle is no longer considered superior [124]. An award winning paper based on a comparative study between techniques found that anatomic SB reconstruction resulted in better antero-posterior and rotational stability than classic SB reconstruction but the results of the anatomic DB were superior to both. However, the difference was significant only between anatomic DB and conventional SB, but in this particular study, the authors did not account for the individual footprint variability [125].

Hence, the most commonly listed indications for DB ACL reconstructions according to Musahl et al. are [126]:

- large insertion sites (18 mm tibial ACL anteroposterior diameter),
- wide notch width (12 mm),
- high-grade pivot shift, and
- revision ACL reconstruction

Established contraindications for double-bundle ACL reconstruction are:

- multi-ligament injuries,
- open physes,
- degenerative OA,
- small insertion sites (12 mm tibial anterior–posterior diameter), and
- small notch width (12 mm)

To perform individualized reconstruction, the footprints of the insertion are measured (Fig. 3.27). These can also be sized on the preoperative MRI so that adequate graft choices can be made (Fig. 3.28).

The individualized approach takes into account each ACL footprint size [127]. Depending on the tibial insertion length, the recommended reconstruction technique is either SB, DB or both:

- <14 mm with a notch width <12 mm – SB
- 14–18 mm with a notch width >12 mm – SB or DB
- >18 mm – DB

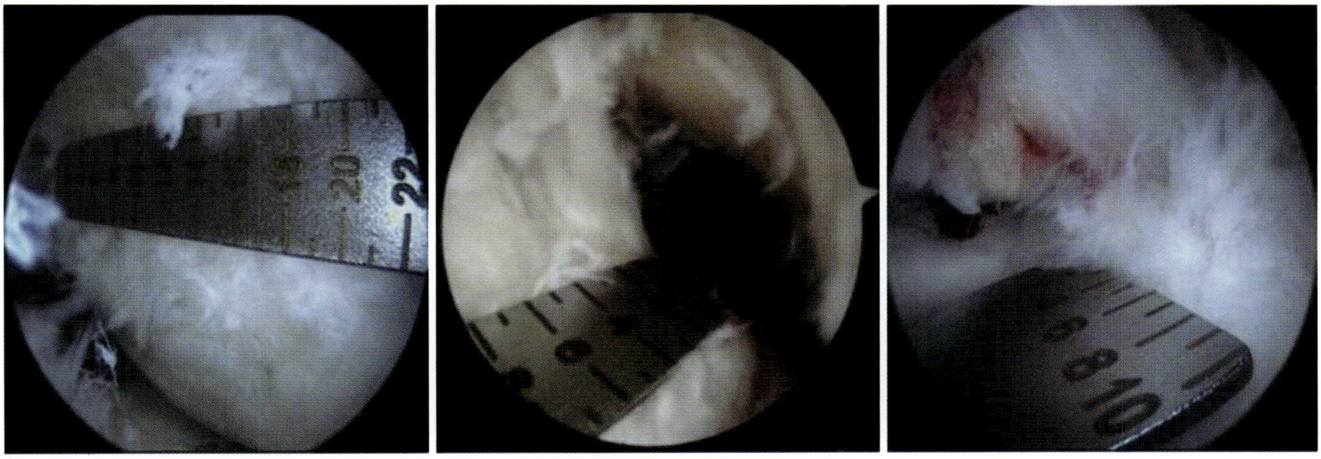

Fig. 3.27 Anteromedial portal measurement of the femoral insertion length on the lateral condyle using a ruler. Anterolateral views of the tibial footprint, measured for length and width. Based on these measurements, an anatomic SB reconstruction was chosen

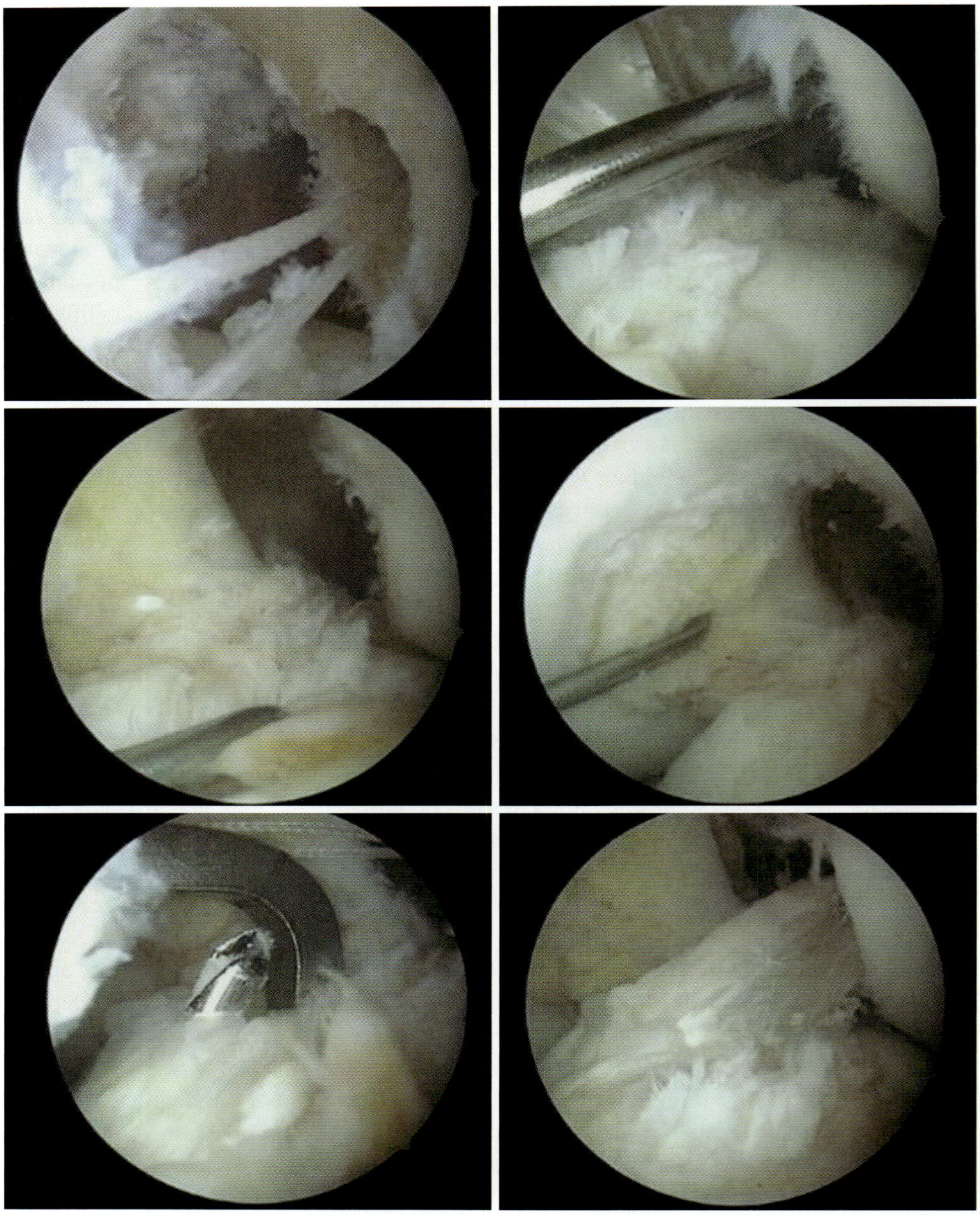

Fig. 3.28 Anatomic SB reconstruction. The femoral and tibial footprints are identified: posterior to the lateral condylar ridge with the tunnel drilled through the anteromedial bundle; the tibial insertion, medial to the anterior horn of the lateral meniscus, anterior to the PCL, in the center of the remnant stump. The final graft in place, views from the anterolateral portals (Gruia)

3.5.5 Single Bundle Augmentation

If clinically important instability is absent, partial tears usually have favorable outcomes with conservative treatment (Fig. 3.29). Approximately one-quarter will develop a positive pivot shift and might require reconstruction. When arthroscopic confirmation of the partial tear is obtained, selective bundle reconstruction can be successfully performed, although it can be challenging with a torn PL and preserved AM (Fig. 3.30) [128].

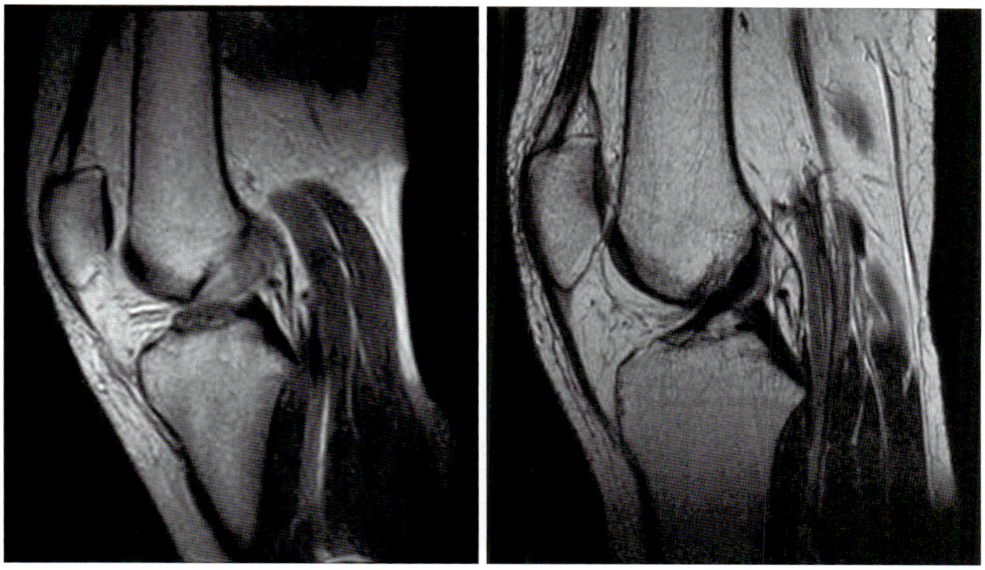

Fig. 3.29 Partial tear of the ACL that healed with conservative treatment as seen on repeat MRI after 2 years

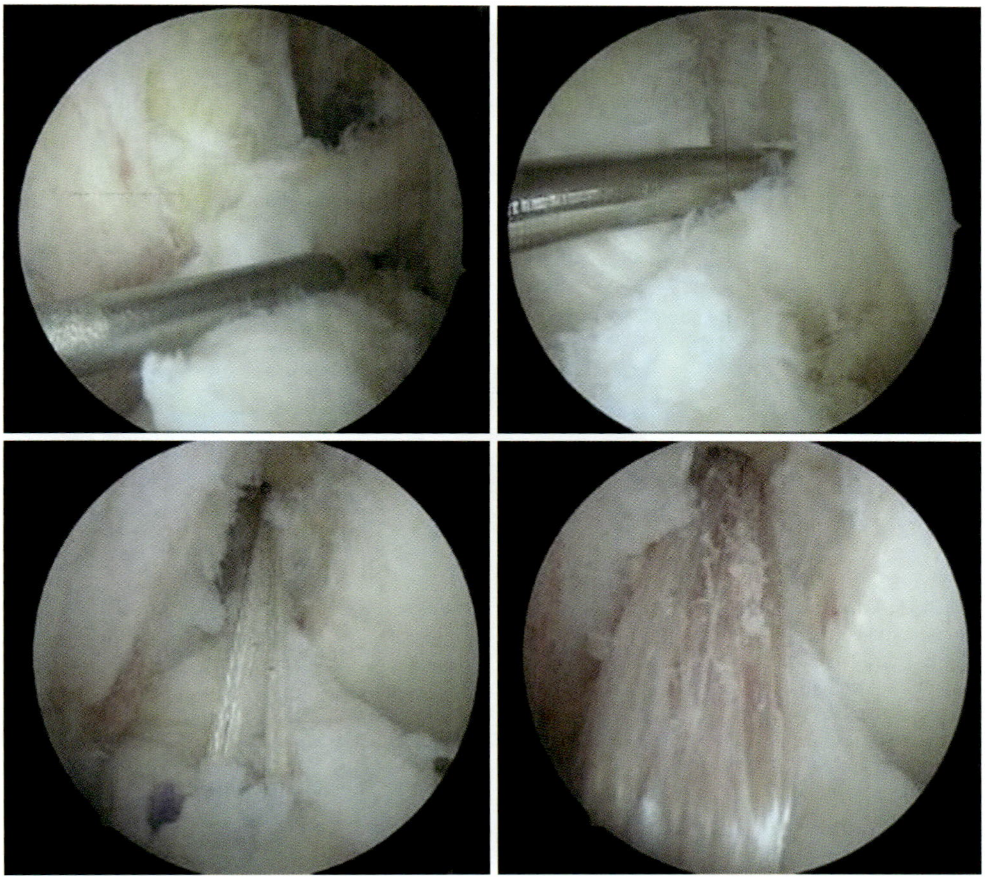

Fig. 3.30 Anterolateral portal views of the left knee. The torn AM bundle was removed and the PL tautness is checked by pulling with the probe. The location of the AM insertion is identified, deeper and higher than the PL with the knee flexed. The guide wire is passed and the tunnel reamed to size 6. The AM graft (doubled semiT) is pulled through, seen from the anteromedial and anterolateral portals

3.5.6 Potential Pitfalls

- Camera and hardware malfunction, incomplete instrument sets and missing sizes for the fixation system – always have alternatives for backup.
- Undiagnosed associated instabilities: PLC, PCL, MCL – start with examination under anesthesia.
- The Tourniquet is too distal or the femoral tunnel is too vertical and the guide wire will pierce the band – check and reposition.
- Iatrogenic medial condyle reaming with the femoral drill – more knee flexion or the anteromedial portal is too deep (medial) (Fig. 3.31).
- The femoral guide pin direction is too horizontal, resulting in a short tunnel with improper external cortical thickness for button fixation – more knee flexion is required or alternative fixation with a screw.
- The femoral tunnel aperture is too posterior and the direction too oblique from shallow to deep, resulting in posterior cortex blow-out: a serious complication, very difficult to correct – cortical button fixation and limited postoperative range of motion; use the offset guide to place the pin entrypoint.
- The femoral drilling is blind because the Hoffa pad obstructs the view from the lateral portal during flexion – shave the tissue, decrease the flexion angle, use an alternative central or accessory antero-medial portal.
- The tibial tunnel is drilled with the aperture misplaced – a small adjustment can be made between the first and last sequential reaming by changing the position of the guide wire (Fig. 3.32).
- The graft is dropped on the floor before fixation – be careful when handling, keep in disinfectant solution and lavage abundantly with saline; monitor for early signs of infection.
- The graft is too lose after fixation – unscrew the tibial side and stabilize under appropriate tension.
- A short graft is found in the tibial tunnel after femoral fixation or the traction sutures are cut during tibial screw fixation with the short graft inside the tunnel – remove femoral fixation and check tunnel lengths when using short grafts.
- Surgical site infection, usually at the tibial tunnel – debride and even use small vacuum; check that the graft is cut flush to the cortex and the fixation hardware is not protruding; lavage the debris before careful layered closure.
- Large and painful early postoperative effusion – needle aspiration, rest, ice and compressive bandage; suspicion of septic arthritis require early (and possibly repeated) arthroscopic lavage and antibiotics even before positive cultures are obtained; if the graft is not necrotic it can be left in place.
- Important pain and edema of the lower limb – exclude deep vein thrombosis (Doppler ultrasound), use compressive stockinettes, rest and nonsteroidal anti-inflammatory medication, adjust the rehabilitation regimen (NSAIDs).
- Extension deficit – allow early range of motion exercises, confirm patient adherence to an adequate rehabilitation program, exclude arthrofibrosis, cyclop lesion and tunnel malposition, check and document (arthroscopic pictures) the absence of roof impingement at the end of the surgery.
- Arthrofibrosis – a rare but unfortunate complication; use continuous passive motion (CPM) machines in the immediate postoperative period, avoid unnecessarily performing surgery during the acute phase, assure patient is compliant to the postoperative rehabilitation program, evaluate full range of motion at 10 and 30 days postoperatively,

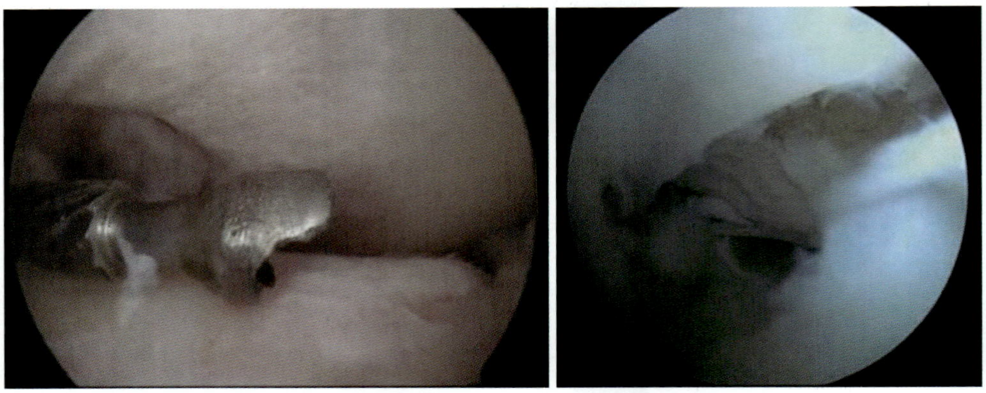

Fig. 3.31 Intraarticular instrument breakage (bone shaver). Iatrogenic osteochondral lesion on the weight bearing surface of the medial condyle during femoral tunnel drilling

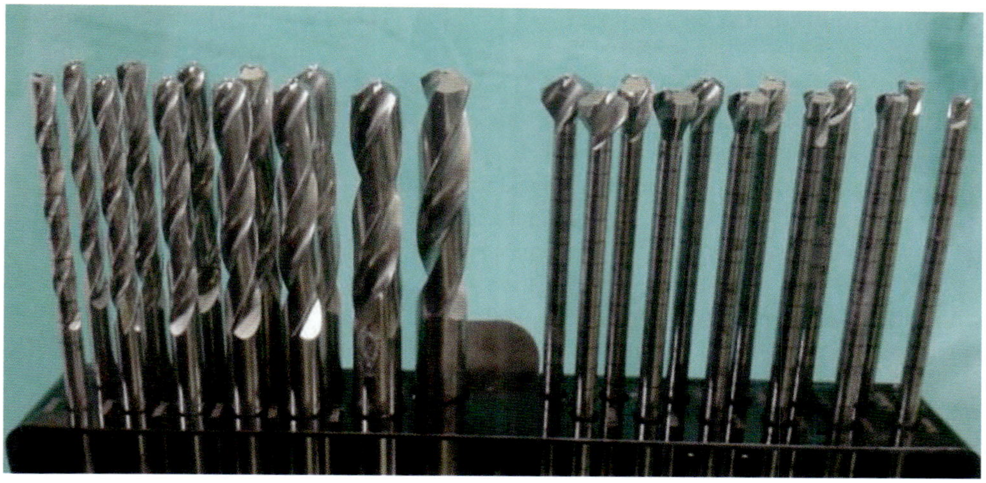

Fig. 3.32 Compared to the tibial (*left*) the femoral drills (*right*) have a thin rounded body and a short reaming tip. This shape is used to protect the medial condyle

3.6 ACL Fixation Systems

The ideal fixation device should provide anatomical fixation, should be biocompatible and MRI safe with a easy, safe and reproducible insertion technique, low risk for complications, allow for easy revision and have a low cost. That said, to date there is no proven gold standard for the femoral fixation of the ACL graft [129], different fixation methods are used that provide a secure fixation of the graft withstanding a minimum of 200–250N in the immediate postoperative phase such as suspensory fixation devices (button type devices), joint line fixation with interference screws (titanium and bioabsorbable) and transfemoral fixation with crosspins being the most popular devices in clinical practice with others having seen much less use such as Femoral Intrafix, bone wedge or bone block in the so called "implant free" ACL fixation technique that uses no implant whatsoever in fixing the ACL graft with very good and excellent reported results by some authors [130–133]and hybrid fixation that uses more than one fixation method in one or both sites. Strong fixation of the graft is necessary for using current rehabilitation protocols, which allow for early weightbearing, full ROM, and return of neuromuscular function [134].

3.6.1 Interference Screws

The first reported use of a intraarticular screw to fix an ACL graft is from Wittek in 1927 [135]. Traditionally the method of fixation of choice was the titanium screw joint line fixation used widely from the 1980s worldwide. The screws are different for the femoral and the tibial side, in diameter and in shape, the femoral ones are of smaller diameter and their articular end is rounded, while the screws used for the tibial fixation are flat ended. In more recent years a transition was made from titanium to bioabsorbable screws made from PLLA (poly-L-lactic acid) or composite material (PLLA combined with beta tricalcium phosphate – β TCP, or hydroxyapatite – HA) that would theoretically transform into bone in a period of time of up to 2 years. This was not at all caused by the lack of fixation strength for these titanium screws as they provide excellent bone purchase and are very good for fixing BTB grafts to the bone but rather by the increased popular demand generated by the bony integration of the screw and also because of the gradual decline in the popularity of the BTB graft in favor of the hamstrings graft for whose fixation they are better suited due to the softer material and the blunter, wider, thread that doesn't cut as deep and much in the substance of the graft

The bioabsorbable interference screw had a very good fixation strength with both the patellar tendon BTB graft and the hamstrings graft, comparable with that of the titanium interference screw [136]. While a properly sized and good quality screw would provide excellent femoral fixation at the bone level on the femur and compression of the graft to the bone providing extra fixation and faster and better integration of the graft with no tunnel widening [136, 137] they tend to cause laceration of graft during implantation and can cause a rotation of the graft in the femoral canal placing it on an undesirable, non ideal position Offerhaus et al. concluding that the use of a standard right threaded screw can cause a systematic placement error in right knees causing significant postoperative laxity [138] and Musgrove et al. performed fixation in right knees with reverse threaded femoral screws in 44 knees and compared them with a group of 36 knees where they used standard right threaded screws and on their group had a statistically significant reduction in laxity (Lachmann test, not for pivot shift, or Lysholm scores) for the reverse thread group at 12 months postoperative (Fig. 3.33) [139].

The clinical results with titanium and PLLA screws seem to be equivalent according to a 7 year follow-up study with BTB grafts by Drogset et al. [140] and with no statistical differences in a hamstring study by Myers et al. [141] while a meta-analysis by Shen et al. found that there was no significant difference in measurement results of knee joint stability or knee joint function outcome between bioabsorbable and metallic interference screws [142].

The resorption of PLLA screws has been tested and followed by both MRI and second look arthroscopy in cases where it was indicated. In our experience we found traces of PLLA in ACL revisions at 2.7 years after the initial surgery (Fig. 3.34). This has been confirmed in literature, different authors citing traces of unresorbed PLLA as far as 5 years after the initial surgery [143–143]. This led to the use of other materials such as polyglycolic acid (PGA), poly L/D lactide (PLDLA) and polylactide carbonate (PLC) which was deemed insecure due to the high number of postoperative complications in 59 patients [145]. Biocomposite screws, PLLA-HA and PLLA-β TCP were developed to increase the osteoconductivity of the screw, Barber et al. found that the screws did indeed resorb at a maximum of 4 years after the initial surgery [147–149], while Herrera et al. established that even the shortest biocomposite PLLA-HA screw of 9×23 mm had a mean load to failure of 295N.

Other properties of biocomposite screws regard their increased plasticity, making them less susceptible to intraoperative shear rupture and also creating the theoretical possibility of bone defect grafting by filling a previous malpositioned tunnel. The nature of the PLLA material makes it quite breakable, postoperative migration of broken implant parts has also been reported [150]. And as all the screws have the advantage of the joint line fixation, titanium screws have been found to have the smallest bacterial adherence out of all the screw types used for ACL reconstruction [151], and their reduced cost and excellent clinical results made for a renewed interest and a wider overall adoption among surgeons. Different variations of the screw have been marketed such as the Delta screw (a BCP – biphasic calcium phosphate and PLDLA screw with a 1.5 mm taper) and the Retro screw (a BCP – PLDLA with an retrograde all inside insertion technique) [152].

Disadvantages of screw fixation should be mentioned as is the operative technique that requires a hyperflexed knee (>110°) to be maintained while drilling, sizing, notching (an extra operative step) and inserting the screw, something that can be quite difficult in a large patient while using the broken table operative setup. The nytinol guide wire can become trapped between the fibers of the graft and the constant pressure that must be maintained on the graft and the implant for the period of insertion of the screw can also pose some difficulties. The single most important factor to be considered when choosing a screw for the femoral fixation is the risk of posterior wall blowout.

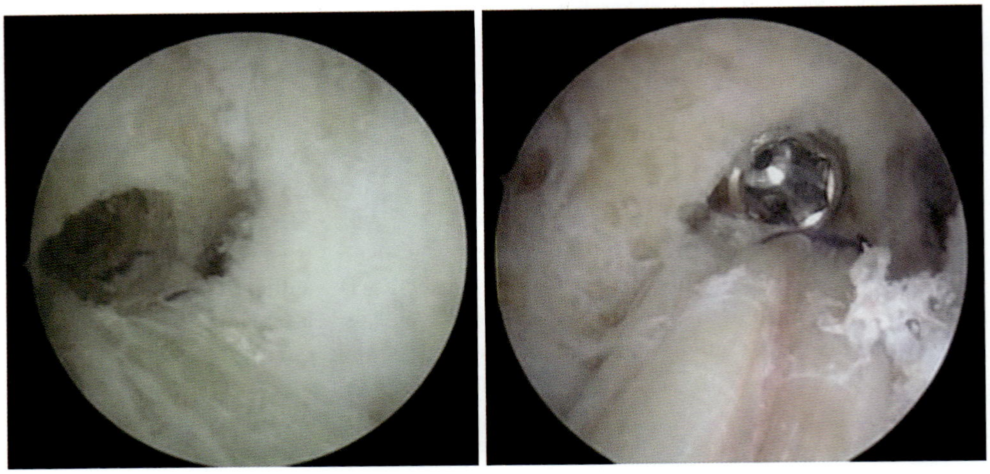

Fig. 3.33 PLLA and titanium screw fixating the femoral end of a soft tissue graft – right knee

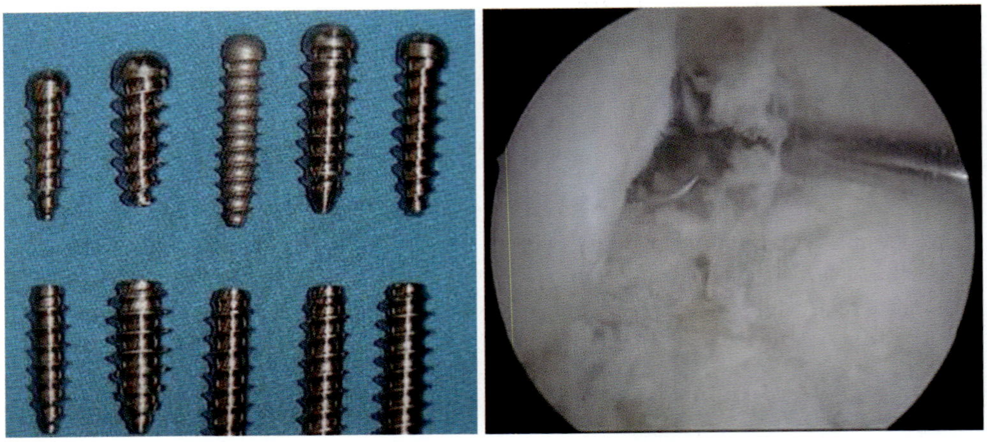

Fig. 3.34 Titanium ACL screws. Note the rounded end of the femoral screws and the sharp edges of the thread; PLLA screw residue in a revision case at 2.7 years after the initial reconstruction

3.6.2 Button and Loop Cortical Fixation

The increased popularity of the soft tissue grafts (mainly hamstrings) lateralization and horizontalization of the femoral tunnel in anatomic ACL reconstruction as well as the advent of the double bundle technique created the necessity of a new class of femoral fixation devices with a simpler, more straightforward surgical technique and fewer intraoperative complications. Suspensory fixation with different devices such as the EndoButton (Smith and Nephew, Andover, MA), the RetroButton (Arthrex) or the ACL TightRope RT (Arthrex), ToggleLoc (Biomet), XO Button (Conmed, Largo, FL) plus many others are that widely available on the market that have been found to provide a excellent fixation of the graft at the femoral site.

All these are basically an evolution of the suture button (a round titanium button with four holes through which the surgeon would pass the sutures and make the knots on top). They involve a tiny strip of titanium 12–18 mm long and 2 mm wide with a continuous suture loop passed through the middle 15–25 mm long. There are few devices that have a self-locking loop that has a self-adjusting feature in relation to the femoral tunnel length as the free ends of the loop are pulled after the button is fixed on the lateral femoral cortex, advancing the graft in the femoral canal (TightRope, ToggleLoc). Technically they use a retrograde introduction technique. A femoral tunnel 4 or 5 mm in diameter is drilled trough the lateral cortex and the femoral tunnel for the graft is overdrilled on the same guide wire. The sutures are passed in an inside out technique with a guide wire. The button is then advanced trough the cortical tunnel and once it exits on the lateral cortex it is flipped so that it lays flat on the cortical surface. The flipping of the button has different technical approaches, the EndoButton has suture loops trough each of the sides of the button making it easier to check for the flipping (Fig. 3.35).

The Retrobutton, TightRope and ToggleLoc on the other hand have only one suture loop trough one side of the button and the flip is made by pulling the graft backwards once the button has emerged on the lateral cortex, the free end of the button hooking on the cortical bone and the whole button flipping on the central loop, which serves as the pivotal point and the back pressure aiding it to seat flat on the lateral cortex. Once flipping is done, trough either technique, a constant pressure must be maintained on the button by pulling on the tibial end so that the button doesn't move. The implants with a self locking loop (TightRope, ToggleLoc) can be visualized trough the medial portal as they advance in the femoral canal and the flip can be made under optical control (Figs. 3.36 and 3.37). Another step described by Nag et al. was to gently push the TightRope button past the guide pin hole with a drill guide [153] and after that to visually check it for flipping and seating.

Another use for buttons would be on the tibia as well as on the femur trough the "all inside" technique with retrograde inside-out drilling of the tibial tunnel and fixation with buttons at both ends of the graft. Double fixation is also a possibility, in case of an unsure flip of the button or of a failed femoral fixation with a button or an clinically unsatisfactory hold on the femoral side one can always insert a femoral screw to augment the fixation, this making button suspensory fixation much more safe as it leaves the option of screw fixation open in case of need.

Several studies exist that compare the mechanical and biomechanical properties of different fixation devices of the tendinous graft. Milano et al. found corticocancellous fixation was superior to two 2.7-mm crosspins and interference screws in terms of fixation strength and stiffness and amount of graft elongation [136, 154]. The authors attributed the poorer performance of the interference screws to the lack of cortical purchase. Ahmad et al. found greater graft slippage with two 2.7-mm crosspins and interference screws when compared with suspensory fixation or one 5-mm crosspin. The interference screw had a lower load to failure than suspensory fixation and both the one 5-mm crosspin and the two 2.7-mm crosspins. Failures were attributed to weakness of the graft-screw interface [129].

The extra-articular fixation techniques such as a flip button strategy provides high fixation strength, which is even superior to the stability of patella-tendon bone grafts fixed with an interference screw but also has its potential downsides. Due to the fact that these fixation devices consist of a suture loop and a titanium button their stiffness is very low. A "bungee effect" may result whereby the graft moves longitudinally within the tunnel. Hoher et al. observed up to 3 mm of hamstring graft motion in the tunnel with loading in a cadaver model. They tested 15, 25 and 35 mm loops and found less motion of the graft with shorter loops and greater motion with longer loops. They also hypothesized that early stress on the graft with rehabilitation activities could cause large graft-tunnel motion but under cyclic loading, suspensory fixation, two 2.7-mm crosspins, and interference screws allow for similar amounts of displacement of the graft [155]. Sagittal graft motion, known as the windshield wiper effect, can also occur [156–158]. Thus, there is no clear biomechanical advantage to one method of fixation versus another.

While the surgical technique of joint line femoral fixation with a screw is more challenging due to the hyperflexed position of the knee and the prolonged insertion time of the implant and the constant pressure that has to be exerted on the graft during implant insertion it is also the established technique of femoral fixation for ACL grafts. Sometimes depending on individual knee anatomy (small notch) the insertion site can be difficult to visualize during screw insertion. Other difficulties or intraoperative incidents that can appear are the laceration of the graft by the screw thread or the rotation of the implant on the screw causing it o be implanted in a less than ideal position.

Button type implants are easier to insert, from a technical point of view after a small learning curve. When selecting a Retrobutton size we always try to use the smallest size of the loop possible (15–20 mm) to minimize the risk of bungee effect [155]. Of the two implants the ACL TightRope RT has the advantage of an adjustable, self locking loop that can be used successfully in situations where the cortical distance measured intraoperatively and the resulting femoral tunnel is short (25 mm) combined with larger diameter graft. However there are reports of loop lengthening with the use of adjustable length cortical suspension devices, Barrow et al. tested comparatively the TightRope RT (Arthrex) and the ToggleLoc (Biomet) to the Endobutton CL (Smith and Nephew, Andover, MA). They found that the total displacement after 4,500 cycles of tensioning at variable loads was significantly higher for the TightRope RT (42.45 ± 7.01 mm) compared to the ToggleLoc (5.76 ± 0.35 mm) and the EndoButton CL Ultra (1.34 ± 0.03 mm) and the Arthrex TightRope reached clinical failure of 3 mm lengthening after fewer cycles. There was also a significant difference in ultimate load between the TightRope and the other 2 constructs [159]. Petre et al. studied comparatively the same implants and the XO Button (Conmed, Largo, FL) and concluded that all implants have the necessary biomechanical properties with regard to ultimate failure strength, displacement, and stiffness for initial fixation of soft tissue grafts in the femoral tunnel for ACL reconstruction only the ToggleLoc crossed over the 3.0-mm clinical failure threshold for cyclic displacement [160]. Other clinical and experimental research has confirmed this data [161–163].

We found button implants to be easier to use in smaller knees with a smaller native ACL femoral footprint and/or a small notch. This is especially because there is no need for notching of the femoral tunnel that is needed for the screw insertion and no risk of subsequent damage to the articular surface of the medial femoral condyle by extra hardware. Although there is more tunnel widening cited in literature and more graft movement due to a less rigid fixation than the bioabsorbable screw we have found the short and medium term clinical results to be similar.

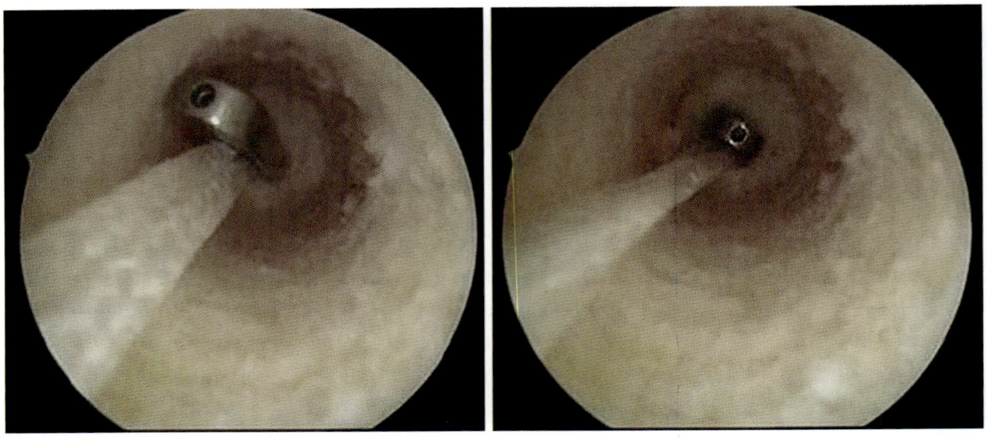

Fig. 3.35 TightRope (Arthrex) inserted in the femoral canal and passing trough the cortical tunnel (medial portal view)

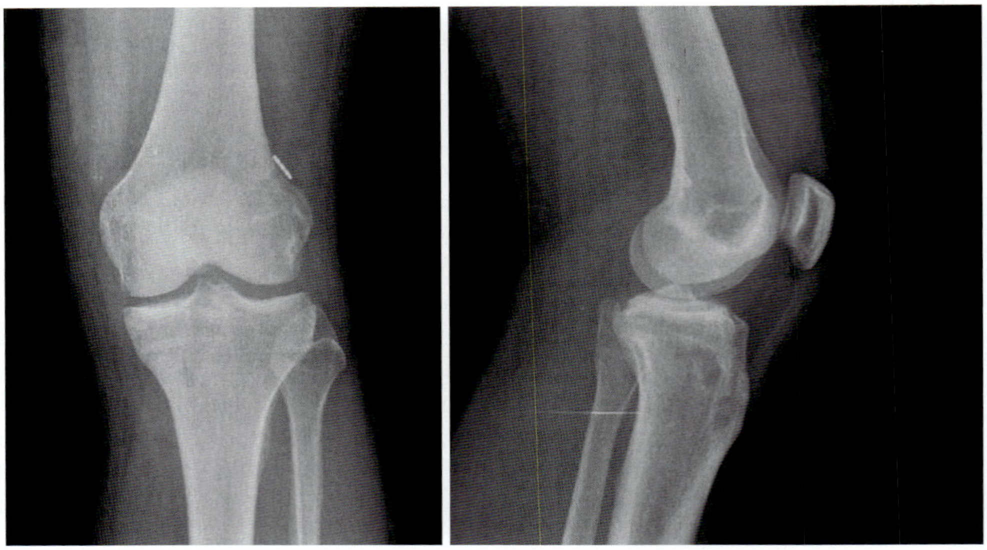

Fig. 3.36 Postoperative AP and lateral X-Rays showing an Endobutton (Smith and Nephew, Andover, MA) on the lateral femoral cortical wall in a correct position, right above the lateral condyle, in the posterior part of it. The tibial and femoral tunnels can also be visualized

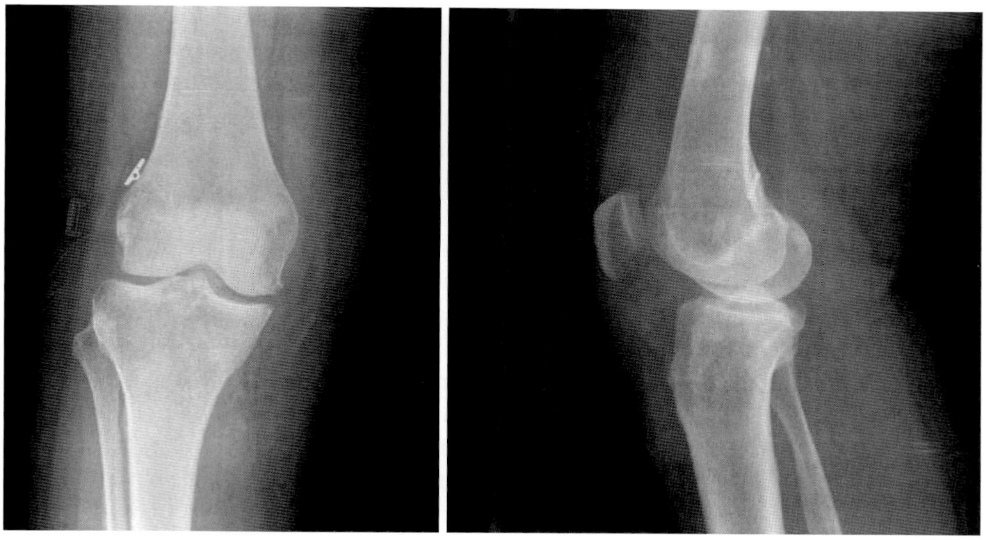

Fig. 3.37 Postoperative AP and lateral X-Rays showing an ToggleLoc (Biomet) in correct position

3.6.3 Crosspins – Transfemoral Fixation

Cross-pins were developed as an alternative to the joint line fixation and the cortical suspensory fixation. The aim was to improve on potential problems associated with interference screw and button fixation methods. They consist of one or two titanium or bioabsorbable pins (PLLA, PLLA-HA) that are inserted through the lateral femoral cortex and cross the proximal end femoral tunnel, the pins either penetrate the 4-strand graft or the 2 strands of the hamstring wrap 180° around the pin to create a quadrupled graft [164]. Various devices exist on the market developed by different companies each with slight variations on the original technique and fixation concept such as RigidFix (De Puy Mitek, Raynham, MA), PINN-ACL (Conmed, Largo, FL), TransFix/Bio-TransFix (Arthrex), Cross Screw (Stryker, Mahwah, NJ) to name just a few.

The idea behind the development of cross-pins was to have an alternative fixation method to the intraarticular screws that had all the advantages of the suspensory fixation that the button devices provided but to decrease the potential shortcomings such as the tunnel widening [165]. Because the anchor point is closer to the articular aperture of the femoral tunnel it has been reported that tunnel widening less commonly occurs with the cross pin system, [166–168] but further research has revealed equal widening in Endobutton CL and cross-pin groups.[169] There has also been a documented tendency in breaking of the bioabsorbable cross-pins postoperatively but without any modification regarding the clinical outcomes [170, 171]. A metaanalysis by Han et al. determined that intratunnel fixation (screw) had earlier full weight bearing and jogging/running, but the groups did not differ in return-to-sports timing or objective IKDC [172].

3.6.4 Implant Free Fixation

There has also been an increased interest in some groups regarding implant free primary ACL reconstructions. This was achieved by either looping the graft trough two femoral tunnels and fixing it in a single tibial tunnel with a screw [173], or fixing the bone plug of the graft by press-fit within the tibial metaphysis and its ligamentous part in the metaphysis by harvested cancellous bone blocks driven into the joint line from the outside [131]. Similar results were obtained in implant-free press-fit ACL reconstruction using hamstring tendon soft tissue grafts [174] and its proponents argue that the importance of the anatomical reconstruction of the ACL was proven since the beginning of the twentieth century and that implant free reconstructions have already been proven successful and as such the postoperative results depend more on a correct technique than in the choice of the femoral fixation device [130]. A 1999 experimental study on 40 human cadaver knees compared bone-block press-fit to screw fixation for BTB grafts and found 570N average for the implant free group and a 402N average for the screw group [132]. Frenzel et al. concluded that implant-free replacement of ACLs is cheaper, and achieves functional results for fixation which are comparable to ACL reconstructions with implants in both BTB and soft tissue grafts [175].

3.6.5 Complications

Screw fixation, as mentioned above is poised to graft malposition due to the rotation of the graft around the screw (Fig. 3.38). Graft laceration is also a serious issue for titanium femoral screws used on soft tissue grafts. Degradation of the screw is also possible, PLLA screws have a tendency towards transversal shearing while biocomposite screws are stiffer and can crack longitudinally (Fig. 3.39). This is a very serious complication, as it can be very difficult to remove the proximal part of the screw that is still inserted in the femoral tunnel especially without damaging the graft. The aim is to accurately test the quality of the remnant femoral fixation and if it is considered sufficient it should be left in place. How much is sufficient is rather difficult to quantize in a clinical situation. The aim is that it should resist a minimum of 200N to have a stable enough fixation but this is difficult to measure intraoperatively. A graft-tensioning device can be used to some success to estimate around 20 kgf (200N = 20.39 kgf) but this is not a truly replicable method, more of a salvage one. The nytinol guide wire can become entrapped in the fibers of the ACL graft and if the femoral screw is fully inserted it may be impossible to remove or it can even break in the femoral canal. Tibial screws can penetrate into the articular space if they are overinserted, something that could be simply resolved by pulling them back but this can detension the graft causing a loose postoperative knee or they can cause an iatrogenic fracture of the internal tibial plateau right at the edge of the tibial spine (Fig. 3.40).

Button fixation, although less technically demanding, can create its own set of intraoperative incidents. One of the important steps of button fixation is the drilling of the femoral tunnel which should be done up to the cortical bone, but not past it. The button exits trough a smaller tunnel 4 or 5 mm in diameter. Overdrilling a 7–8 mm tunnel past the lateral cortex, the so called cortical blowout, can greatly diminish the strength of fixation for button devices that regularly have 10–12 mm of length. If this happens, two options are available, either the use of an implant with a longer button like the Xtendobutton (Smith and Nephew, Andover, MA) or the Retrobutton XL (Arthrex, Nalpes, FL) to enlarge the footprint of the button or use supplementary femoral fixation with a screw [176]. The last option is in our experience the better one but it does imply a higher cost. Flipping the button can also create issues sometimes and intraoperative fluoroscopy should be used to assess the position of the button every time there are some doubts about its position. If a fixed loop device is being used the lateral cortex – femoral tunnel distance can be too big. The graft must be removed and the femoral tunnel should be measured and redrilled with great care not to blow the lateral cortex and the graft reinserted. The button can also become entrapped in the femoral canal or the periosteum either performing an incomplete flip or not flipping at all, but remaining stuck, without the possibility of removing and adjusting the graft (Fig. 3.41). Double fixation with a femoral screw should be performed in all cases where femoral fixation is not 100 % satisfactory. Excessive force when pulling a self locking loop device can cause the button to pass the bone, periosteum, iliotibial band where it can flip and become attached or it can even be pulled out through the skin. In this case a small incision over the button is probably the best option the surgeon has, with dissection of the soft tissues to the bone and placing the button on the lateral cortex under direct visualization and then advancing the graft in the femoral tunnel. Supplementary fixation is usually not necessary in this case, however the patient should be informed of the reason and the nature of the extra incision on the superolateral side of the knee. Direct visualization of the button should be carried out routinely but even so a too tight or to large cortical tunnel can cause this event [153].

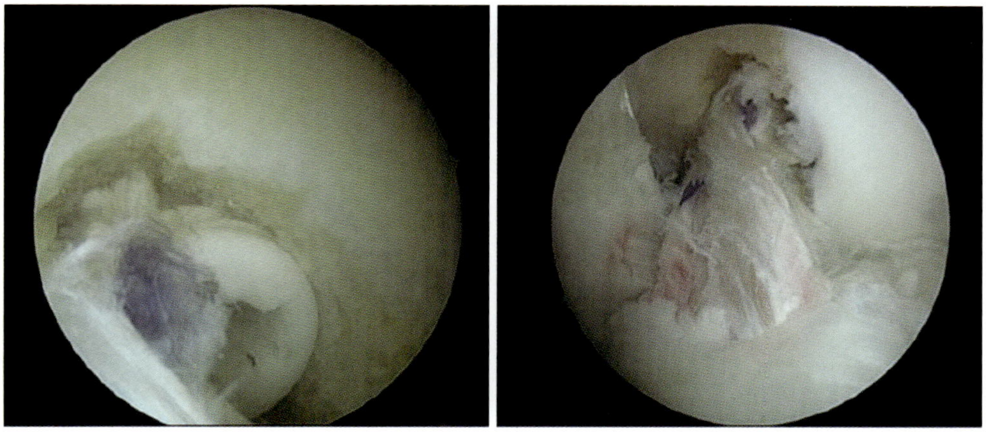

Fig. 3.38 A biocomposite PLLA-HA screw with a longitudinal crack and a rotated graft in a left knee. Medial and lateral portal views

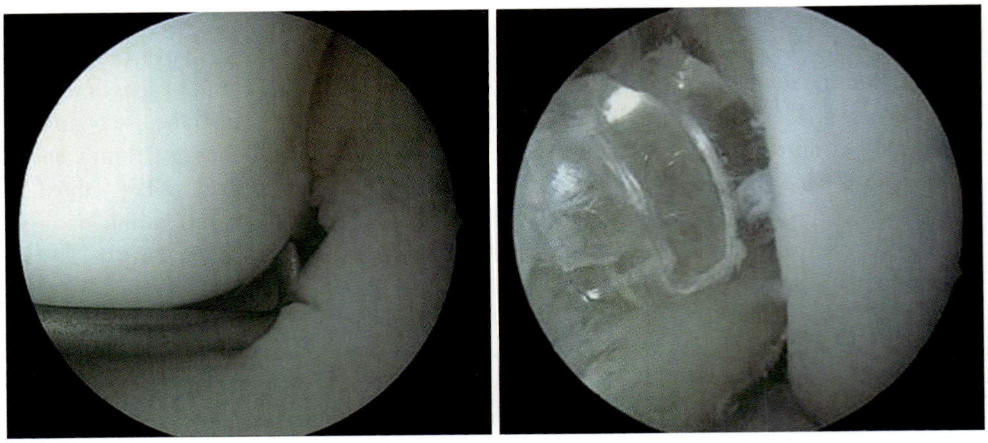

Fig. 3.39 Fracture of the tibial spine due to an overinserted tibial screw. A broken femoral screw floating free in the notch

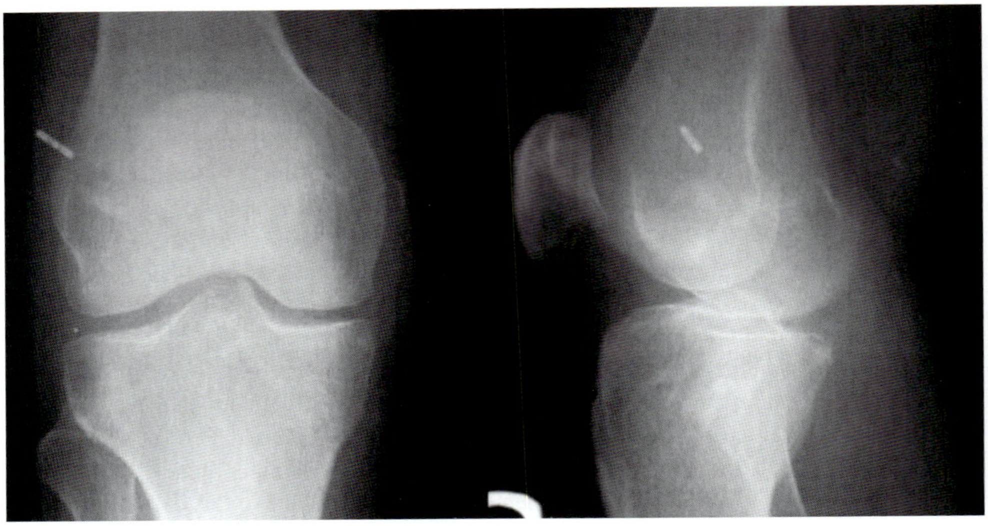

Fig. 3.40 Postoperative AP and lateral X-Rays showing a Retrobutton (Arthrex, Nalpes, FL) that has not exited the femoral canal and has not flipped. A femoral screw was applied in this case

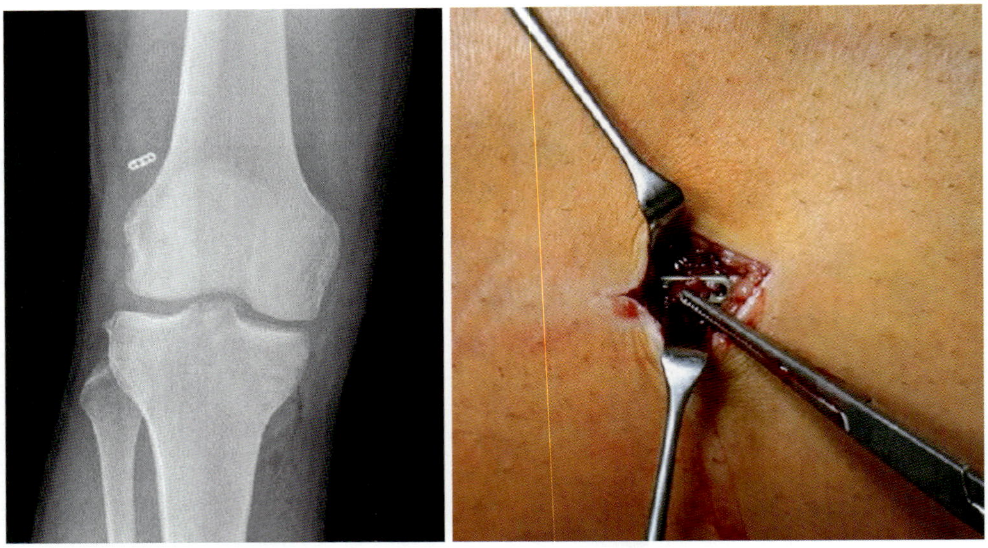

Fig. 3.41 The button has passed through the iliotibial band and is trapped in the soft tissues. A minimal incision identifies the button and then seats it on the femur under direct visualization

3.7 ACL Graft Choices

There are many techniques available for ACL reconstructions that use autografts and allografts as well as artificial grafts. Currently, the most popular and widely used are autografts – hamstrings, followed by patellar tendon (see Sect. 3.6.1). The ipsilateral middle third patellar tendon graft, with bone plugs at each end has traditionally been the standard choice for ACL reconstruction. The relatively high incidence of kneeling pain related to donor site morbidity, as well as the spread of double bundle (DB) procedures saw the advent of semitendinosus (ST) and gracilis (G) as the grafts most preferred.

Several literature reviews have compared hamstrings and patellar tendon autografts (BPTB) [176–179]. There is agreement that BPTB produces more anterior knee pain, especially while kneeling and a more statically stable knee. There are no differences for anterior knee sensory deficit, clinical outcome (Tegner – Lysholm, International Knee Documentation Committee scores), function (single leg hop test), re-rupture and return to sports. The hamstrings graft is associated with inferior knee flexion strength at higher angles and more tunnel widening while the patellar tendon disturbs the extensor apparatus and leads to loss of knee extension range of motion and strength. However, none of these appear be clinically relevant and they gradually disappear with time.

3.7.1 Hamstrings Autograft

We harvest both ST and G. The tendons are approached through a small 3 cm incision approximately 2 cm distal and medial to the tibial tubercle (Fig. 3.42) [180]. The same incision is also used to drill the tibial tunnel. In thin patients, the tendons and their distal insertion can be palpated. If this is difficult, one should remember that the upper border of the gracilis is located approximately 5.5 cm below the anteromedial joint line [181]. The aim is to center the incision over the pes anserine and extend in medially and proximally. The oblique orientation allows better access along the length of the tendons and protects the superficial branches of the saphenous nerve by lying parallel to their course. The subcutaneous tissue is dissected and nerve branches are respected if possible. These sensory terminals have a variable location but their trajectory in this area is 45° oblique [182]. Transection of these fibers leads to a sensory loss on the lateral aspect of the thigh, mainly distal to the incision which gradually attenuates over time.

The entire hamstrings harvest is performed with the knee in 90° of flexion. This position sets the tendons in a straight line from their insertion to the muscle body and origin on the ischial tuberosity. Thus it facilitates tendon mobilization, passage of the stripper and may reduce the risk of injury to the saphenous nerve as it crosses the gracilis tendon. The investigating fascia is incised parallel to the superior border of the gracilis tendon to avoid inadvertently cutting them. The tendon insertion can be palpated through the investigating fascia. A small curved overholt forceps is then used to hook the tendons one at a time. The gracilis lies superior (more proximal) and the ST is just below. The gracilis and ST fuse an average of 3 cm from their insertion. Therefore, if identification is difficult the tendons should be explored more proximally from the insertion since here they are better defined as separate structures. A loop of No. 2 non absorbable braided suture is passed over each tendon. These traction sutures are used to mobilize the tendons anteriorly during harvesting. A langenbeck retractor is placed medially to allow deeper visualization. Comfortable access to the tendons is important since these are firmly adherent to the sartorius and have tendon slips that insert separately into the tibia or the crural fascia [180, 181]. By pulling out on the tendons, the accessory insertions are better visualized and palpated with the index finger. We perform progressive release with curved scissors and the tip pointing medially to prevent accidentally transecting the tendons. The ST has a main accessory insertion to the medial gastrocnemius (77 %) which should be searched for and cut [180]. Failure to adequately release these structures could result in cutting the tendons too short.

After the tendons have been freed from accessory slips the surgeon should be able to significantly and easily mobilize them anteriorly through the incision. Also, they should incompletely retract from this point on. Our standard procedures are performed under spinal or epidural anesthesia. We have sometimes observed incomplete relaxation of the ST and gracilis muscles. We also routinely use a closed stripper which requires dethatching the tendons from their insertion prior to harvesting (Fig. 3.42). With incomplete muscle relaxation, if the tendons are slipped they can retract deep into the posterior compartment and become very difficult if not impossible to find. Therefore, if significant elastic resistance is encountered during harvesting, careful dethatching and handling or the use of an open stripper is advised. An open stripper is more prone to produce short grafts. Closable open strippers ale available but they tend to be rather thick and bulky. The two tendons are separated as distally as possible by pulling apart on the traction sutures (Fig. 3.43). This maximizes the usable length of the tendons and prevents accidentally cutting both tendons at once. One at a time the tendons are freed from the tibia with a scalpel while holding them in tension by pulling on the sutures. The free end of the leading sutures is passed through the closed stripper and grasped with an arthroscopy forceps. The tendon is pulled through the stripper, held between the index and the thumb with a surgical gauze pad for better grip. The stripper is pushed deeper towards the ischial tuberosity while the tendon is held tensioned. We harvest the gracilis first and the ST second. When it passes beneath the semimembranosus the ST is isolated by a deep fascia sling which opposes resistance during harvesting [183].

The tendons are prepared on the back table by an assistant, while the surgeon deals with tunnel placement and associated lesions. The average usable lengths of the ST and the gracilis tendons are considered to be 23.5 and 20 cm respectively. All muscle is removed from the tendons. For SB reconstruction, the grafts are doubled and sized in four strands and 0.5 increments. The best 20 cm are chosen and the rest is discarded. The grafts are placed under tension one on top of the other on the preparation station. Absorbable No. 1 braided leading sutures are attached at each end, approximately 4 rows in a continuous or Krackow fashion. The appropriately sized cortical button fixation is opened and the graft passed through the loop. The graft is then pretensioned, a mark is made to the level of the expected femoral tunnel length and supplemental sutures can be placed on the tibial free ends (Fig. 3.44). If the diameter is less than 7 mm or the patient is heavy with large notch and native footprints and the tendons are of sufficient length, a six strand neoligament is prepared (Fig. 3.45). We feel comfortable if a minimum of 8 cm long final graft is obtained, from 24 cm tendons. If the gracilis is too short it can be double looped and only the ST placed in three strands. When a five or six configuration is chosen, the proximal end of the tendon is first sutured to the button loop using No. 2 nonabsorbable sutures. The tendons are then passed through the loop and preparation is continued in the same fashion as described above. Doubling and tripling the ST and G (four/six strands) leads to a graft that has a greater diameter than the 10 mm wide BPTB [184]. For DB reconstruction, 19 and 17 cm long tendons from the ST and gracilis are prepared as looped to obtain double strand AM and PL bundles respectively (Fig. 3.46).

The ST and G tendon have been shown to regenerate. However, the new tendons originate within the appropriate muscles but have a more proximal insertion, near the semimembranosus, as well as altered histological composition, with regions that resemble scar tissue. They are thus deemed inappropriate for tendon reharvest and do not compensate the deep flexion and internal tibia rotation strength deficit [185].

The most common complication associate with hamstrings harvest is cutting the tendons to short. Many factors contribute, out of which inappropriate release of accessory insertions is the most important. Donor site morbidity is uncommon and manifests as postero-medial thigh pain and antero-lateral knee anesthesia. The authors have had one case of extensive postoperative hematoma (Fig. 3.45)

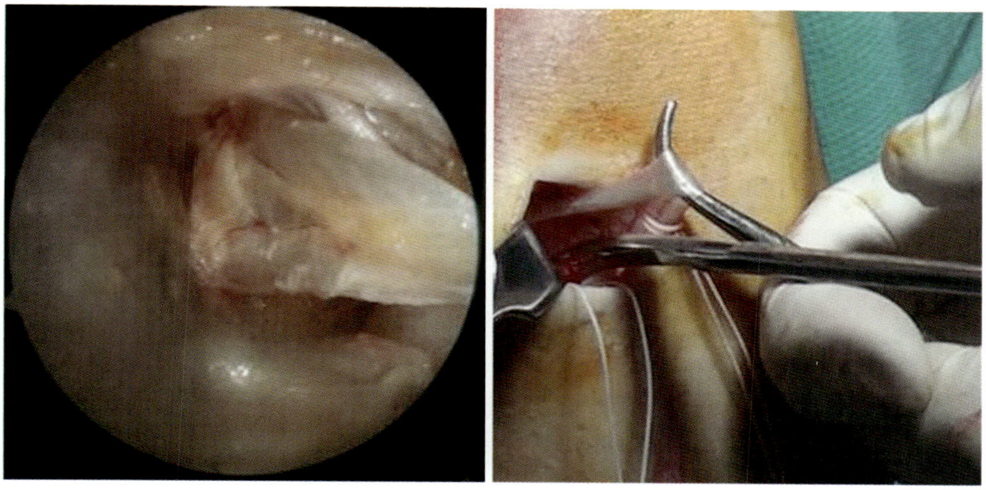

Fig. 3.42 Tendon slips insert separately into the tibia or the crural fascia. The ST has a main accessory insertion to the medial gastrocnemius which should be always identified and cut. By pulling out on the tendons, the accessory insertions are better visualized. We perform progressive release with curved scissors and the tip pointing medially to prevent accidentally transecting the tendons

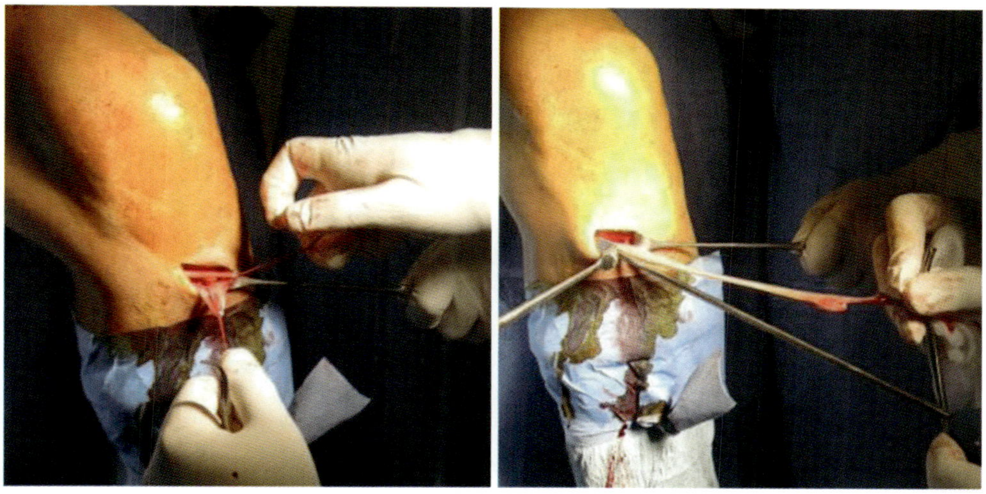

Fig. 3.43 A loop of No. 2 non absorbable braided suture is passed over each tendon. These traction sutures are used to mobilize the tendons anteriorly during harvesting. The two tendons are separated as distally as possible by pulling apart on the traction sutures. A langenbeck retractor is placed medially to allow deeper visualization

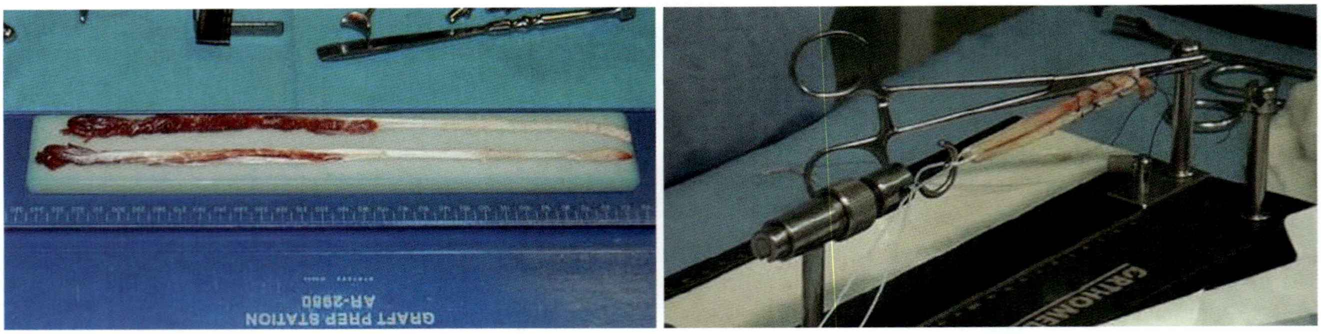

Fig. 3.44 All muscle is removed from the tendons. The graft is pretensioned on the preparation station

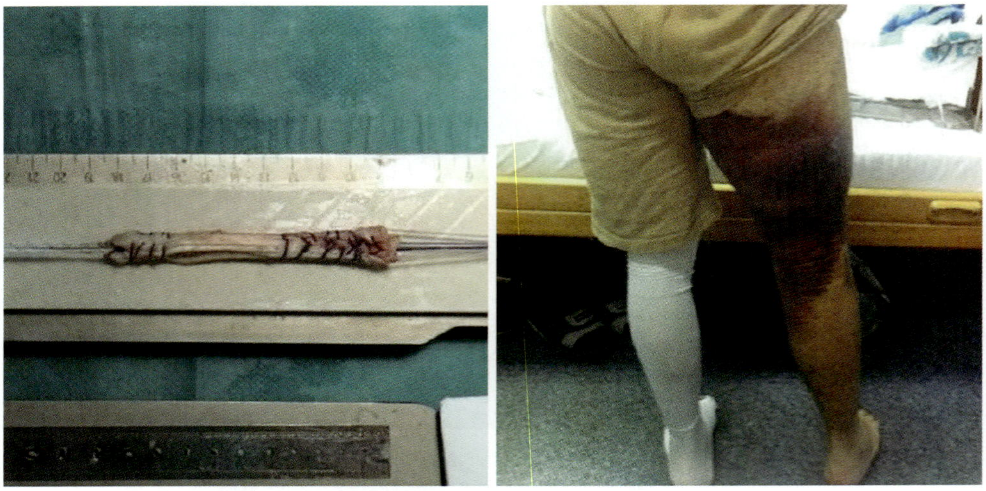

Fig. 3.45 A six strand 9/95 mm hamstrings graft over ToggleLock. Extensive postoperative hematoma after hamstrings harvest

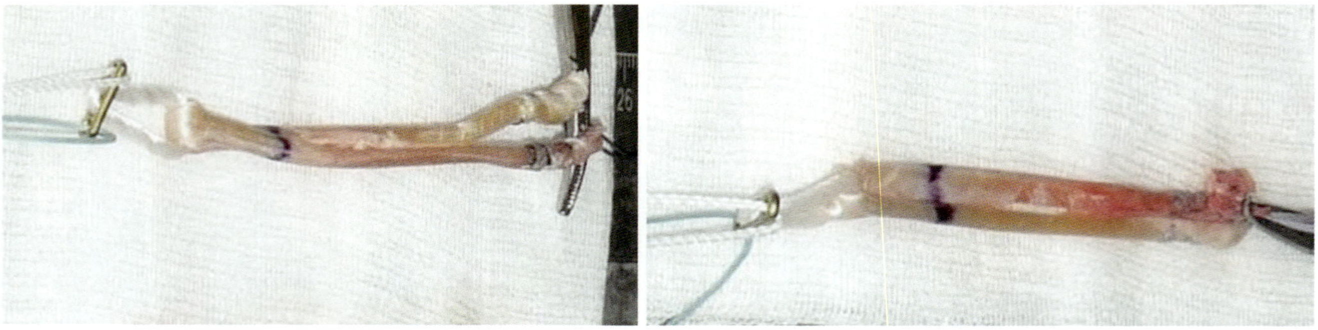

Fig. 3.46 AM (double strand ST) and PL (double strand gracilis) bundles over EndoButtons for DB reconstruction

3.7.2 Bone-Patellar Tendon-Bone

The ipsilateral middle third BPTB autograft has been the benchmark to compare all other choices. A vertical incision in made over the central part of the tendon, spanning from the inferior pole of the patella to the tibial tuberosity. A separate small (1 cm) incision is made for the tibial tunnel, anterior to the medial collateral ligament (MCL) border. Alternatively, the same incision can be made on the medial border of the patellar tendon to provide access for tibial tunnel placement. The subcutaneous tissue is dissected and if possible, the infrapatellar branches of the saphenous nerve are protected. These are usually two (60 %) oriented horizontally with high variability. The distance from the inferior pole of the patella to the most proximal branch and from the tibial tubercle to the most distal branch is approximately 3 cm [186].

The peritendon is incised longitudinally and a 1 cm wide section from the middle third of the patellar tendon is isolated with a scalpel or scissors on its entire length, in line with the fibers (Fig. 3.47). An oscillating saw is used to cut 1 cm wide and 2 cm long bone blocks at each end. A small drill or K wire can be used to mark the corners of the bone block on the patella. This prevents stress shielding and can reduce the already rare incidence of patellar fracture, associated with this graft harvest. Keeping the depth of the bone block to less than 1/3 of the thickness of the patella also reduces the likelihood of fracture. This can be achieved by using a depthmark of the oscillating blade. If a fracture does occur (very rare and unlikely situation), osteosynthesis is performed in a standard fashion using screws or K wires and cerclage wire. The direction of the cut with the oscillating saw is slightly angled so that it is not perpendicular to the anterior cortex but all three converge in depth. The final bone block is lifted with a small chisel. Keeping the knee flexed during patellar procedures puts the extensor mechanism under tension and helps stabilize the patella during harvesting. The same is then performed on the tibial tuberosity. The peritendon is closed with No. 2/0 absorbable sutures.

The graft is then transferred to the back table for final adjustments. The periosteum is removed from the anterior cortex of the patellar block. Any other soft tissue is also debrided using a small rongeur. The bone plugs are shaped circular to fit the bone tunnels. This usually requires downsizing to 9 mm in diameter by removing excess bone from the lateral margins of the bone plugs cortex. Care should be taken not to fracture them. A hole is drilled in the middle of both bone plugs, perpendicular to the cortex, using a small K wire (1.5 mm). No. 2 nonabsorbable braided traction sutures are passes through (Fig. 3.47) and the graft is finally sized. The graft is then pulled through the tibial and femoral tunnels, usually with the patellar end first. The graft can also be twisted 90° before the tibial fixation so that the fibers orientation will closer resemble the double bundle configuration. The cancellous side of the bone plug is introduced so that is facing superior and anterior, in order to accommodate the interference screw (Fig. 3.47). The entire bone plug must introduced in the femoral tunnel. Interference screw fixation on both the femur and the tibia (see Sect. 3.6.1) is the most widely used anchorage system for BPTB grafts. Tensioning of the graft for tibial fixation is performed in the same manner as for hamstrings (see Sect. 3.5.2.1). The inrtaarticular tendon is integrated through the ligamentization process (see Sect. 3.4). The bone plugs consolidate within the tunnels, as opposed to the Sharpey fibers connection of the soft tissue grafts.

Harvesting the central third of the patellar tendon has been significantly associated with anterior knee pain especially during kneeling. The symptoms fade over time but can be clinically present for up to 2 years. The pathophysiology of the phenomenon is not entirely understood. Scaring of the tendon, infrapatellar fat pad and surrounding tissues probably have an important role. A MRI study showed that the size of the donor site gap decreases for up to 6 years, while the thickness and the width of the tendon are increased up to 2 years. Reharvesting of the patellar tendon is therefore not recommended [187]. An alternative to the central strip is the use on the medial third of the patellar tendon. Small patellar tracking changes (mainly lateral displacement) are noted with this technique but have not proved clinically significant [188].

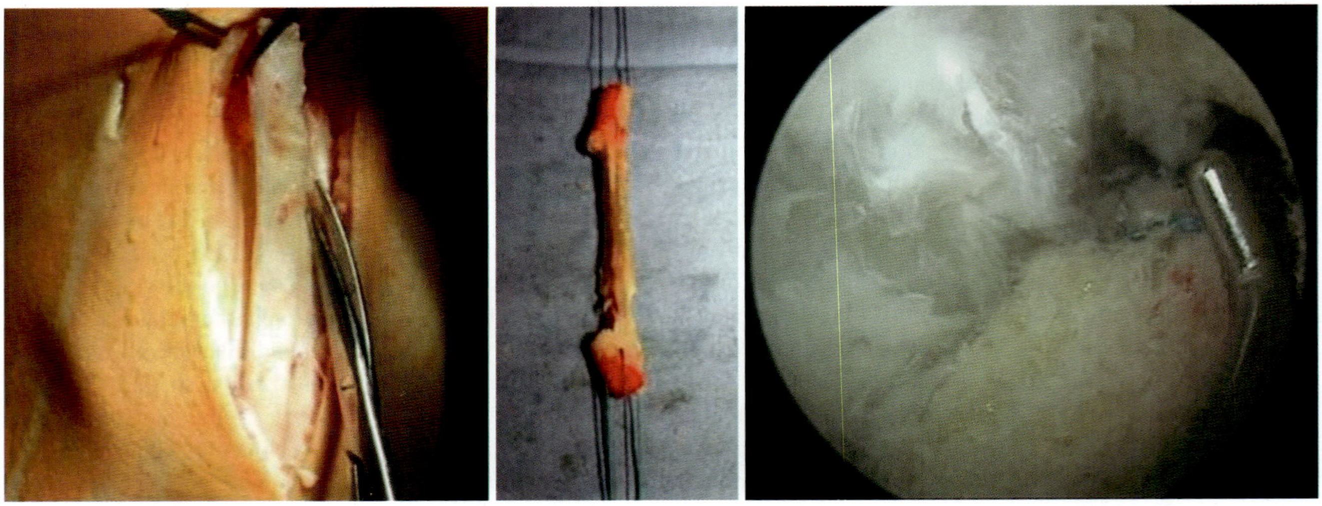

Fig. 3.47 A vertical incision in made over the central part of the tendon, spanning from the inferior pole of the patella to the tibial tuberosity. A 1 cm wide section from the middle third of the patellar tendon is isolated on its entire length, in line with the fibers. An oscillating saw is used to cut 1 cm wide and 2 cm long bone blocks at each end. Final graft prepared with traction sutures in place. The cancellous side of the bone plug is introduced so that is facing superior and anterior, in order to accommodate the interference screw

3.7.3 Quadriceps Tendon

The central portion of the quadriceps tendon (QTB) is an autograft choice that gained popularity over the last years. Harvesting is easier than for hamstrings with fewer complications. A minimum of four stand ST and gracilis, the central portions of the patellar tendon and the middle strip of the quadriceps all provide grafts with tensile strength higher than the native ACL [189–189]. The versatility and reliability of the has also been proved in vivo. Compared to the BPTB, it offered similar stability with less kneeling pain, donor site morbidity and sensory [192].

A longitudinal incision is centered over the middle portion of the quadriceps tendon, starting at the superior border of the patella and continued proximally. The subcutaneous tissue is dissected and the tendon exposed. A 10 mm wide strip from the middle portion is isolated with a scalpel and continued proximally until the muscle attachment, in line with the fibers. Close to the patella, the dissection should be kept shallow to the deep layers, to prevent articular penetration. The deep layer that covers the articular capsule can be bluntly dissected from the graft (Fig. 3.48). With experience, a shorter incision can be made above the patella, the dissection continued blindly proximal and the end cut made through a separate transversal stab incision. The quadriceps graft can also be harvested without the bone block but there is some concern regarding adequate length. Furthermore, there is no apparent advantage not to harvest with the bone plug. A 2 cm long and 1 cm wide bone block is dethatched from the proximal border of the patella in the same way as for BPTB tendon (described above). In this area, the patellar bone is denser and the patella wider which reduces the risk of fracture. The mid tendon defect is repaired with No. 2 absorbable suture.

The bone block is prepared in the same way as for BPTB, described above (Fig. 3.48). The bone plug is usually prepared to be completely introduced into a 9 mm diameter femoral tunnel. A No. 2 traction suture is used to pull the graft through the tunnels. On the tibial end of the graft, 4 rows of Krackow sutures are placed using No. 2 sutures, that will be used to maintain adequate tensioning during fixation. Interference screw fixation is the system of choice for both sides. The diameters are downsized for the femur and one or two sizes larder on the tibia, depending on bone quality and tunnel/graft size mismatch. Although rare, any excess tendon is cut flush to the tibial cortex. The postoperative regimen is similar to that used for BPTB.

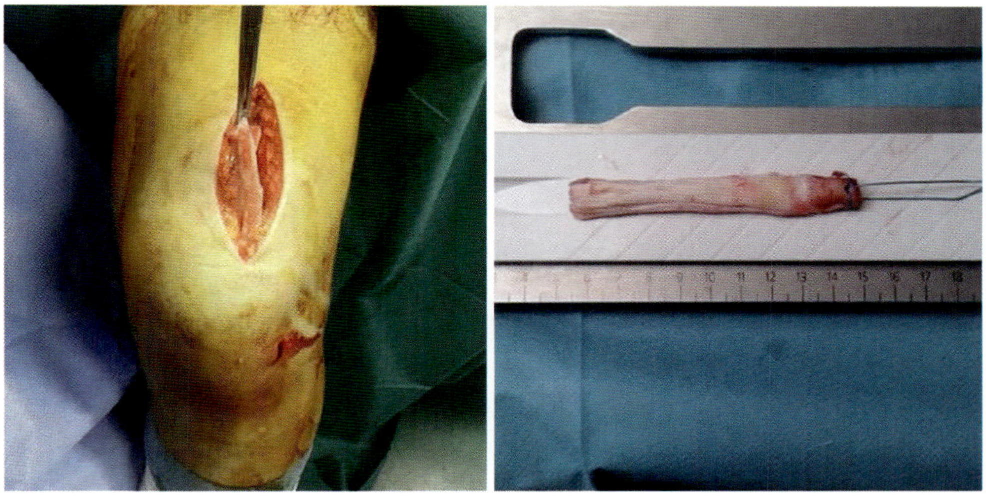

Fig. 3.48 A longitudinal incision is centered over the middle portion of the quadriceps tendon, starting at the superior border of the patella and continued proximally. A 10 mm wide strip from the middle portion is isolated with a scalpel and continued proximally until the muscle attachment, in line with the fibers. The bone block is prepared to be completely introduced into a 9 mm diameter femoral tunnel

3.7.4 Allografts

Allografts may face bioethical and legal concerns but they effectively eliminate donor site morbidity of graft harvest. Even though more expensive than autografts, their use has gained popularity, especially in the USA. In the past, allografts have been associated with an increased incidence of bone tunnel widening and a very small potential risk of viral disease transmission.

A variety of allograft tendons are available. The most commonly used in ACL reconstruction are bone patellar tendon bone, Achilles tendon with bone plug and tibialis anterior tendon. After harvesting from the donors, they are intensely and variably processed to achieve sterilization and preservation. The more aggressive this preparation is, the weaker the graft becomes. In addition, compared to BPTB and hamstrings autografts, allograft use leads to higher postoperative anterior tibial translation. Even though most are in the normal range, there is a three times higher rate for knees with abnormal stability, which is usually an expression of failure [193].

Just as well as chemical processing, high dose radiation has proved to significantly alter the mechanical strength. Even with the use of crio and radiation protective agents, new methods are needed to provide sterility and preserve resistance. Replacing gamma with electron beam radiation, using doses lower than 2.5 Mrad on fresh frozen might offer better clinical results [194–196]. It is therefore important to always use allografts in lieu of their processing method, donor age, shelf life and source of origin to guarantee predictable and safe results.

3.7.5 Artificial Grafts

Synthetic grafts were initially very popular due to lack of harvest site morbidity, graft strength and early start of rehabilitation and return to sports. However a high rate of complications soon emerged. These grafts underwent partial or total degradation due to mechanical abrasion against the notch walls which led to massive foreign-body synovitis. Furthermore, the artificial scaffolds did not function as inductive scaffolds for cell proliferation, collagen fiber apposition and biological integration.

Currently, the third generation Ligament Augmentation and Reconstruction System (LARS) is the most commonly used artificial graft. Animal models have showed less tissue ingrowth compared to autografts and important mechanical abrasion but with a very low tendency for synovitis [197]. It appears to be a viable short and midterm solution with good biological tolerance [198].

3.7.6 Infections

Anterior cruciate ligament reconstructions have very low infection rates, between 0.48 and 0.6 %. Approximately half are superficial, at the hamstrings harvest / tibial tunnel incision. Most occur between 2 and 3 weeks postoperatively. The most common pathogens are coagulase-negative staphylococci and staphylococcus aureus. The later are more aggressive, can lead to graft removal and loss of flexion and required more days of antibiotherapy [199, 200]. Fungal infections are also encountered and more difficult to diagnose (Fig. 3.49).

Hamstring tendon autografts have a higher incidence of infection (1.44 %) than BPTB autografts or allografts and show a trend toward more common need for graft removal due to deep infections (8 times higher) [199, 201]. The prevalence of septic arthritis might also be higher in professional athletes [202].

Early arthroscopic irrigation and debridement is the treatment of choice. Coupled with intravenous antibiotics, this management usually allows for graft retention. The most important decisional moment for graft removal is done during arthroscopic exploration, for a reported incidence of 14 %. A stable neoligament without deep necrosis can be meticulously debrided and left in place. The arthroscopic irrigation and debridement is usually performed once or twice (repeat after a few days) [203].

Dropping or contaminating the autograft during reconstruction is reported to happen in high volume centers. Most authors would clean the graft and continue with implantation. There has not been yet reported even a single case of septic arthritis after such practice. Solutions of chlorhexidine, antibiotics, povidoneiodine or combinations can be used for graft decontamination [204, 205].

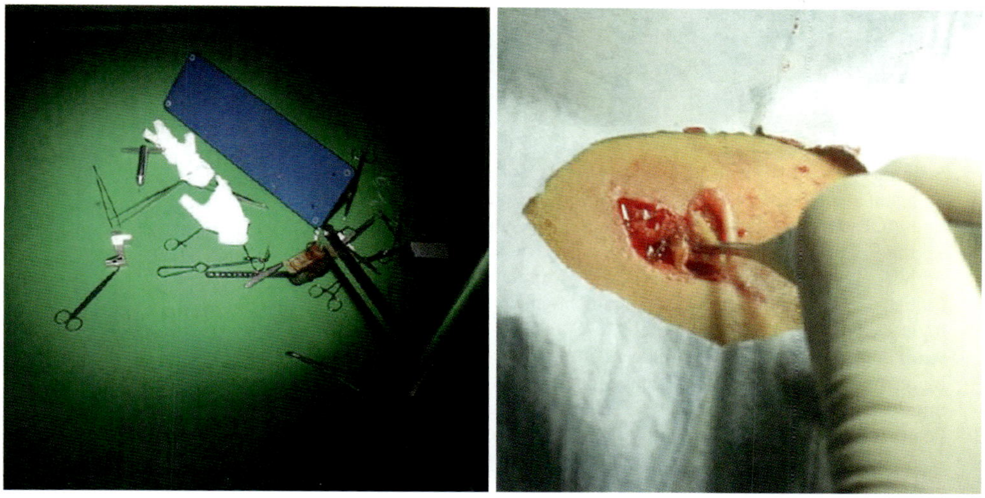

Fig. 3.49 Overthrown back table with the autograft. Surgical site infection at the hamstrings harvest/tibial tunnel incision which required debridement and led to premature (6 weeks) interference screw removal

References

1. Granan LP, Forssblad M, Lind M, Engebretsen L. The Scandinavian ACL registries 2004–2007: baseline epidemiology. Acta Orthop. 2009;80(5):563–7.
2. Ahldén M, Samuelsson K, Sernert N, Forssblad M, Karlsson J, Kartus J. The Swedish National Anterior Cruciate Ligament Register: a report on baseline variables and outcomes of surgery for almost 18,000 patients. Am J Sports Med. 2012;40(10):2230–5.
3. Nordenvall R, Bahmanyar S, Adami J, Stenros C, Wredmark T, Felländer-Tsai L. A population-based nationwide study of cruciate ligament injury in Sweden, 2001–2009: incidence, treatment, and sex differences. Am J Sports Med. 2012;40(8):1808–13.
4. Magnussen RA, Granan LP, Dunn WR, Amendola A, Andrish JT, Brophy R, Carey JL, Flanigan D, Huston LJ, Jones M, Kaeding CC, McCarty EC, Marx RG, Matava MJ, Parker RD, Vidal A, Wolcott M, Wolf BR, Wright RW, Spindler KP, Engebretsen L. Cross-cultural comparison of patients undergoing ACL reconstruction in the United States and Norway. Knee Surg Sports Traumatol Arthrosc. 2010;18(1):98–105.
5. Maletis GB, Granan LP, Inacio MC, Funahashi TT, Engebretsen L. Comparison of community-based ACL reconstruction registries in the U.S. and Norway. J Bone Joint Surg Am. 2011;93 Suppl 3:31–6.
6. Prodromos CC, Han Y, Rogowski J, Joyce B, Shi K. A meta-analysis of the incidence of anterior cruciate ligament tears as a function of gender, sport, and a knee injury-reduction regimen. Arthroscopy. 2007;23(12):1320–5.e6.
7. Schindler OS. Historical aspects on surgery for anterior cruciate ligament deficiency. In: Sanchis-Alfonso V, Monllau JC, editors. The ACL-deficient knee. A problem solving approach. London: Springer; 2013.
8. Ferretti M, Levicoff EA, Macpherson TA, Moreland MS, Cohen M, Fu FH. The fetal anterior cruciate ligament: an anatomic and histologic study. Arthroscopy. 2007;23(3):278–83.
9. Amis AA, Dawkins GP. Functional anatomy of the anterior cruciate ligament. Fibre bundle actions related to ligament replacements and injuries. J Bone Joint Surg Br. 1991;73(2):260–7.
10. Petersen W, Zantop T. Anatomy of the anterior cruciate ligament with regard to its two bundles. Clin Orthop Relat Res. 2007;454:35–47.
11. Zantop T, Herbort M, Raschke MJ, Fu FH, Petersen W. The role of the anteromedial and posterolateral bundles of the anterior cruciate ligament in anterior tibial translation and internal rotation. Am J Sports Med. 2007;35(2):223–7.
12. Claes S, Vereecke E, Maes M, Victor J, Verdonk P, Bellemans J. Anatomy of the anterolateral ligament of the knee. J Anat. 2013; 223(4):321–8.
13. Ferretti M, Ekdahl M, Shen W, Fu FH. Osseous landmarks of the femoral attachment of the anterior cruciate ligament: an anatomic study. Arthroscopy. 2007;23(11):1218–25.
14. Kopf S, Pombo MW, Szczodry M, Irrgang JJ, Fu FH. Size variability of the human anterior cruciate ligament insertion sites. Am J Sports Med. 2011;39(1):108–13.
15. Edwards A, Bull AM, Amis AA. The attachments of the anteromedial and posterolateral fibre bundles of the anterior cruciate ligament. Part 2: femoral attachment. Knee Surg Sports Traumatol Arthrosc. 2008;16(1):29–36.
16. Edwards A, Bull AM, Amis AA. The attachments of the anteromedial and posterolateral fibre bundles of the anterior cruciate ligament: Part 1: tibial attachment. Knee Surg Sports Traumatol Arthrosc. 2007;15(12):1414–21.
17. Odensten M, Gillquist J. Functional anatomy of the anterior cruciate ligament and a rationale for reconstruction. J Bone Joint Surg Am. 1985;67(2):257–62.
18. Amis AA. The functions of the fibre bundles of the anterior cruciate ligament in anterior drawer, rotational laxity and the pivot shift. Knee Surg Sports Traumatol Arthrosc. 2012;20(4):613–20.
19. Petersen W, Tillmann B. Structure and vascularization of the cruciate ligaments of the human knee joint. Anat Embryol (Berl). 1999;200(3):325–34.
20. Arnoczky SP. Anatomy of the anterior cruciate ligament. Clin Orthop Relat Res. 1983;(172):19–25.
21. DeMorat G, Weinhold P, Blackburn T, Chudik S, Garrett W. Aggressive quadriceps loading can induce noncontact anterior cruciate ligament injury. Am J Sports Med. 2004;32(2):477–83.
22. Myers CA, Torry MR, Shelburne KB, Giphart JE, LaPrade RF, Woo SL, Steadman JR. In vivo tibiofemoral kinematics during 4 functional tasks of increasing demand using biplane fluoroscopy. Am J Sports Med. 2012;40(1):170–8.
23. Markolf KL, Burchfield DM, Shapiro MM, Shepard MF, Finerman GA, Slauterbeck JL. Combined knee loading states that generate high anterior cruciate ligament forces. J Orthop Res. 1995;13(6):930–5.
24. Quatman CE, Kiapour AM, Demetropoulos CK, Kiapour A, Wordeman SC, Levine JW, Goel VK, Hewett TE. Preferential loading of the ACL compared with the MCL during landing: a novel in sim approach yields the multiplanar mechanism of dynamic valgus during ACL injuries. Am J Sports Med. 2014;42(1):177–86.
25. Oh YK, Lipps DB, Ashton-Miller JA, Wojtys EM. What strains the anterior cruciate ligament during a pivot landing? Am J Sports Med. 2012;40(3):574–83.
26. Wall SJ, Rose DM, Sutter EG, Belkoff SM, Boden BP. The role of axial compressive and quadriceps forces in noncontact anterior cruciate ligament injury: a cadaveric study. Am J Sports Med. 2012;40(3):568–73.
27. Meyer EG, Haut RC. Anterior cruciate ligament injury induced by internal tibial torsion or tibiofemoral compression. J Biomech. 2008;41(16):3377–83.
28. Olsen OE, Myklebust G, Engebretsen L, Bahr R. Injury mechanisms for anterior cruciate ligament injuries in team handball: a systematic video analysis. Am J Sports Med. 2004;32(4):1002–12.
29. Nagano Y, Ida H, Akai M, Fukubayashi T. Gender differences in knee kinematics and muscle activity during single limb drop landing. Knee. 2007;14(3):218–23.
30. Lipps DB, Oh YK, Ashton-Miller JA, Wojtys EM. Morphologic characteristics help explain the gender difference in peak anterior cruciate ligament strain during a simulated pivot landing. Am J Sports Med. 2012;40(1):32–40.
31. Wordeman SC, Quatman CE, Kaeding CC, Hewett TE. In vivo evidence for tibial plateau slope as a risk factor for anterior cruciate ligament injury: a systematic review and meta-analysis. Am J Sports Med. 2012;40(7):1673–81.
32. Levine JW, Kiapour AM, Quatman CE, Wordeman SC, Goel VK, Hewett TE, Demetropoulos CK. Clinically relevant injury patterns after an anterior cruciate ligament injury provide insight into injury mechanisms. Am J Sports Med. 2013;41(2):385–95.
33. Zantop T, Brucker PU, Vidal A, Zelle BA, Fu FH. Intraarticular rupture pattern of the ACL. Clin Orthop Relat Res. 2007;454:48–53.
34. Griffin LY, Kercher J. Risk and gender factors for noncontact anterior cruciate ligament injury. In: Prodromos CC, editor. The anterior cruciate ligament reconstruction, Expert Consult series. Saunders; 2008
35. Maffulli N, Binfield PM, King JB, Good CJ. Acute haemarthrosis of the knee in athletes. A prospective study of 106 cases. J Bone Joint Surg Br. 1993;75(6):945–9.
36. Kim SJ, Kim HK. Reliability of the anterior drawer test, the pivot shift test, and the Lachman test. Clin Orthop Relat Res. 1995;317:237–42.

37. Ahn JH, Bae TS, Kang KS, Kang SY, Lee SH. Longitudinal tear of the medial meniscus posterior horn in the anterior cruciate ligament-deficient knee significantly influences anterior stability. Am J Sports Med. 2011;39(10):2187–93.
38. Rangger C, Daniel DM, Stone ML, Kaufman K. Diagnosis of an ACL disruption with KT-1000 arthrometer measurements. Knee Surg Sports Traumatol Arthrosc. 1993;1(1):60–6.
39. Prodromos CC. Diagnosis of anterior cruciate ligament tear. In: Prodromos CC, editor. The anterior cruciate ligament reconstruction, Expert Consult series. Saunders; 2008.
40. Jakob RP, Stäubli HU, Deland JT. Grading the pivot shift. Objective tests with implications for treatment. J Bone Joint Surg Br. 1987;69:294–9.
41. Jonsson H, Riklund-Ahlström K, Lind J. Positive pivot shift after ACL reconstruction predicts later osteoarthrosis: 63 patients followed 5–9 years after surgery. Acta Orthop Scand. 2004;75(5):594–9.
42. Ayeni OR, Chahal M, Tran MN, Sprague S. Pivot shift as an outcome measure for ACL reconstruction: a systematic review. Knee Surg Sports Traumatol Arthrosc. 2012;20(4):767–77.
43. Kuroda R, Hoshino Y, Araki D, Nishizawa Y, Nagamune K, Matsumoto T, Kubo S, Matsushita T, Kurosaka M. Quantitative measurement of the pivot shift, reliability, and clinical applications. Knee Surg Sports Traumatol Arthrosc. 2012;20(4):686–91.
44. Patel SA, Hageman J, Quatman CE, Wordeman SC, Hewett TE. Prevalence and location of bone bruises associated with anterior cruciate ligament injury and implications for mechanism of injury: a systematic review. Sports Med. 2014;44(2):281–93.
45. Shelbourne KD, Wilckens JH, Mollabashy A, DeCarlo M. Arthrofibrosis in acute anterior cruciate ligament reconstruction. The effect of timing of reconstruction and rehabilitation. Am J Sports Med. 1991;19(4):332–6.
46. Marcacci M, Zaffagnini S, Iacono F, Neri MP, Petitto A. Early versus late reconstruction for anterior cruciate ligament rupture. Results after five years of follow-up. Am J Sports Med. 1995;23(6):690–3.
47. Laxdal G, Kartus J, Ejerhed L, Sernert N, Magnusson L, Faxén E, Karlsson J. Outcome and risk factors after anterior cruciate ligament reconstruction: a follow-up study of 948 patients. Arthroscopy. 2005;21(8):958–64.
48. Noyes FR, Barber SD, Mooar LA. A rationale for assessing sports activity levels and limitations in knee disorders. Clin Orthop. 1989;246:238–49.
49. Lohmander LS, Englund PM, Dahl LL, Roos EM. The long-term consequence of anterior cruciate ligament and meniscus injuries: osteoarthritis. Am J Sports Med. 2007;35(10):1756–69.
50. Kessler MA, Behrend H, Henz S, Stutz G, Rukavina A, Kuster MS. Function, osteoarthritis and activity after ACL-rupture: 11 years follow-up results of conservative versus reconstructive treatment. Knee Surg Sports Traumatol Arthrosc. 2008;16(5):442–8.
51. Marcacci M, Zaffagnini S, Giordano G, Iacono F, Presti ML. Anterior cruciate ligament reconstruction associated with extra-articular tenodesis: a prospective clinical and radiographic evaluation with 10- to 13-year follow-up. Am J Sports Med. 2009;37(4):707–14.
52. Li RT, Lorenz S, Xu Y, Harner CD, Fu FH, Irrgang JJ. Predictors of radiographic knee osteoarthritis after anterior cruciate ligament reconstruction. Am J Sports Med. 2011;39(12):2595–603.
53. Spindler KP, Huston LJ, Wright RW, Kaeding CC, Marx RG, Amendola A, Parker RD, Andrish JT, Reinke EK, Harrell FE Jr; MOON Group, Dunn WR. The prognosis and predictors of sports function and activity at minimum 6 years after anterior cruciate ligament reconstruction: a population cohort study. Am J Sports Med. 2011;39(2):348–59.
54. Barenius B, Ponzer S, Shalabi A, Bujak R, Norlén L, Eriksson K. Increased risk of osteoarthritis after anterior cruciate ligament reconstruction: a 14-year follow-up study of a randomized controlled trial. Am J Sports Med. 2014;18.
55. Desai N, Björnsson H, Samuelsson K, Karlsson J, Forssblad M. Outcomes after ACL reconstruction with focus on older patients: results from The Swedish National Anterior Cruciate Ligament Register. Knee Surg Sports Traumatol Arthrosc. 2014;22(2):379–86.
56. Chalmers PN, Mall NA, Moric M, Sherman SL, Paletta GP, Cole BJ, Bach Jr BR. Does ACL reconstruction alter natural history?: a systematic literature review of long-term outcomes. J Bone Joint Surg Am. 2014;96(4):292–300.
57. Hefti F, Muller W, Jakob RP, Staubli HU. Evaluation of knee ligament injuries with the IKDC form. Knee Surg Sports Traumatol Arthrosc. 1993;1(3–4):226–34.
58. Kocher MS, Saxon HS, et al. Management and complications of anterior cruciate ligament injuries in skeletally immature patients: survey of the Herodicus Society and The ACL Study Group. J Pediatr Orthop. 2002;22(4):452–7.
59. Lawrence JT, Argawal N, et al. Degeneration of the knee joint in skeletally immature patients with a diagnosis of an anterior cruciate ligament tear: is there harm in delay of treatment? Am J Sports Med. 2011;39(12):2582–7.
60. Dumont GD, Hogue GD, et al. Meniscal and chondral injuries associated with pediatric anterior cruciate ligament tears: relationship of treatment time and patient-specific factors. Am J Sports Med. 2012;40(9):2128–33.
61. Gebhard F, Ellermann A, et al. Multicenter-study of operative treatment of intraligamentous tears of the anterior cruciate ligament in children and adolescents: comparison of four different techniques. Knee Surg Sports Traumatol Arthrosc. 2006; 14(9):797–803.
62. Vavken P, Murray MM. Treating anterior cruciate ligament tears in skeletally immature patients. Arthroscopy. 2011;27(5):704–16.
63. Moksnes H, Engebretsen L, et al. The current evidence for treatment of ACL injuries in children is low: a systematic review. J Bone Joint Surg Am. 2012;94(12):1112–9.
64. Hărăguş H, Prejbeanu R, Vermeşan D, Damian G, Vermeşan S. Pediatric ACL reconstructions using transphyseal hamstrings. J Pediatr. 2012;XV(59–60):37–41. ISSN 2065-4855.
65. Courvoisier A, Grimaldi M, et al. Good surgical outcome of transphyseal ACL reconstruction in skeletally immaturepatients using four-strand hamstring graft. Knee Surg Sports Traumatol Arthrosc. 2011;19(4):588–91.
66. McIntosh AL, Dahm DL, et al. Anterior cruciate ligament reconstruction in the skeletally immature patient. Arthroscopy. 2006;22(12):1325–30.
67. Streich NA, Barié A, et al. Transphyseal reconstruction of the anterior cruciate ligament in prepubescent athletes. Knee Surg Sports Traumatol Arthrosc. 2010;18(11):1481–6.
68. Redler LH, Brafman RT, et al. Anterior cruciate ligament reconstruction in skeletally immature patients with transphyseal tunnels. Arthroscopy. 2012;28(11):1710–7.
69. Shea KG, Apel PJ, et al. The anatomy of the proximal tibia in pediatric and adolescent patients: implications for ACL reconstruction and prevention of physeal arrest. Knee Surg Sports Traumatol Arthrosc. 2007;15(4):320–7.
70. Shea KG, Belzer J, et al. Volumetric injury of the physis during single-bundle anterior cruciate ligament reconstruction in children: a 3-dimensional study using magnetic resonance imaging. Arthroscopy. 2009;25(12):1415–22.
71. Xerogeanes JW, Hammond KE, et al. Anatomic landmarks utilized for physeal-sparing, anatomic anterior cruciate ligament reconstruction: an MRI-based study. J Bone Joint Surg Am. 2012;94(3):268–76.

72. Nwachukwu BU, McFeely ED, et al. Arthrofibrosis after anterior cruciate ligament reconstruction in children and adolescents. J Pediatr Orthop. 2011;31(8):811–7.
73. Frosch KH, Stengel D, et al. Outcomes and risks of operative treatment of rupture of the anterior cruciate ligament in children and adolescents. Arthroscopy. 2010;26(11):1539–50.
74. Kaeding CC, Flanigan D, et al. Surgical techniques and outcomes after anterior cruciate ligament reconstruction in preadolescent patients. Arthroscopy. 2010;26(11):1530–8.
75. van Eck CF, Lesniak BP, Schreiber VM, Fu FH. Anatomic single- and double-bundle anterior cruciate ligament reconstruction flowchart. Arthroscopy. 2010;26(2):258–68.
76. Amiel D, Kleiner JB, Roux RD, Harwood FL, Akeson WH. The phenomenon of "ligamentization": anterior cruciate ligament reconstruction with autogenous patellar tendon. J Orthop Res. 1986;4(2):162–72.
77. Kleiner JB, Amiel D, Harwood FL, Akeson WH. Early histologic, metabolic, and vascular assessment of anterior cruciate ligament autografts. J Orthop Res. 1989;7(2):235–42.
78. Papalia R, Franceschi F, Vasta S, Di Martino A, Maffulli N, Denaro V. Sparing the anterior cruciate ligament remnant: is it worth the hassle? Br Med Bull. 2012;104:91–111.
79. Arnoczky SP, Tarvin GB, Marshall JL. Anterior cruciate ligament replacement using patellar tendon. An evaluation of graft revascularization in the dog. J Bone Joint Surg Am. 1982;64(2):217–24.
80. Johnson LL. The outcome of a free autogenous semitendinosus tendon graft in human anterior cruciate reconstructive surgery: a histological study. Arthroscopy. 1993;9(2):131–42.
81. Claes S, Verdonk P, Forsyth R, Bellemans J. The "ligamentization" process in anterior cruciate ligament reconstruction: what happens to the human graft? A systematic review of the literature. Am J Sports Med. 2011;39(11):2476–83.
82. Denti M, Monteleone M, Berardi A, Panni AS. Anterior cruciate ligament mechanoreceptors. Clin Orthop Relat Res. 1994;308:29–32.
83. Barrack RL, Lund PJ, Munn BG, Wink C, Happel L. Evidence of reinnervation of free patellar tendon autograft used for anterior cruciate ligament reconstruction. Am J Sports Med. 1997;25:196–202.
84. Georgoulis AD, Pappa L, Moebius U, Malamou-Mitsi V, Pappa S, Papageorgiou CO, Agnantis NJ, Soucacos PN. The presence of proprioceptive mechanoreceptors in the remnants of the ruptured ACL as a possible source of re-innervation of the ACL autograft. Knee Surg Sports Traumatol Arthrosc. 2001;9:364–8.
85. Dhillon MS, Bali K, Vasistha RK. Immunohistological evaluation of proprioceptive potential of the residual stump of injured anterior cruciate ligaments. Int Orthop. 2010;34:737–41.
86. Gohil S, Annear PO, Breidahl W. Anterior cruciate ligament reconstruction using autologous double hamstrings: a comparison of standard versus minimal debridement techniques using MRI to assess revascularisation. A randomised prospective study with a one-year follow-up. J Bone Joint Surg Br. 2007;89(9):1165–71.
87. Lee BI, Kwon SW, Kim JB, Choi HS, Min KD. Comparison of clinical results according to amount of preserved remnant in arthroscopic anterior cruciate ligament reconstruction using quadrupled hamstring graft. Arthroscopy. 2008;24(5):560–8.
88. Lee BI, Min KD, Choi HS, Kwon SW, Chun DI, Yun ES, Lee DW, Jin SY, Yoo JH. Immunohistochemical study of mechanoreceptors in the tibial remnant of the ruptured anterior cruciate ligament in human knees. Knee Surg Sports Traumatol Arthrosc. 2009;17:1095–101.
89. Bali K, Dhillon MS, Vasistha RK, Kakkar N, Chana R, Prabhakar S. Efficacy of immunohistological methods in detecting functionally viable mechanoreceptors in the remnant stumps of injured anterior cruciate ligaments and its clinical importance. Knee Surg Sports Traumatol Arthrosc. 2012;20:75–80.
90. Del Valle ME, Harwin SF, Maestro A, Murcia A, Vega JA. Immunohistochemical analysis of mechanoreceptors in the human posterior cruciate ligament: a demonstration of its proprioceptive role and clinical relevance. J Arthroplasty. 1998; 13:916–22.
91. Lee BI, Min KD, Choi HS, Kim JB, Kim ST. Arthroscopic anterior cruciate ligament reconstruction with the tibial-remnant preserving technique using a hamstring graft. Arthroscopy. 2006;22(3): 340.e1–7.
92. Löcherbach C, Zayni R, Chambat P, Sonnery-Cottet B. Biologically enhanced ACL reconstruction. Orthop Traumatol Surg Res. 2010;96(7):810–5.
93. Cha J, Choi SH, Kwon JW, Lee SH, Ahn JH. Analysis of cyclops lesions after different anterior cruciate ligament reconstructions: a comparison of the single-bundle and remnant bundle preservation techniques. Skeletal Radiol. 2012;41(8):997–1002.
94. Howell SM, Barad SJ. Knee extension and its relationship to the slope of the intercondylar roof. Implications for positioning the tibial tunnel in anterior cruciate ligament reconstructions. Am J Sports Med. 1995;23(3):288–94.
95. Yagi M, Wong EK, Kanamori A, Debski RE, Fu FH, Woo SL. Biomechanical analysis of an anatomic anterior cruciate ligament reconstruction. Am J Sports Med. 2002;30(5):660–6.
96. Arnold MP, Kooloos J, van Kampen A. Single-incision technique misses the anatomical femoral anterior cruciate ligament insertion: a cadaver study. Knee Surg Sports Traumatol Arthrosc. 2001;9(4):194–9.
97. Hantes ME, Zachos VC, Liantsis A, Venouziou A, Karantanas AH, Malizos KN. Differences in graft orientation using the transtibial and anteromedial portal technique in anterior cruciate ligament reconstruction: a magnetic resonance imaging study. Knee Surg Sports Traumatol Arthrosc. 2009;17(8):880–6.
98. Marchant BG, Noyes FR, Barber-Westin SD, Fleckenstein C. Prevalence of nonanatomical graft placement in a series of failed anterior cruciate ligament reconstructions. Am J Sports Med. 2010;38(10):1987–96.
99. Bowers AL, Bedi A, Lipman JD, Potter HG, Rodeo SA, Pearle AD, Warren RF, Altchek DW. Comparison of anterior cruciate ligament tunnel position and graft obliquity with transtibial and anteromedial portal femoral tunnel reaming techniques using high-resolution magnetic resonance imaging. Arthroscopy. 2011;27(11):1511–22.
100. Kopf S, Forsythe B, Wong AK, Tashman S, Irrgang JJ, Fu FH. Transtibial ACL reconstruction technique fails to position drill tunnels anatomically in vivo 3D CT study. Knee Surg Sports Traumatol Arthrosc. 2012;20(11):2200–7.
101. Bedi A, Musahl V, Steuber V, Kendoff D, Choi D, Allen AA, Pearle AD, Altchek DW. Transtibial versus anteromedial portal reaming in anterior cruciate ligament reconstruction: an anatomic and biomechanical evaluation of surgical technique. Arthroscopy. 2011;27(3):380–90.
102. Ayerza MA, Múscolo DL, Costa-Paz M, Makino A, Rondón L. Comparison of sagittal obliquity of the reconstructed anterior cruciate ligament with native anterior cruciate ligament using magnetic resonance imaging. Arthroscopy. 2003;19(3):257–61.
103. Ahn JH, Lee SH, Yoo JC, Ha HC. Measurement of the graft angles for the anterior cruciate ligament reconstruction with transtibial technique using postoperative magnetic resonance imaging in comparative study. Knee Surg Sports Traumatol Arthrosc. 2007;15(11):1293–300.
104. Ahn JH, Lee SH, Choi SH, Lim TK. Magnetic resonance imaging evaluation of anterior cruciate ligament reconstruction using quadrupled hamstring tendon autografts: comparison of remnant bundle preservation and standard technique. Am J Sports Med. 2010;38(9):1768–77.

105. Fujimoto E, Sumen Y, Deie M, Yasumoto M, Kobayashi K, Ochi M. Anterior cruciate ligament graft impingement against the posterior cruciate ligament: diagnosis using MRI plus three-dimensional reconstruction software. Magn Reson Imaging. 2004;22(8):1125–9.
106. Iwahashi T, Shino K, Nakata K, Otsubo H, Suzuki T, Amano H, Nakamura N. Direct anterior cruciate ligament insertion to the femur assessed by histology and 3-dimensional volume-rendered computed tomography. Arthroscopy. 2010;26(9 Suppl):S13–20.
107. Lertwanich P, Martins CA, Asai S, Ingham SJ, Smolinski P, Fu FH. Anterior cruciate ligament tunnel position measurement reliability on 3-dimensional reconstructed computed tomography. Arthroscopy. 2011;27(3):391–8.
108. Han Y, Kurzencwyg D, Hart A, Powell T, Martineau PA. Measuring the anterior cruciate ligament's footprints by three-dimensional magnetic resonance imaging. Knee Surg Sports Traumatol Arthrosc. 2012;20(5):986–95.
109. Kopf S, Musahl V, Tashman S, Szczodry M, Shen W, Fu FH. A systematic review of the femoral origin and tibial insertion morphology of the ACL. Knee Surg Sports Traumatol Arthrosc. 2009;17(3):213–9.
110. Hantes ME, Tsarouhas A, Giakas G, Spiropoulos G, Sideris V, Christel P, Malizos KN. Effect of fatigue on tibial rotation after single- and double-bundle anterior cruciate ligament reconstruction: a 3-dimensional kinematic and kinetic matched-group analysis. Am J Sports Med. 2012 Sep;40(9):2045–51.
111. Ziegler CG, Pietrini SD, Westerhaus BD, Anderson CJ, Wijdicks CA, Johansen S, Engebretsen L, LaPrade RF. Arthroscopically pertinent landmarks for tunnel positioning in single-bundle and double-bundle anterior cruciate ligament reconstructions. Am J Sports Med. 2011;39(4):743–52.
112. Hensler D, Working ZM, Illingworth KD, Thorhauer ED, Tashman S, Fu FH. Medial portal drilling: effects on the femoral tunnel aperture morphology during anterior cruciate ligament reconstruction. J Bone Joint Surg Am. 2011;93(22):2063–71.
113. Nakamura M, Deie M, Shibuya H, Nakamae A, Adachi N, Aoyama H, Ochi M. Potential risks of femoral tunnel drilling through the far anteromedial portal: a cadaveric study. Arthroscopy. 2009;25(5):481–7.
114. Kopf S, Martin DE, Tashman S, Fu FH. Effect of tibial drill angles on bone tunnel aperture during anterior cruciate ligament reconstruction. J Bone Joint Surg Am. 2010;92(4):871–81.
115. Geeslin AG, Jansson KS, Wijdicks CA, Chapman MA, Fok AS, LaPrade RF. Tibial tunnel aperture irregularity after drilling with 5 reamer designs: a qualitative micro-computed tomography analysis. Am J Sports Med. 2011;39(4):825–31.
116. Yamazaki S, Yasuda K, Tomita F, Minami A, Tohyama H. The effect of intraosseous graft length on tendon-bone healing in anterior cruciate ligament reconstruction using flexor tendon. Knee Surg Sports Traumatol Arthrosc. 2006;14(11):1086–93.
117. Zantop T, Ferretti M, Bell KM, Brucker PU, Gilbertson L, Fu FH. Effect of tunnel-graft length on the biomechanics of anterior cruciate ligament-reconstructed knees: intra-articular study in a goat model. Am J Sports Med. 2008;36(11): 2158–66.
118. Arneja S, McConkey MO, Mulpuri K, Chin P, Gilbart MK, Regan WD, Leith JM. Graft tensioning in anterior cruciate ligament reconstruction: a systematic review of randomized controlled trials. Arthroscopy. 2009;25(2):200–7.
119. Muneta T, Sekiya I, Yagishita K, Ogiuchi T, Yamamoto H, Shinomiya K. Two-bundle reconstruction of the anterior cruciate ligament using semitendinosus tendon with Endobuttons: operative technique and preliminary results. Arthroscopy. 1999;15(6):618–24.
120. Colombet P, Robinson J, Jambou S, Allard M, Bousquet V, de Lavigne C. Two-bundle, four-tunnel anterior cruciate ligament reconstruction. Knee Surg Sports Traumatol Arthrosc. 2006;14(7):629–36.
121. Vermesan D, Prejbeanu R, Laitin S, Georgianu V, Haragus H, Nitescu S, Tatullo M, Tattoli M, Caprio M, Cagiano R. Meniscal tears left in situ during anatomic single bundle anterior cruciate ligament reconstruction. Eur Rev Med Pharmacol Sci. 2014; 18(2):252–6.
122. Neuman P, Englund M, Kostogiannis I, Fridén T, Roos H, Dahlberg LE. Prevalence of tibiofemoral osteoarthritis 15 years after nonoperative treatment of anterior cruciate ligament injury: a prospective cohort study. Am J Sports Med. 2008;36(9): 1717–25.
123. Georgoulis AD, Papadonikolakis A, Papageorgiou CD, Mitsou A, Stergiou N. Three-dimensional tibiofemoral kinematics of the anterior cruciate ligament-deficient and reconstructed knee during walking. Am J Sports Med. 2003;31(1):75–9.
124. Siebold R. The concept of complete footprint restoration with guidelines for single- and double-bundle ACL reconstruction. Knee Surg Sports Traumatol Arthrosc. 2011;19(5): 699–706.
125. Hussein M, van Eck CF, Cretnik A, Dinevski D, Fu FH. Prospective randomized clinical evaluation of conventional single-bundle, anatomic single-bundle, and anatomic double-bundle anterior cruciate ligament reconstruction: 281 cases with 3- to 5-year follow-up. Am J Sports Med. 2012;40(3):512–20.
126. Musahl V, Becker R, Fu FH, Karlsson J. New trends in ACL research. Knee Surg Sports Traumatol Arthrosc. 2011;19 Suppl 1:S1–3.
127. Rabuck SJ, Middleton KK, Maeda S, Fujimaki Y, Muller B, Araujo PH, Fu FH. Individualized anatomic anterior cruciate ligament reconstruction. Arthrosc Tech. 2012;1(1):e23–9.
128. Pujol N, Colombet P, Cucurulo T, Graveleau N, Hulet C, Panisset JC, Potel JF, Servien E, Sonnery-Cottet B, Trojani C, Djian P, French Arthroscopy Society (SFA). Natural history of partial anterior cruciate ligament tears: a systematic literature review. Orthop Traumatol Surg Res. 2012;98(8 Suppl):S160–4.
129. Ahmad CS, Gardner TR, Groh M, Arnouk J, Levine WN. Mechanical properties of soft tissue femoral fixation devices for anterior cruciate ligament reconstruction. Am J Sports Med. 2004;32(3):635–40.
130. Pässler HH. History of implant-free anterior cruciate ligament reconstruction. Unfallchirurg. 2010;113(7):524–31. Springer-Verlag.
131. Hertel P, Behrend H. Implant-free anterior cruciate ligament reconstruction with the patella ligament and press-fit double bundle technique. Unfallchirurg. 2010;113(7):540–8. Springer-Verlag.
132. Kühne JH, Fottner M, Plitz W. Experimental stability of a new implant-free fixation technique in ACL replacement. Unfallchirurg. 1999;102(10):791–6. Springer-Verlag.
133. Geiges B, von Falck C, Knobloch K, Haasper C, Meller R, Krettek C, et al. Biodegradable screw versus a press-fit bone plug fixation for ACL reconstruction: a prospective randomized study. Unfallchirurg. 2013;116(2):109–17.
134. Colvin A, Sharma C, Parides M, Glashow J. What is the best femoral fixation of hamstring autografts in anterior cruciate ligament reconstruction?: a meta-analysis. Clin Orthop Relat Res. 2011;469(4):1075–81.
135. Sanchis-Alfonso V, Monllau JC. The ACL-deficient knee. Springer; 2012. p. 1.
136. Milano G, Mulas PD, Ziranu F, Piras S, Manunta A, Fabbriciani C. Comparison between different femoral fixation devices for ACL reconstruction with doubled hamstring tendon graft: a biomechanical analysis. Arthroscopy. 2006;22(6):660–8.

137. McGuire DA, Barber FA, Elrod BF, Paulos LE. Bioabsorbable interference screws for graft fixation in anterior cruciate ligament reconstruction. Arthroscopy. 1999;15(5):463–73.
138. Offerhaus C, Balke M, Braas M, Pennig D, Gick S, Höher J. Knee laxity in anterior cruciate ligament reconstruction: the influence of graft rotation using interference screw fixation. Unfallchirurg. 2014;117(9):822–8.
139. Musgrove TP, Salmon LJ, Burt CF, Pinczewski LA. The influence of reverse-thread screw femoral fixation on laxity measurements after anterior cruciate ligament reconstruction with hamstring tendon. Am J Sports Med. 2000;28(5):695–9.
140. Drogset JO, Straume LG, Bjørkmo I, Myhr G. A prospective randomized study of ACL-reconstructions using bone-patellar tendon-bone grafts fixed with bioabsorbable or metal interference screws. Knee Surg Sports Traumatol Arthrosc. 2011;19(5):753–9. Springer-Verlag.
141. Myers P, Logan M, Stokes A, Boyd K, Watts M. Bioabsorbable versus titanium interference screws with hamstring autograft in anterior cruciate ligament reconstruction: a prospective randomized trial with 2-year follow-up. Arthroscopy. 2008;24(7):817–23. Elsevier.
142. Shen C, Jiang S-D, Jiang L-S, Dai L-Y. Bioabsorbable versus metallic interference screw fixation in anterior cruciate ligament reconstruction: a meta-analysis of randomized controlled trials. Arthroscopy. 2010;26(5):705–13.
143. Bergsma J. Late degradation tissue response to poly(?-lactide) bone plates and screws. Biomaterials. 1995;16(1):25–31.
144. Martinek V, Seil R, Lattermann C, Watkins SC, Fu FH. The fate of the poly-L-lactic acid interference screw after anterior cruciate ligament reconstruction. Arthroscopy. 2001;17(1):73–6.
145. American Orthopaedic Society for Sports Medicine. Magnetic resonance imaging analysis of bioabsorbable interference screws used for fixation of bone-patellar tendon-bone autografts in endoscopic reconstruction of the anterior cruciate ligament. Am J Sports Med. 2006;34(7):1164–9.
146. Konan S, Haddad FS. The unpredictable material properties of bioabsorbable PLC interference screws and their adverse effects in ACL reconstruction surgery. Knee Surg Sports Traumatol Arthrosc. 2009;17(3):293–7.
147. Barber FA, Dockery WD. Long-term absorption of beta-tricalcium phosphate poly-L-lactic acid interference screws. Arthroscopy. 2008;24(4):441–7.
148. Barber FA, Dockery WD, Hrnack SA. Long-term degradation of a poly-lactide co-glycolide/β-tricalcium phosphate biocomposite interference screw. Arthroscopy. 2011;27(5):637–43.
149. Barber FA, Hrnack SA. Poly L-lactide co-glycolide/β-tricalcium phosphate interference screw fixation for bone-patellar tendon bone anterior cruciate ligament reconstruction. J Knee Surg. 2013;26(6):423–8.
150. Baums MH, Zelle BA, Schultz W, Ernstberger T, Klinger H-M. Intraarticular migration of a broken biodegradable interference screw after anterior cruciate ligament reconstruction. Knee Surg Sports Traumatol Arthrosc. 2006;14(9):865–8.
151. Masini BD, Stinner DJ, Waterman SM, Wenke JC, Gerlinger TL. Bacterial adherence to titanium, poly-L-lactic acid, and composite hydroxyapatite and poly-L-lactic acid interference screws. J Surg Orthop Adv. 2012;21(4):237–41.
152. Rhee PC, Dahm DL, Stuart MJ, Thoreson A, An K-N, Levy BA. Delta screw versus RetroScrew tibial fixation for ACL reconstruction. Knee Surg Sports Traumatol Arthrosc. 2011;19 Suppl 1(S1):S94–100.
153. Nag HL, Gupta H. Seating of TightRope RT button under direct arthroscopic visualization in anterior cruciate ligament reconstruction to prevent potential complications. Arthrosc Tech. 2012;1(1):e83–5. Elsevier.
154. McGuire DA, Barber FA, Milchgrub S, Wolchok JC. A postmortem examination of poly-L lactic acid interference screws 4 months after implantation during anterior cruciate ligament reconstruction. Arthroscopy. 2001;17(9):988–92.
155. Höher J, Livesay GA, Ma CB, Withrow JD, Fu FH, Woo SL. Hamstring graft motion in the femoral bone tunnel when using titanium button/polyester tape fixation. Knee Surg Sports Traumatol Arthrosc. 1999;7(4):215–9.
156. Kousa P, Järvinen TLN, Vihavainen M, Kannus P, Järvinen M. The fixation strength of six hamstring tendon graft fixation devices in anterior cruciate ligament reconstruction. Part I: femoral site. Am J Sports Med. 2003;31(2):174–81.
157. Halder AM. Arthroscopic reconstruction of anterior cruciate ligament with press-fit technique. Unfallchirurg. 2010;113(8):635–40.
158. Lenschow S, Herbort M, Strässer A, Strobel M, Raschke M, Petersen W, et al. Structural properties of a new device for graft fixation in cruciate ligament reconstruction: the shim technique. Arch Orthop Trauma Surg. 2011;131(8):1067–72.
159. Barrow AE, Pilia M, Guda T, Kadrmas WR, Burns TC. Femoral suspension devices for anterior cruciate ligament reconstruction: do adjustable loops lengthen? Am J Sports Med. 2014;42(2):343–9.
160. Petre BM, Smith SD, Jansson KS, de Meijer P-P, Hackett TR, LaPrade RF, et al. Femoral cortical suspension devices for soft tissue anterior cruciate ligament reconstruction: a comparative biomechanical study. Am J Sports Med. 2013;41(2):416–22.
161. Eguchi A, Ochi M, Adachi N, Deie M, Nakamae A, Usman MA. Mechanical properties of suspensory fixation devices for anterior cruciate ligament reconstruction: comparison of the fixed-length loop device versus the adjustable-length loop device. Knee. 2014;21(3):743–8. Elsevier.
162. Conner CS, Perez BA, Morris RP, Buckner JW, Buford WL, Ivey FM. Three femoral fixation devices for anterior cruciate ligament reconstruction: comparison of fixation on the lateral cortex versus the anterior cortex. Arthroscopy. 2010;26(6):796–807.
163. Papachristou G, Kalliakmanis A, Papachristou K, Magnissalis E, Sourlas J, Plessas S. Comparison of fixation methods of double-bundle double-tibial tunnel ACL reconstruction and double-bundle single-tunnel technique. Int Orthop. 2008;32(4):483–8.
164. Marx RG, Spock CR. Complications following hamstring anterior cruciate ligament reconstruction with femoral cross-pin fixation. Arthroscopy. 2005;21(6):762–3. Elsevier.
165. Clark R, Olsen RE, Larson BJ, Goble EM, Farrer RP. Cross-pin femoral fixation: a new technique for hamstring anterior cruciate ligament reconstruction of the knee. Arthroscopy. 1998;14(3):258–67.
166. Kuskucu SM. Comparison of short-term results of bone tunnel enlargement between EndoButton™ CL and cross-pin fixation systems after chronic anterior cruciate ligament reconstruction with autologous quadrupled hamstring tendons. J Int Med Res. 2008;36(1):23–30. SAGE Publications.
167. Baumfeld JA, Diduch DR, Rubino LJ, Hart JA, Miller MD, Barr MS, et al. Tunnel widening following anterior cruciate ligament reconstruction using hamstring autograft: a comparison between double cross-pin and suspensory graft fixation. Knee Surg Sports Traumatol Arthrosc. 2008;16(12):1108–13. Springer-Verlag.
168. Sabat D, Kundu K, Arora S, Kumar V. Tunnel widening after anterior cruciate ligament reconstruction: a prospective randomized computed tomography – based study comparing 2 different femoral fixation methods for hamstring graft. Arthroscopy: The Journal of Arthroscopic & Related Surgery. 2011;27(6):776–83. Elsevier.
169. Kong C-G, In Y, Kim G-H, Ahn C-Y. Cross pins versus Endobutton femoral fixation in hamstring anterior cruciate ligament reconstruction: minimum 4-year follow-up. Knee Surg Relat Res. 2012;24(1):34.
170. Ahn JH, Lee SA, Choi S-H, Wang JH, Yoo JC, Lee SS, et al. Femoral cross-pin breakage and its effects on the results of anterior cruciate ligament reconstruction using a hamstring autograft. Arthroscopy. 2012;28(12):1826–32. Elsevier.

171. Bakhru P, Park B, Umans H, DiFelice GS, Tobin K. MRI of broken bioabsorbable crosspin fixation in hamstring graft reconstruction of the anterior cruciate ligament. Skeletal Radiol. 2011;40(6):737–43.
172. Han DLY, Nyland J, Kendzior M, Nawab A, Caborn DNM. Intratunnel versus extratunnel fixation of hamstring autograft for anterior cruciate ligament reconstruction. Arthroscopy. 2012;28(10):1555–66.
173. Prado RK, Ntagiopoulos PG, Fucs PMB, Severino NR, Dejour D. A new technique in double-bundle anterior cruciate ligament reconstruction using implant-free femoral fixation. Int Orthop. 2012;36(7):1479–85. Springer-Verlag.
174. Pässler HH. Anatomic anterior cruciate ligament reconstruction with hamstrings using press-fit fixation without hardware: operative technique and long-term results of a prospective and randomized study. Unfallchirurg. 2010;113(7):555–60. Springer-Verlag.
175. Frenzel G, Wuschech H, Felmet G, Ingenhoven E, Schmidt M, Ziesche JJ. Cost analysis of implant-free replacement of anterior cruciate ligament. Unfallchirurg. 2010;113(8):615–20.
176. Poolman RW, Abouali JA, Conter HJ, Bhandari M. Overlapping systematic reviews of anterior cruciate ligament reconstruction comparing hamstring autograft with bone-patellar tendon-bone autograft: why are they different? J Bone Joint Surg Am. 2007;89(7):1542–52.
177. Spindler KP, Kuhn JE, Freedman KB, Matthews CE, Dittus RS, Harrell Jr FE. Anterior cruciate ligament reconstruction autograft choice: bone-tendon-bone versus hamstring: does it really matter? A systematic review. Am J Sports Med. 2004;32(8):1986–95.
178. Samuelsson K, Andersson D, Karlsson J. Treatment of anterior cruciate ligament injuries with special reference to graft type and surgical technique: an assessment of randomized controlled trials. Arthroscopy. 2009;25(10):1139–74.
179. Mohtadi NG, Chan DS, Dainty KN, Whelan DB. Patellar tendon versus hamstring tendon autograft for anterior cruciate ligament rupture in adults. Cochrane Database Syst Rev. 2011;9, CD005960.
180. Pagnani MJ, Warner JJ, O'Brien SJ, Warren RF. Anatomic considerations in harvesting the semitendinosus and gracilis tendons and a technique of harvest. Am J Sports Med. 1993;21(4):565–71.
181. Ivey M, Prud'homme J. Anatomic variations of the pes anserinus: a cadaver study. Orthopedics. 1993;16(5):601–6.
182. Kerver AL, Leliveld MS, den Hartog D, Verhofstad MH, Kleinrensink GJ. The surgical anatomy of the infrapatellar branch of the saphenous nerve in relation to incisions for anteromedial knee surgery. J Bone Joint Surg Am. 2013;95(23):2119–25.
183. Ferrari JD, Ferrari DA. The semitendinosus: anatomic considerations in tendon harvesting. Orthop Rev. 1991;20(12):1085–8.
184. Tohyama H, Beynnon BD, Johnson RJ, Nichols CE, Renström PA. Morphometry of the semitendinosus and gracilis tendons with application to anterior cruciate ligament reconstruction. Knee Surg Sports Traumatol Arthrosc. 1993;1(3–4):143–7.
185. Carofino B, Fulkerson J. Medial hamstring tendon regeneration following harvest for anterior cruciate ligament reconstruction: fact, myth, and clinical implication. Arthroscopy. 2005;21(10):1257–65.
186. Kartus J, Ejerhed L, Eriksson BI, Karlsson J. The localization of the infrapatellar nerves in the anterior knee region with special emphasis on central third patellar tendon harvest: a dissection study on cadaver and amputated specimens. Arthroscopy. 1999;15(6):577–86.
187. Svensson M, Kartus J, Ejerhed L, Lindahl S, Karlsson J. Does the patellar tendon normalize after harvesting its central third?: a prospective long-term MRI study. Am J Sports Med. 2004;32(1):34–8.
188. Moebius UG, Georgoulis AD, Papageorgiou CD, Papadonikolakis A, Rossis J, Soucacos PN. Alterations of the extensor apparatus after anterior cruciate ligament reconstruction using the medial third of the patellar tendon. Arthroscopy. 2001;17(9):953–9.
189. Prodromos CC, Joyce BT. The relative strengths of anterior cruciate ligament autografts and allografts. In: Prodromos CC, editor. The anterior cruciate ligament reconstruction, Expert Consult series. Saunders; 2008.
190. Stäubli HU, Schatzmann L, Brunner P, Rincón L, Nolte LP. Mechanical tensile properties of the quadriceps tendon and patellar ligament in young adults. Am J Sports Med. 1999;27(1):27–34.
191. Sasaki N, Farraro KF, Kim KE, Woo SL. Biomechanical evaluation of the quadriceps tendon autograft for anterior cruciate ligament reconstruction: a cadaveric study. Am J Sports Med. 2014;42(3):723–30.
192. Lund B, Nielsen T, Faunø P, Christiansen SE, Lind M. Is quadriceps tendon a better graft choice than patellar tendon? A prospective randomized study. Arthroscopy. 2014;30(5):593–8.
193. Prodromos C, Joyce B, Shi K. A meta-analysis of stability of autografts compared to allografts after anterior cruciate ligament reconstruction. Knee Surg Sports Traumatol Arthrosc. 2007;15(7):851–6. Epub 2007 Apr 17.
194. Hoburg AT, Keshlaf S, Schmidt T, Smith M, Gohs U, Perka C, Pruss A, Scheffler S. Effect of electron beam irradiation on biomechanical properties of patellar tendon allografts in anterior cruciate ligament reconstruction. Am J Sports Med. 2010;38(6):1134–40.
195. Lamblin CJ, Waterman BR, Lubowitz JH. Anterior cruciate ligament reconstruction with autografts compared with non-irradiated, non-chemically treated allografts. Arthroscopy. 2013; 29(6):1113–22.
196. Park SS, Dwyer T, Congiusta F, Whelan DB, Theodoropoulos J. Analysis of irradiation on the clinical effectiveness of allogenic tissue when used for primary anterior cruciate ligament reconstruction. Am J Sports Med. Epub 2014 Jan 29.
197. Viateau V, Manassero M, Anagnostou F, Guérard S, Mitton D, Migonney V. Biological and biomechanical evaluation of the ligament advanced reinforcement system (LARS AC) in a sheep model of anterior cruciate ligament replacement: a 3-month and 12-month study. Arthroscopy. 2013;29(6):1079–88.
198. Newman SD, Atkinson HD, Willis-Owen CA. Anterior cruciate ligament reconstruction with the ligament augmentation and reconstruction system: a systematic review. Int Orthop. 2013;37(2):321–6.
199. Barker JU, Drakos MC, Maak TG, Warren RF, Williams 3rd RJ, Allen AA. Effect of graft selection on the incidence of postoperative infection in anterior cruciate ligament reconstruction. Am J Sports Med. 2010;38(2):281–6.
200. Wang C, Lee YH, Siebold R. Recommendations for the management of septic arthritis after ACL reconstruction. Knee Surg Sports Traumatol Arthrosc. 2014;22(9):2136–44.
201. Maletis GB, Inacio MC, Reynolds S, Desmond JL, Maletis MM, Funahashi TT. Incidence of postoperative anterior cruciate ligament reconstruction infections: graft choice makes a difference. Am J Sports Med. 2013;41(8):1780–5.
202. Sonnery-Cottet B, Archbold P, Zayni R, Bortolletto J, Thaunat M, Prost T, Padua VB, Chambat P. Prevalence of septic arthritis after anterior cruciate ligament reconstruction among professional athletes. Am J Sports Med. 2011;39(11):2371–6.
203. Saper M, Stephenson K, Heisey M. Arthroscopic irrigation and debridement in the treatment of septic arthritis after anterior cruciate ligament reconstruction. Arthroscopy. 2014;30(6):747–54. doi:10.1016/j.arthro.2014.02.015. pii: S0749-8063(14)00126-1.
204. Izquierdo Jr R, Cadet ER, Bauer R, Stanwood W, Levine WN, Ahmad CS. A survey of sports medicine specialists investigating the preferred management of contaminated anterior cruciate ligament grafts. Arthroscopy. 2005;21(11):1348–53.
205. Plante MJ, Li X, Scully G, Brown MA, Busconi BD, DeAngelis NA. Evaluation of sterilization methods following contamination of hamstring autograft during anterior cruciate ligament reconstruction. Knee Surg Sports Traumatol Arthrosc. 2013;21(3): 696–701.

4 Revision ACL Surgery

Horia Haragus, Radu Prejbeanu, and Florin Ramadani

4.1 Incidence and Importance

The fact that the anterior cruciate ligament (ACL) is the most commonly reconstructed ligament in the human body has led to a high prevalence in the general population. Since this has addressed the physically active adults, an inherent result has been a rising incidence in the requirement of revision surgery. The shift from the transtibial vertical reconstructions, as well as the popularization of ACL reconstructions in emerging markets has led to many variables and challenges regarding the surgical techniques, outcomes and resource utilization.

Lessons learned from total joint arthroplasty has spawned interest in gathering comprehensive data in the form of national or corporate registries. During 2005–2010 many such endeavors have collected large amount of information from multicenter reports. The incidence of revision ACL reconstructions has therefore been reported with reliable evidence but relative variability. Maletis et al. have compared registries in Norway and the U.S. Kaiser Permanente and found a revision rate per follow-up year of 0.9 % in the first and 1.5 % in the second respectively [1]. A further follow-up report of community based registry showed that 7.2 % of the ACL reconstructions performed were revisions. Sixty-four percent of patients were male and the mean age for both primary and revision surgeries were 29.5. Cartilage injuries were noted in a quarter of primary and over a third of revision reconstructions. There was a 3.7 % rate of had subsequent surgery on the ACL reconstructed knee and 1.7 % on the contralateral. The overall yearly revision was 1.7 % [2].

The Danish ACL reconstruction registry report has found a rate of revision ACL reconstruction of 4.1 %. Revisions occurred most frequently in the first 2 years postoperatively. Furthermore, the rate of re-revision after 5 years was 5.4 % [3]. The Swedish National Anterior Cruciate Ligament Register reported a male: female ratio of approximately 1.3 for both primary and revision reconstructions. 4.1% of the patients underwent a revision reconstruction of the index knee and 5.0 % a contralateral ACL reconstruction. The corresponding figure for 15–18 year old female soccer players was 22.0 % [4].

In the Multicenter Orthopedic Outcomes Network (MOON) cohort there was a similar (3.0 %) risk of contralateral anterior cruciate ligament injury as for the reconstructed knee at 2 years [5]. When patients were observed for longer periods, this ratio continued to be in the same range, although minor differences have emerged. At 6-year follow-up, 7.7 % of reconstructed knees were revised and 6.4 % had injured the contralateral ACL. There was a high (18.9 %) percentage of subsequent surgeries on the reconstructed knee, mainly for cartilage procedures [6]. The MOON cohort was coupled with the Multicenter ACL Revision Study (MARS). The demographics of this specific target group also had a slight higher prevalence of men, a median age of 26 years with females being younger. For the majority the reconstruction was the first revision. Most were more than 2 years from their last reconstruction and only one-quarter returned to the same surgeon [7]. A later systematic review led by the same author found a slightly older mean age (30.6 years) and also a preponderance of males (66 %). The interval from primary to revision ACL reconstruction averaged 4.6 years [8].

Further reported values fall relatively in the same range, weather 4 % in a literature review [9] or 8.2 % in panel discussions [10]. A Canadian survey reported a revision rate

H. Haragus, MD, PhD (✉) • R. Prejbeanu, MD, PhD
Department of Orthopedics and Trauma,
University of Medicine and Pharmacy 'Victor Babes' Timisoara,
2 Eftimie Murgu Square, Timisoara 300041, Romania

I-st Clinic of Orthopedics and Trauma,
Emergency Clinical County Hospital Timisoara,
10 Iosif Bulbuca Blvd, Timisoara 300736, Romania
e-mail: horia.haragus@yahoo.com; raduprejbeanu@gmail.com

F. Ramadani, MD, PhD
Unfallchirurgie, Klinikum Wels-Grieskirchen,
42 Grieskirchner St, Wels A-4600, Austria

University of Medicine and Pharmacy 'Victor Babes' Timisoara,
Timisoara, Romania
e-mail: florin.ramadani@liwest.at

R. Prejbeanu (ed.), *Atlas of Knee Arthroscopy*,
DOI 10.1007/978-1-4471-6593-4_4, © Springer-Verlag London 2015

of 2.6 and 4.6 % for primary contralateral reconstructions [11]. Shelbourne et al. reported a 5.3 % of injury to the contralateral and 4.3 % to the reconstructed knee over 5 years. In the same study, women had more injuries (7.8 %) to the contralateral knee than men (3.7 %) but not to the reconstructed ACL (4.3 % versus 4.1 %) [12].

4.2 What Is a Failure of the Reconstruction?

One of the first aspects that should be clarified in symptomatic patients with ACL reconstructions is whether or not the neoligament is functional. This can present certain challenges, especially after new trauma or with associated lesions. There are not definitive criteria to decide if the graft is integrated and even more important if it provides adequate function. However, a consensus can be drawn on key aspects that need to be evaluated, and they all target stability.

Objective failure should be estimated by pivot shift and side to side difference in anterior translation measured by arthrometer (Medmetric, San Diego). Most authors consider a pivot shift grade 2 or 3 to be relevant of clinical insufficiency [7, 8, 13, 14, 16]. The Lachman test can also be used [7, 15, 16]. The KT-1000/2000 arthrometer over 5 mm is a definitive measure of pathologic sagittal stability [7, 8, 13, 14] although some authors set an even smaller significant cutoff value at over 3 mm van [9, 15, 16].

Functional instability is also a key subjective factor with importance in deciding for revision surgery [7, 9, 15, 16]. If the patients has pain and a sensation of instability during daily routine or intense sporting activity and there is also pathological laxity on examination a revision ACL procedure should be highly considered. Stiffness, defined as an extension deficit of more than 10° or flexion under 120° can also be an indirect sign or impingement due to improper tunnel positioning and require revision of the graft [9, 15].

The MRI aspect of the neoligament can pose certain interpretation challenges. Not many radiologists and orthopedic surgeons are familiarized with the MRI aspect due to the relative paucity of patients with ACL reconstructions compared to other routine cases. The normal graft has a homogenous hypointense signal immediately after reconstruction and after 1 year when the integration has been complete. A graft that is missing or ruptured can be relatively easy to diagnose since it appears as a hyperintense interruption. However, there are situations when the neoligament is failing to integrate, elongated or the two bundles heal differently [17]. This is when indirect signs such as a vertical graft, nonanatomic placement of the tunnels or anterior tibial translation can give clues to insufficiency [18]. Only when these situations are corroborated with functional instability on examination a revision surgery can be recommended, since there is poor correlation between clinical findings and MRI aspect of failed grafts [19].

To summarize, a panel consensus has defined failure as functional instability on examination, a need for revision and/or evidence of tear on magnetic resonance imaging (MRI) [10]. Of course, arthroscopic confirmation is an irrefutable evidence of graft failure but this should already be precluded by the preoperative examination.

4.3 Modes of Failure

The most common ways the ACL reconstruction fails are new trauma and technical errors of the primary procedures [20]. Of these, improper femoral tunnel placement is the most common, but overall a nonanatomical position of the graft is what will lead to insufficiency or failure to integrate. Nevertheless, not all non-anatomic vertical grafts will fail or require revision surgery. Some patients have well integrated and competent neoligaments even with non-anatomical positioning that allow them to have an active life and return to sports.

An analysis of the MARS group found a 32 % incidence of traumatic reinjury. For the majority the event was noncontact (cutting or jumping), during sport activities (soccer or basketball) and most affirmed to even hearing a 'pop'. A further 24 % had technical reasons for failure and a small (7 %) number were deemed to have lack of integration. Femoral tunnel malposition was rated as the most common technical failure by far (80 %), followed by tibial tunnel malposition (37 %) but a significant percentage (37 %) also had a combination of these [7]. To summarize, in the MARS database, 24–60 % had a technical cause of failure, with 44.2 % incidence of femoral malposition as the single cause [21]. A subsequent review of the literature also identified a 49.3 % incidence of new trauma, closely followed by technical error (45.8 %) [8]. A single center Danish report also found the causes of failure to be mostly traumatic (30 %), followed by femoral malposition (20 %) [22]. A French multicenter study also showed 50 % technical cause of failure with 36 % femoral and 10 % tibial malposition, 12 % impingement and 30 % of new trauma as etiology for the revision cases [23].

The new traumatic event might explain the higher incidence of neoligament and contralateral ACL ruptures in younger patients. There is a much higher risk of subsequent injury to either knee for patients under 18 years old (17 %) which drops to 7 % for patients aged 18–25 and 4 % for patients over 25 respectively [12]. This situation was also found by other authors, with a relative risk of 2.5 in patients below 20 years of age (8.7 % revision rate) compared to older patients (2.8 %) at the time of index surgery [3, 22]. Nonetheless, early return to sporting activities does not appear to influence the reinjury rates [12].

In addition to young age, graft diameters of less than 8 mm has a revision rate of 16.4 % and are both factors are coupled with an increased risk of revision [24]. Hamstrings autografts larger than 8 mm have decreased revision even in younger patients and also correlate with improved KOOS scores [40]. A different study found young age and the use of allografts to be predictors for graft failure [2]. These findings were reinforced by other authors, who also noted that revision procedure and female gender had no influence [6]. A Canadian experience also noted younger age and the use of allograft increased the risk of revision. Furthermore, there was an increased probability for revision if the index reconstruction was performed at an academic hospital, whereas only age was associated with increased risk of contralateral ACL surgery [11].

The modes of failure of the neoligament also appear to differ from the native ACL. They even differ with regard of the reconstruction technique. Van Eck et al. showed that for single bundle reconstructions (SB) the most common rupture pattern was elongation of the graft (Figs. 4.1, 4.2, and 4.3), followed in decreasing order by proximal (Fig. 4.4), mid-substance (Figs. 4.5, 4.6, 4.7, and 4.8) and distal (Figs. 4.9 and 4.10) rupture of the graft. The elongated graft group had a significantly greater interval between index and revision surgery compared to distal or mid-substance ruptures. Elongated and proximal ruptures were mostly autografts, while 91 % of the mid-substance and distal ruptures were allografts. Patient age and gender, tunnel angle, and etiology of failure did not influence the rupture pattern [26]. For double bundle procedures (DB), the most frequent rupture pattern was mid-substance rupture of both bundles (35 %), followed by proximal or mid-substance rupture of the anteromedial bundle with either elongation or proximal rupture of the posterolateral fascicle. Virtually all tears but only half of elongated grafts were traumatic [27]. Double bundle reconstruction could also result in fewer failures compared to SB even if the stability and osteoarthritic changes are similar [28].

The current trend towards anatomic ACL reconstructions has had a somewhat contradicting situation identified in the Danish Knee Ligament Reconstruction Register, where the use of the anteromedial portal technique increased from 13 % in 2007 to 40 % in 2010. This procedure, aimed at improving placement of the graft was found to have a two to three fold increase in relative risk of revision, sagittal instability and positive pivot shift compared with the older transtibial technique (TT). The authors potentially explain these findings through technical failures from introduction of a new technique or by the higher forces that anatomic placed grafts withstand compared to vertical ones [29]. This leads us to underline that anatomic placement of the graft requires careful analysis of the landmarks and that merely anteromedial drilling of the femoral tunnel might not suffice.

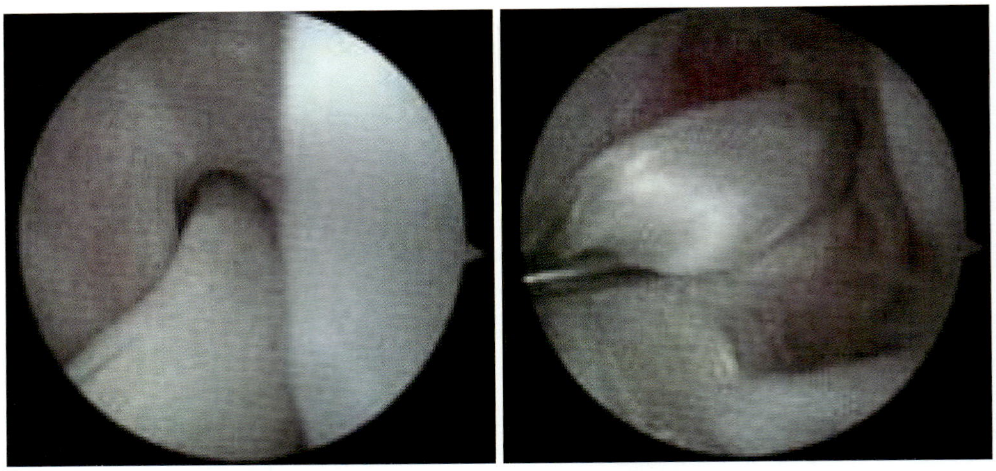

Fig. 4.1 Arthroscopic view through the anterolateral portal of an elongated SB vertical autograft with a high notch roof femoral tunnel aperture

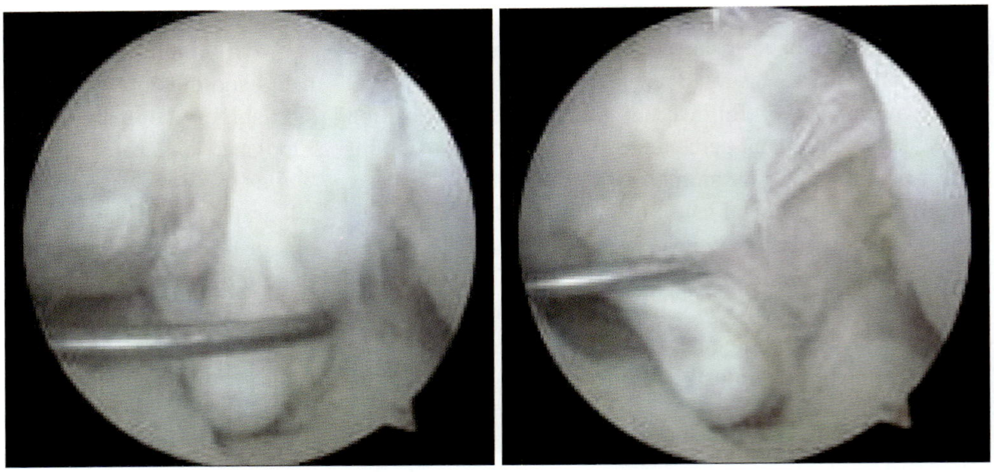

Fig. 4.2 Arthroscopic view through the anterolateral portal of a very elongated, insufficient SB vertical hamstrings autograft, 1 year after reconstruction in a young female handball player

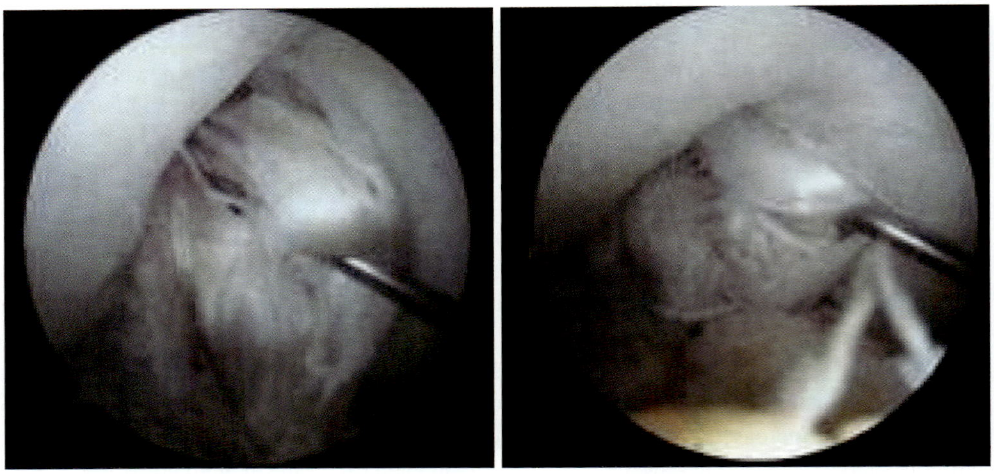

Fig. 4.3 Arthroscopic view through the anterolateral portal of an elongated, insufficient DB hamstrings autograft 1 year after reconstruction in a professional soccer player

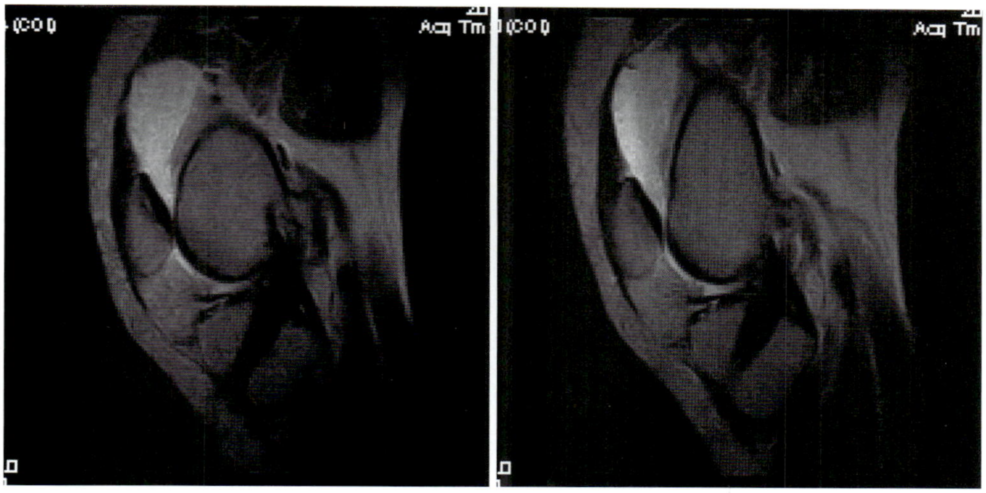

Fig. 4.4 Sagittal T2 MRI 5 years after anatomic SB ACL reconstruction with ipsilateral hamstrings autograft showing a homogenic hypointense aspect of the neoligament with a hyperintense femoral insertion suggestive of partial proximal rupture

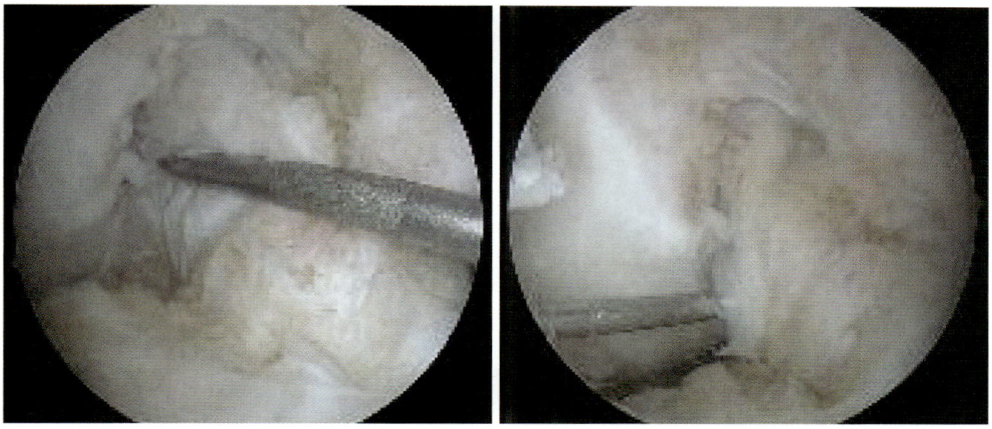

Fig. 4.5 Arthroscopic views of the same case through the anterolateral and anteromedial portals respectively showing a healed and integrated graft; the arthroscopic evaluation was performed in order to perform a partial medial meniscectomy resulting from a recent noncontact sporting injury

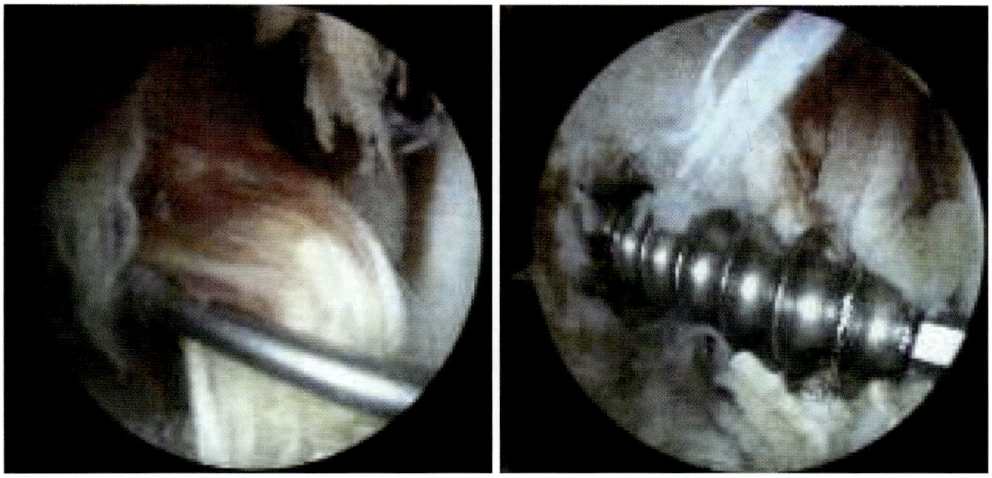

Fig. 4.6 Arthroscopic views through the anterolateral portal showing an elongated, insufficient patellar tendon autograft at the time of revision, 5 years after index surgery; removal of the misplaced metallic femoral interference screw (Fig. 4.18)

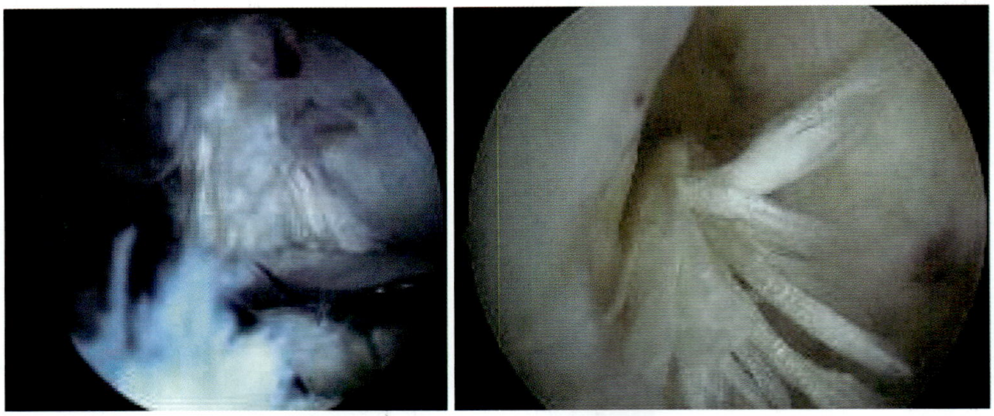

Fig. 4.7 Arthroscopic view of the same case through the anterolateral portal showing the placement of the tibial tunnel aperture at the time of revision; 3 years afterwards, the patient has a midruptured ipsilateral hamstrings autograft (Fig. 4.20)

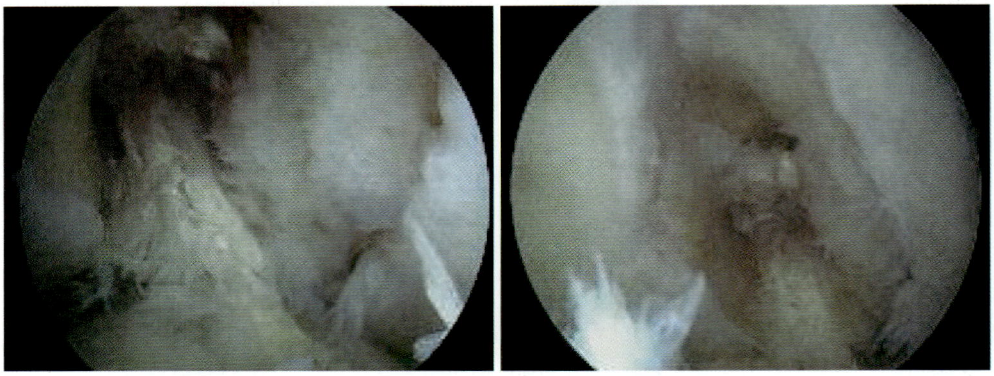

Fig. 4.8 Arthroscopic views of the same case through the anterolateral and anteromedial portals respectively after debridement; the arthroscopic evaluation was performed in order to remove a loose body (a fragment of the femoral biodegradable interference screw)

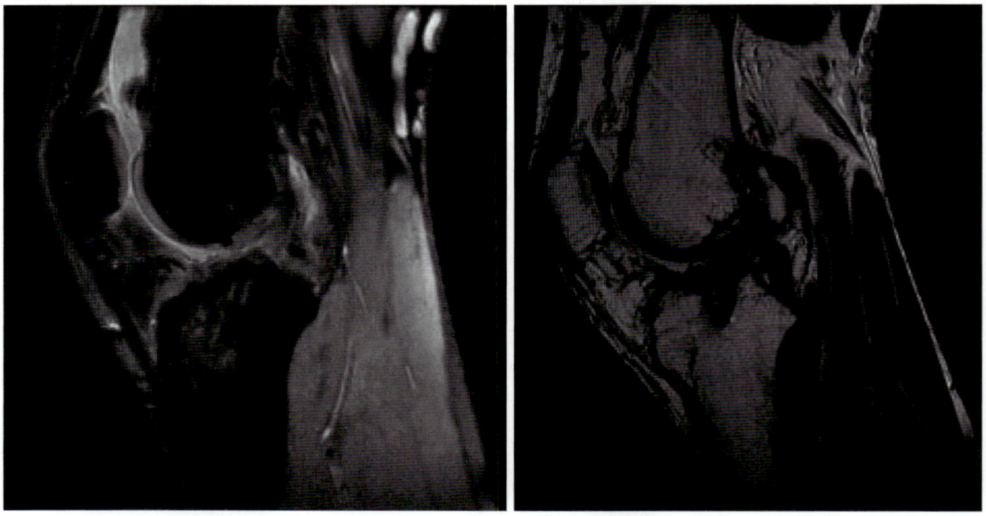

Fig. 4.9 Sagittal PD and T2 MRI of a failed vertical neoligament with distal rupture

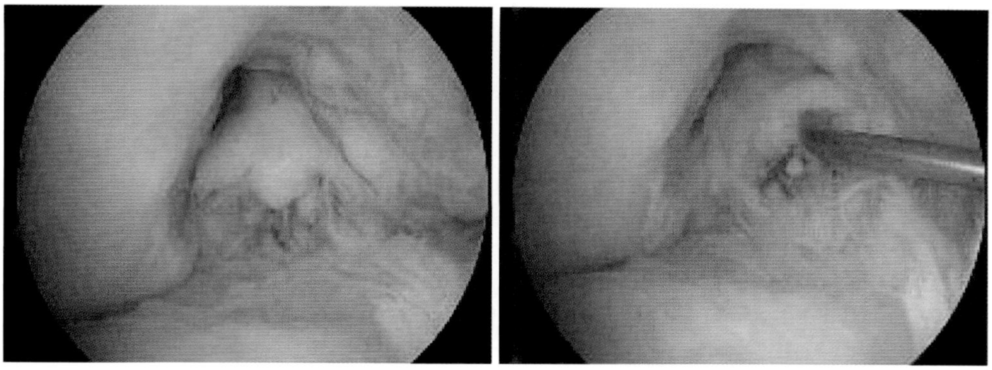

Fig. 4.10 Arthroscopic views of the same case through the anterolateral portal showing a distally ruptured graft; the arthroscopic evaluation was performed in order to perform a partial meniscectomy resulting from a recent injury

4.4 Assessment of Bone Tunnels

Inappropriate tunnel positioning or new trauma account for the majority of cases planned for revision ACL surgery. This leads to different situations for the placement of the new apertures. Standard x-rays are not able to satisfactorily give information regarding the location, size and bone quality in order to adequately perform the preoperative planning. Therefore, the standard imaging modality is now considered computed tomography (CT) with 3D (three dimensional) volume rendering (reconstruction) [30] (Figs. 4.11 and 4.12). The CT also demonstrated excellent intra- and inter-observer reliability compared to plain x-ray and MRI [31].

In addition, the tunnels might also be enlarged and might require graft filling prior to the new reconstruction. Tunnel expansion has been shown to occur predominantly during the first months after surgery, as the bone-tendon interface is more active [32]. However, in the setting of failure to integrate, this process can continue and might be irreversible spontaneously within a reasonable timeframe before revision (Figs. 4.13, 4.14, and 4.15).

When the revision plan is to drill entirely new tunnels, care should be taken to ensure a strong enough bridge between the two. It has been shown that a minimum of 2 mm are required to provide structural stability, which is of particular interest in revision cases, double bundle reconstruction and small knees. In addition, cortical buttons provide superior strength compared to aperture fixation when multiple tunnels are drilled through the lateral femoral condyle [33]. Clock dial, quadrant and anatomic insertion references are used to describe the location of the tunnel apertures [34] and more recently even a proposed standardized 3D CT evaluation of femoral tunnel based on the relationship of the aperture to the lateral intercondylar ridge [35].

The revision ACL reconstruction should not be a planned as a salvage procedure and all efforts should be put into restoring the native function and anatomy. In the MARS study, the most common technique for both index and revision procedures was arthroscopic single-incision transtibial drilling. Bone grafting of dilated tunnels was uncommon (3 %) and rarely performed as a two staged procedure. Unfortunately the prevalence of cartilage or meniscal damage was very high (70 %) [7]. A similar situation was identified by a systematic review. At the time of revision half of patients underwent a meniscectomy and. 15 % a repair, and more than half had chondral damage [8]. The community based register report of Maletis et al. noted cartilage damage in more than one-third of revision procedures and meniscal lesions in more than half respectively. Fixation distribution was similar for primary and revisions with a preponderance use of interference screws [2].

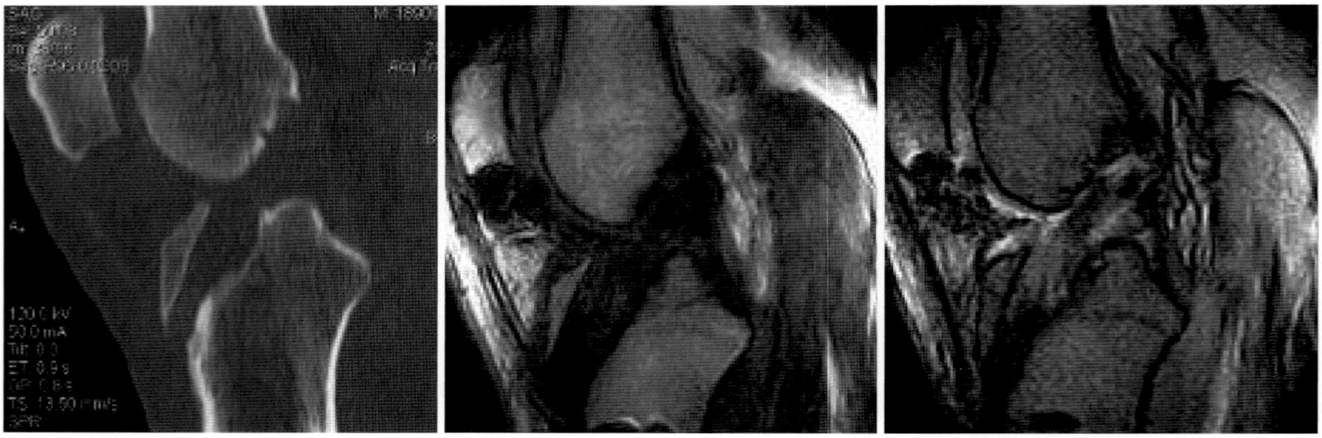

Fig. 4.11 Sagittal CT and T1 and T2 Gradient Echo MRI aspects of tibial tunnel enlargement following ACL reconstruction

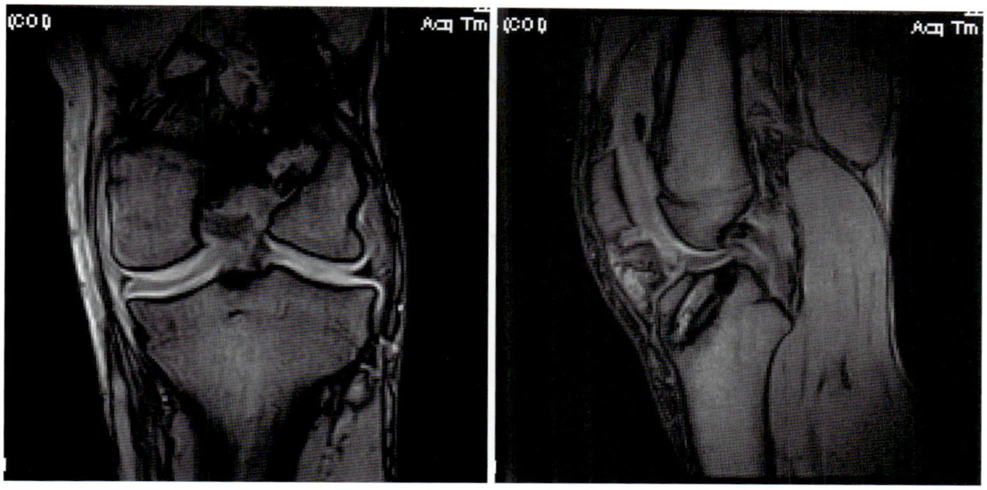

Fig. 4.12 Coronal and sagittal frequency-encoding gradient (GFE) T1 MRI scan of a patient with failed ACL reconstruction and significant tunnel enlargement; bioabsorbable screw fragments are visible in both tunnels

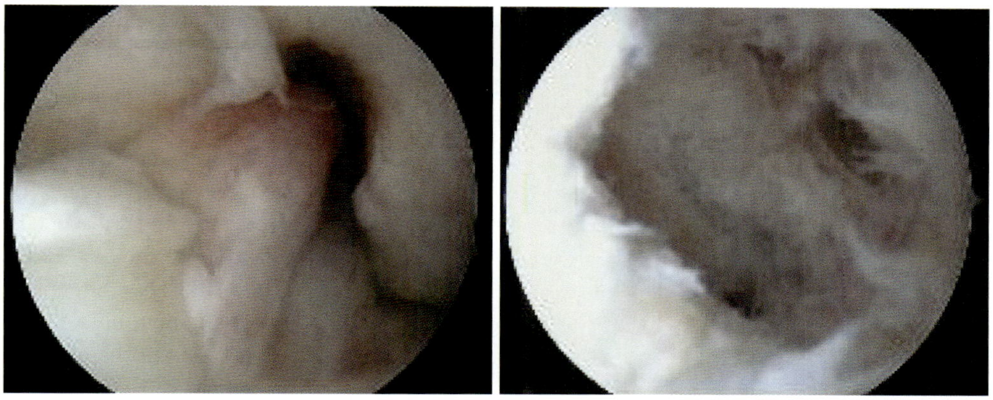

Fig. 4.13 Arthroscopic views of the same case through the anterolateral and anteromedial portals respectively showing a complete proximal discontinuity of the graft, before and after debridement

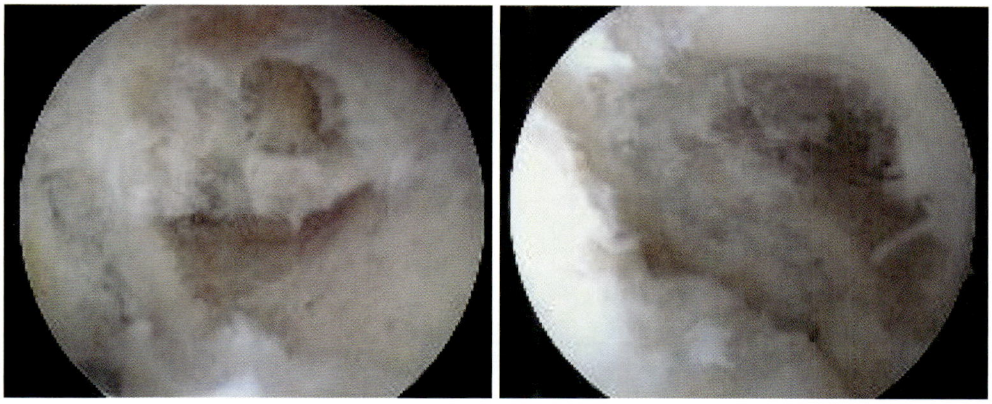

Fig. 4.14 Arthroscopic views of the same case through the anteromedial portal depicting an enlarged but well positioned femoral tunnel aperture

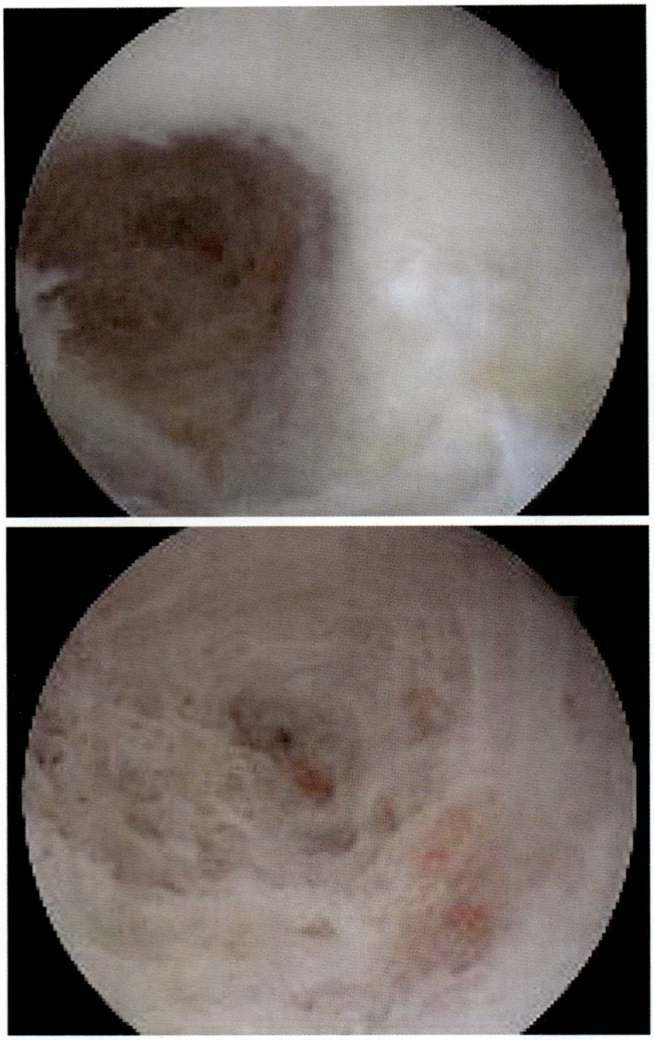

Fig. 4.15 Arthroscopic views of the same case through the anteromedial portal with additional close-up of the femoral tunnel bone structure

4.5 Graft Choices

There are only few differences between graft choice rationale in revisions compared to primary reconstructions. The clinical outcome does not appear to be influenced by graft type [37]. Most commonly the graft choice is determined by what was previously used and the surgeon's preference [7]. Bone patellar tendon bone (B-PT-B) autograft is generally the most commonly used [7, 8, 14, 36]. It has the potential to aid with filling of bone tunnel enlargement when the same tunnel is used.

In the MARS cohort, previous grafts were 70 % autologus and 27 % allograft. Choices for revisions were 45 % auto and 54 % allograft [7]. A systematic review reported the index graft material to be 86.1 % autologus, 5.5 % allograft and 8.5 % synthetic. For revisions, there was a slight increase in the use of autografts 89.4 %. These were mainly B-PT-B (48 %) followed by hamstrings (40 %) and quadriceps tendon (12 %) [8]. Similar data was presented by Trojani et al. with the use for revision of predominantly B-PT-B (50 %) followed by hamstrings (40 %) and quadriceps tendon (10 %). Initial B-PT-B was revised by either B-PT-B (ipsi or contralateral, 45 %), by an ipsilateral hamstrings in 45 % and by quadriceps tendonin 10 %. Primary hamstrings were revised by ipsilateral B-PT-B in 67 %, the contralateral hamstring in 24 % and quadriceps tendonin 9 % [14].

There are also surgeons who prefer either unharvested ipsilateral hamstrings or B-PT-B or Achilles allografts [37]. The contralateral hamstrings [39] or the ipsilateral quadriceps tendon [41] are also options without increased donor site morbidity. Centers with routine use of allografts in primary procedures (42.4 %) tend to also favor them for revisions (78.8 %) [2]. Results with allografts that had not undergone irradiation or chemical sterilization appear to be comparable to those with autografts [38].

4.6 Previous Non Anatomic Placement

At least for now, this is the most common situation for revision. In the presence of improperly positioned tunnels without significant enlargement, the revision allows for new tunnels to be drilled, making it similar to a primary procedure. When the SB femoral tunnel is placed high in the notch, even DB revision reconstruction can be successfully performed [42]. The reverse can also be used. If both initial DB bundles are too anterior (posterolateral PL) and too high (anteromedial AM) there might be sufficient space on the posterior lateral condyle to perform an anatomic SB reconstruction.

Out of all possibilities for non anatomical graft placement, femoral tunnel malpositioning is the most common single cause (76.9 %). In the MARS cohort, this was further evaluated as being mainly too vertical (35.9 %), followed by too anterior (29.9 %) or both (26.5 %) [21]. This is mainly attributable to the transtibial (TT) drilling technique, which tends to place the tibial aperture too posterior and the femoral too anterior and superior, leading to a "vertical" aspect of the neoligament.

On the tibial side, aperture malpositioning varies from 29.7 % (MARS) [21] to 11 % [23] or as little as 6 % [22]. For these reasons, revision usually involves drilling an entirely new femoral with the same optimal tibial aperture (82.1 % and 51.3 % respectively in the MARS report by Morgan et al.) [21].

Case Example

A 25 years old male with elongated B-PT-B graft, bucket handle internal meniscus tear and grade II chondral damage of the medial compartment after a recent trauma. The patient had a history of giving way since index surgery. The clinical exam found antero-posterior instability and KT-1000 side to side difference of 10 mm. CT exam showed improper tunnel positioning (femoral vertical and anterior) and moderate tibial tunnel widening (Fig. 4.16). The sagittal MRI T2 was suggestive for an elongated graft. We performed a one stage revision: arthroscopic exploration, removal of the ruptured border of the internal meniscus, confirmation of the elongated graft and debridement (Fig. 4.17). Ipsilateral semitendinosus and gracilis were harvested and quadrupled into a size 7 neoligament. The new femoral tunnel was drilled in the anatomic footprint through the anteromedial portal. We then drilled a new tibial tunnel, medial to the previous, in the anatomic position (Figs. 4.18 and 4.19). Proper placement of the new ligament does not create notch or posterior cruciate ligament (PCL) impingement (Fig. 4.20). For fixation we used a cortical button for the femur and 9.30 absorbable (PLLA) interference screw on the tibia in 20° of flexion. Proper tunnel positioning can be seen on the postoperative X-rays (Fig. 4.21).

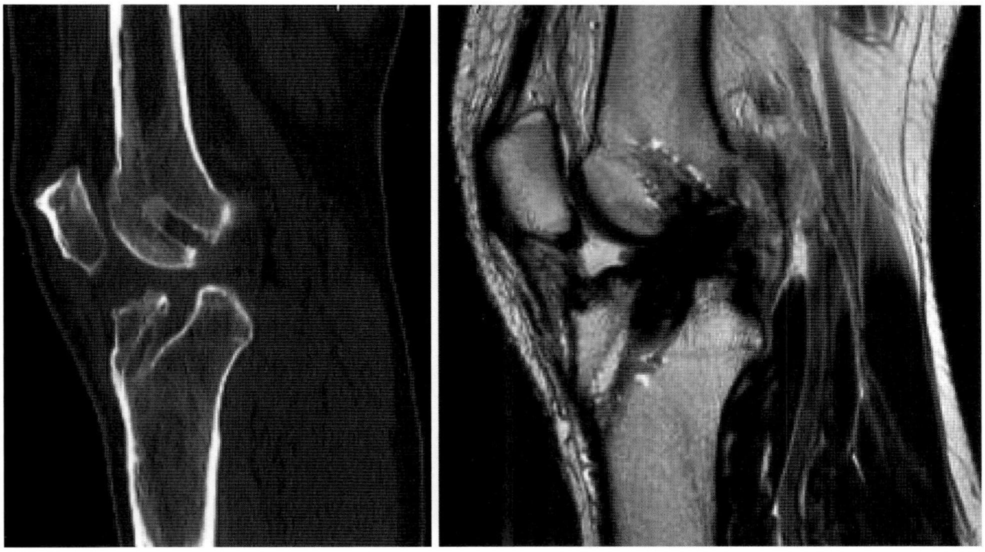

Fig. 4.16 Sagittal CT exam shows improper tunnel positioning (femoral vertical and anterior) and moderate tibial tunnel widening. The sagittal MRI T2 was suggestive for an elongated graft

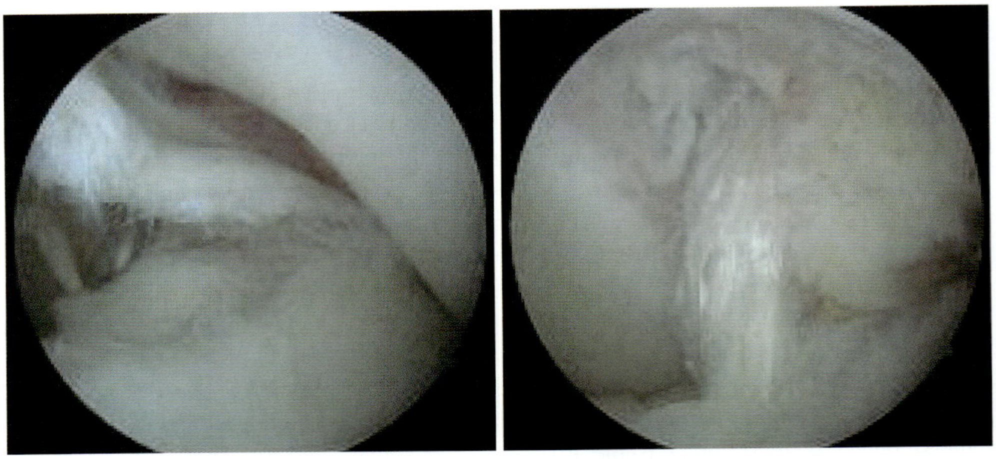

Fig. 4.17 Arthroscopic views through the anteromedial portal showing the internal border of the medial meniscus dislocated in the notch and a vertical graft. a complete proximal discontinuity of the graft, before and after debridement

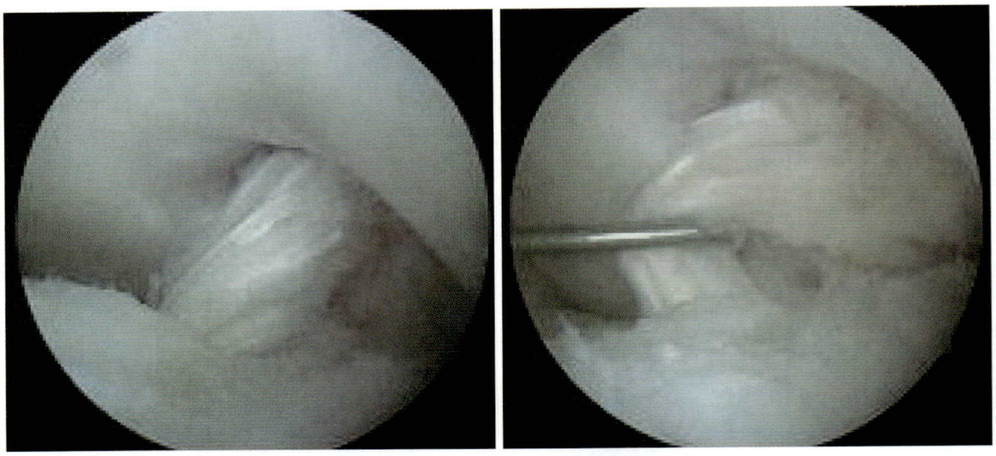

Fig. 4.18 Arthroscopic views through the anteromedial portal showing roof impingement and an insufficient and elongated graft

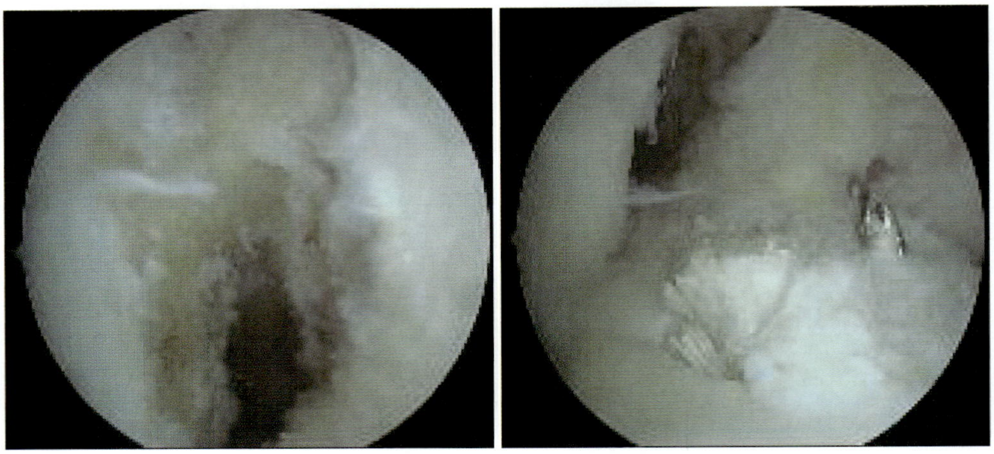

Fig. 4.19 Arthroscopic views through the anterolateral portal showing the correct position of the femoral and tibial apertures: lower and deeper on the lateral condyle and more medial on the tibia respectively

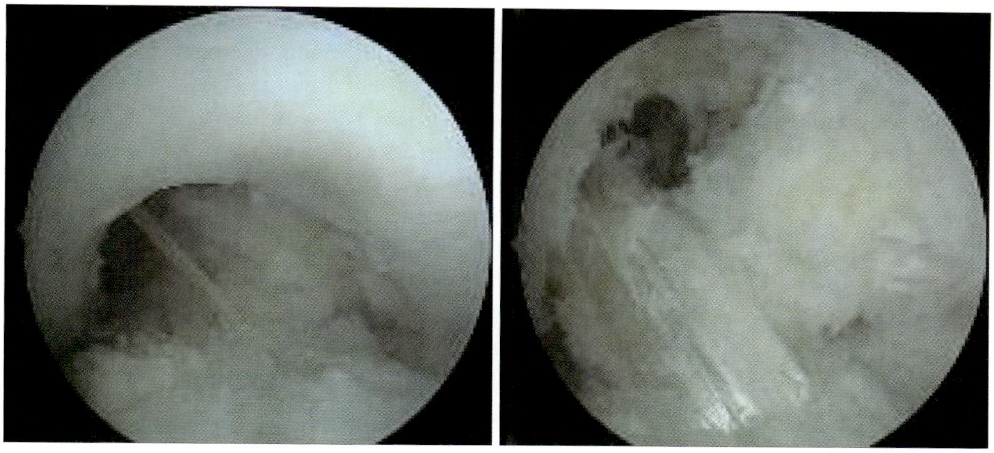

Fig. 4.20 Arthroscopic views through the anterolateral portal showing the correct position of the new ligament which does not create roof or posterior cruciate ligament (PCL) impingement

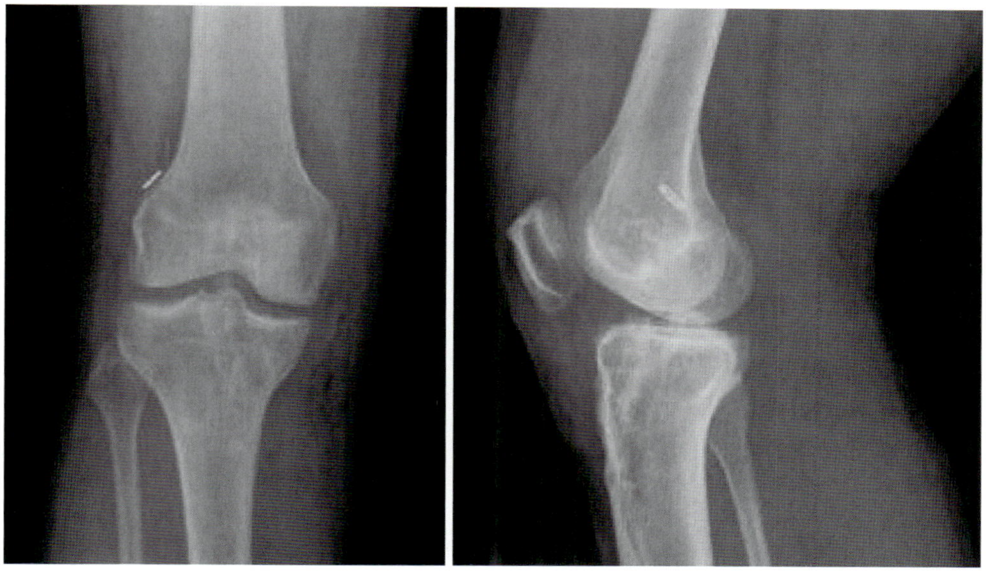

Fig. 4.21 AP (antero-posterior) and lateral postoperative X-rays showing adequate tunnel positioning

Case Example

A 25 years old male presents with elongated B-PT-B graft, extension deficit and grade II chondral damage of the medial compartment. The patient has initially torn his ACL 2 years before. The index reconstruction was performed using the transtibial (TT) technique. The sagittal MRI T2 was suggestive for an elongated graft and the patellar tendon showed signs of tendinitis (Fig. 4.22). The patient had a history of giving way since index surgery. The clinical exam found antero-posterior instability and KT-1000 side to side difference of 7 mm and 5° of extension deficit. CT exam showed improper tunnel positioning (femoral vertical and anterior) and minor tibial tunnel widening (Fig. 4.23). We performed one stage anatomic SB revision. Arthroscopic exploration confirmed the elongated graft with roof impingement and it was debrided wising a shaver and a punch (Fig. 4.24). Ipsilateral semitendinosus and gracilis were harvested and quadrupled into a size 7.5 neoligament. The new femoral tunnel was drilled in the anatomic footprint through the anteromedial portal. We then drilled a new tibial tunnel, more posterior to the previous, in the anatomic position (Fig. 4.25). For fixation we used a cortical button for the femur and 9.35 absorbable (PLLA) interference screw on the tibia in 20° of flexion. Proper placement of the new ligament does not create notch or posterior cruciate ligament (PCL) impingement (Fig. 4.26). Proper tunnel positioning can be seen on the postoperative X-rays (Fig. 4.27).

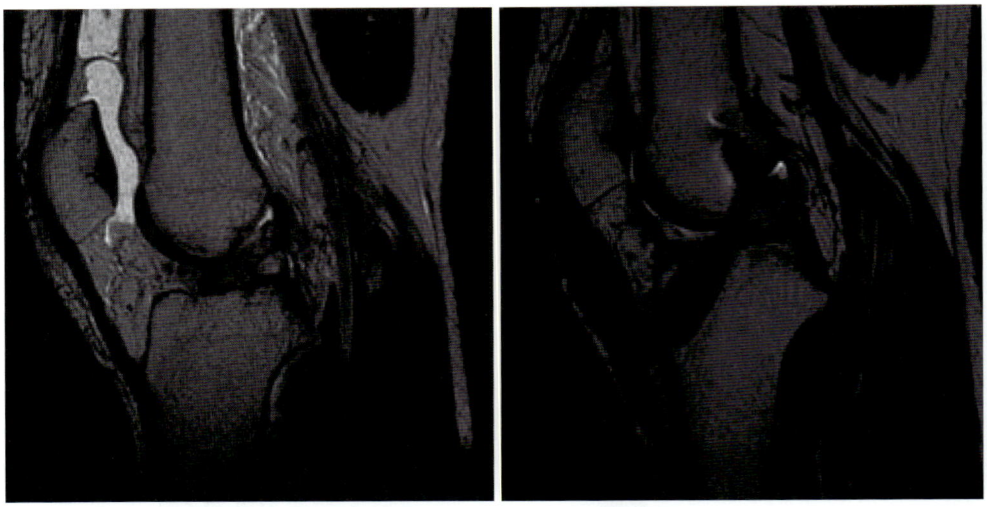

Fig. 4.22 Sagittal MRI T2 soon after the initial injury with a hyperintense, discontinued ACL in the proximal part; 1 year after index reconstruction, the MRI is suggestive for an elongated graft and the patellar tendon is thickened

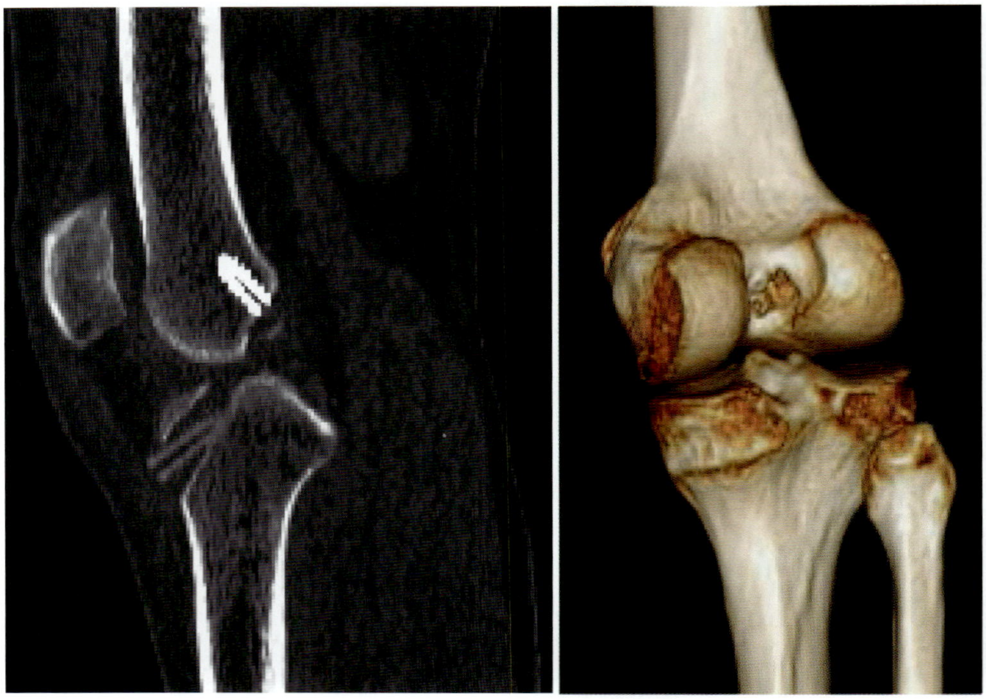

Fig. 4.23 Sagittal CT exam and 3D volume rendering (posteromedial oblique view) showing improper tunnel positioning (femoral vertical and anterior) and minor tibial tunnel widening

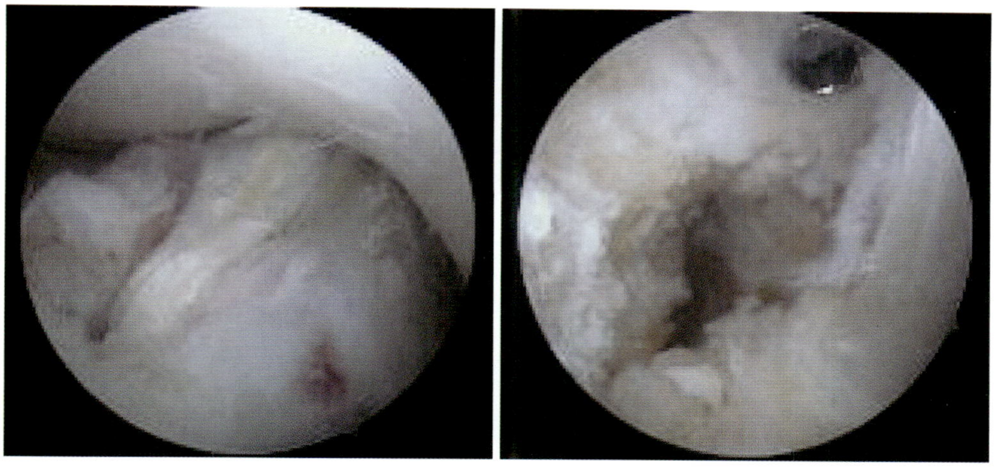

Fig. 4.24 Arthroscopic exploration through the anteromedial portal confirms roof impingement and improper femoral aperture (high)

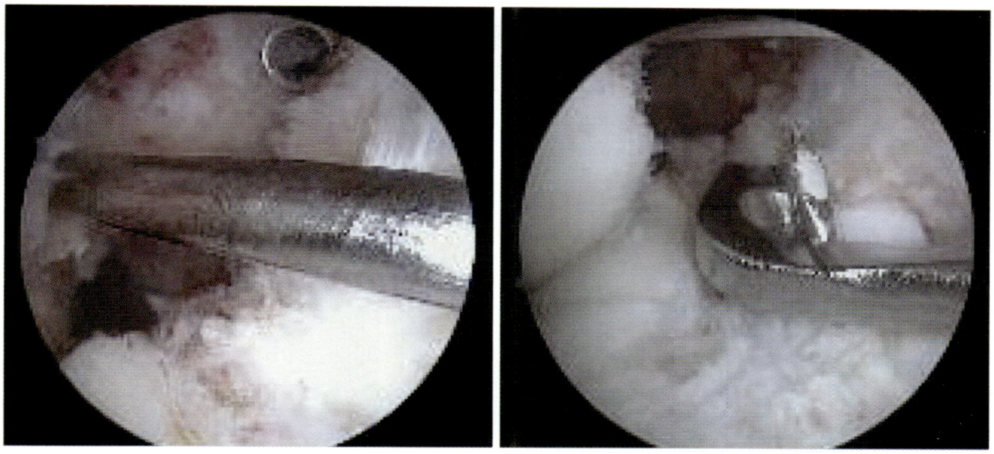

Fig. 4.25 Arthroscopic views through the anterolateral portal showing the correct position of the femoral and tibial apertures: lower and deeper on the lateral condyle and more posterior on the tibia respectively

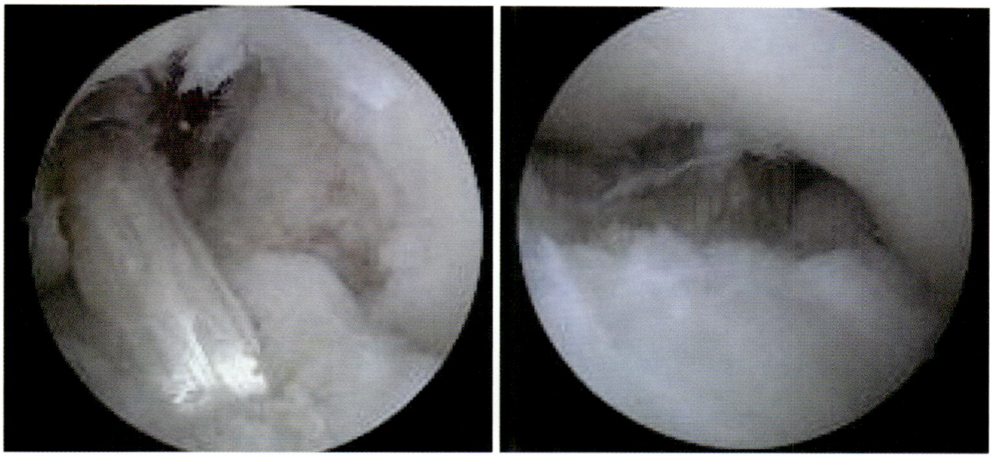

Fig. 4.26 Arthroscopic views through the anterolateral and anteromedial portals respectively, showing the correct position of the new ligament which does not create PCL or roof impingement

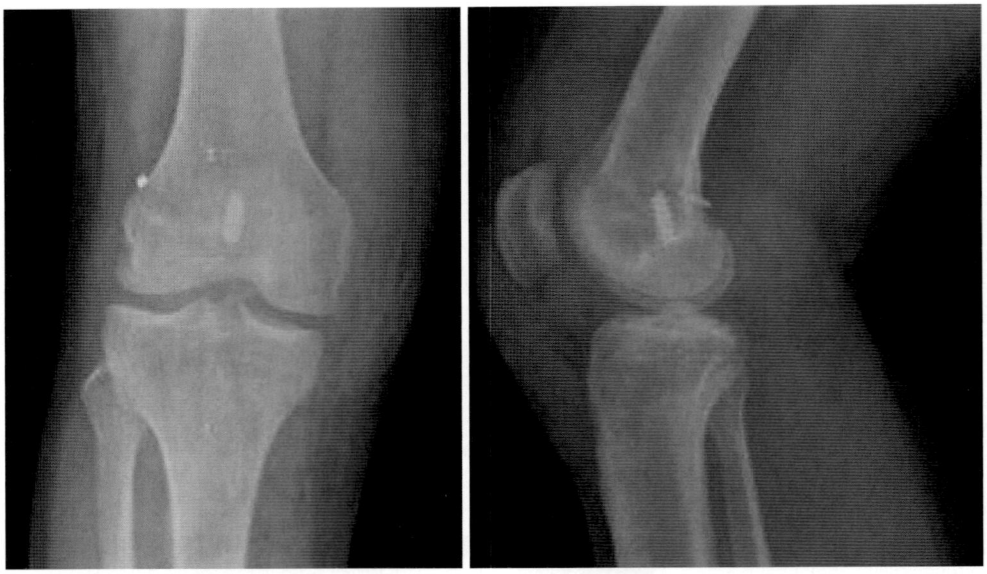

Fig. 4.27 AP and lateral postoperative X-rays showing adequate tunnel positioning compared to the previous femoral tunnel

Case Example

A 30 years old male presented with bilateral ACL reconstructions using B-PT-B grafts and TT techniques. The sagittal MRI T2 of the left knee was suggestive for an elongated and vertical graft (Fig. 4.28). The patient had a history of giving way that was aggravated after a recent trauma. The clinical exam found antero-posterior instability and KT-1000 side to side difference of 3 mm. CT exam showed improper graft positioning (femoral vertical and anterior) and good tunnel bone filling. We performed one stage anatomic SB revision. Arthroscopic exploration confirmed the insufficient graft (Fig. 4.29). After debridement the medial and lateral compartments were explored (Figs. 4.30, 4.31, and 4.32). Ipsilateral semitendinosus and gracilis were harvested and quadrupled into a size 8 neoligament. The new femoral tunnel was drilled in the anatomic footprint through the anteromedial portal (Fig. 4.33). We then drilled a new tibial tunnel converging towards the same aperture. For fixation we used a cortical button for the femur and 9.35 absorbable (PLLA) interference screw on the tibia in 20° of flexion. Proper placement of the new ligament does not create notch or PCL impingement (Fig. 4.34). Proper tunnel positioning can be seen on the postoperative CT and X-rays (Fig. 4.35).

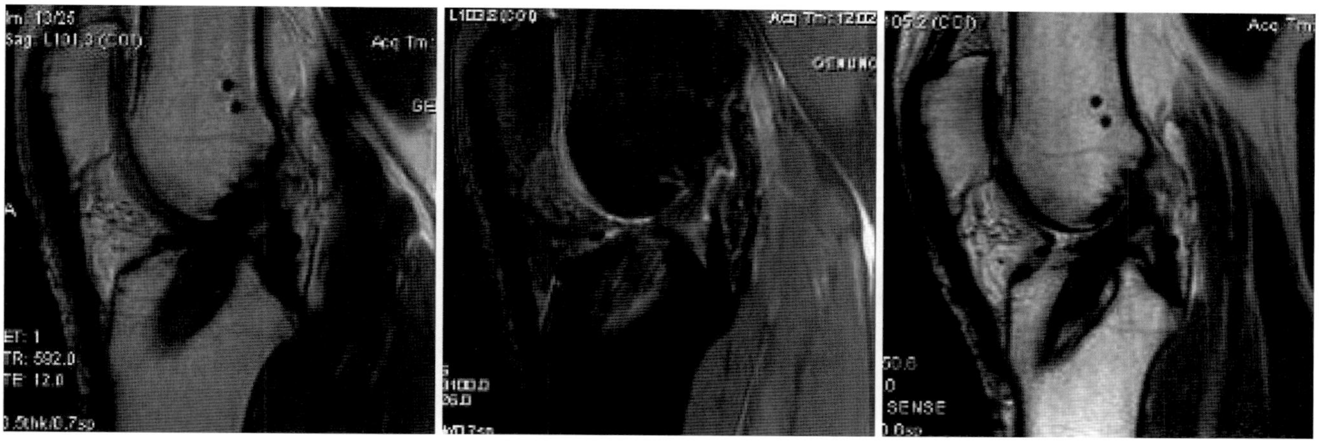

Fig. 4.28 The sagittal MRI T2 of the left knee was suggestive for an elongated and vertical graft

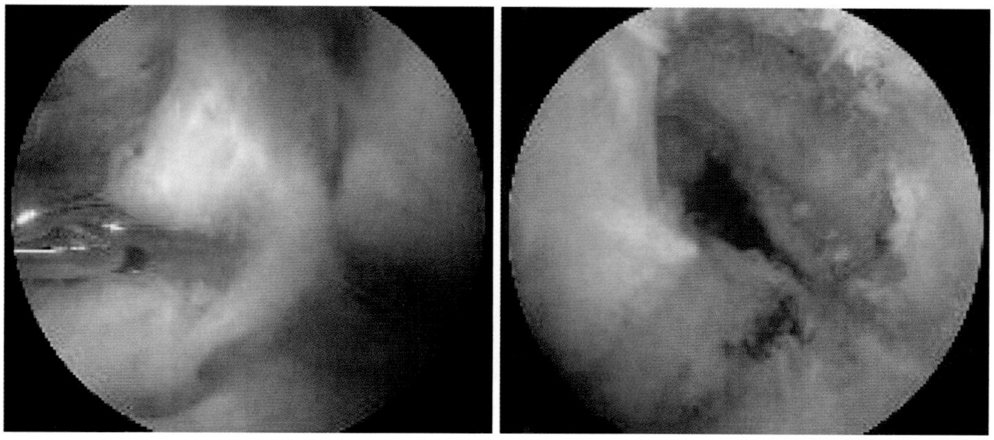

Fig. 4.29 Arthroscopic exploration through the antero lateral and anteromedial portals confirmed the insufficient graft

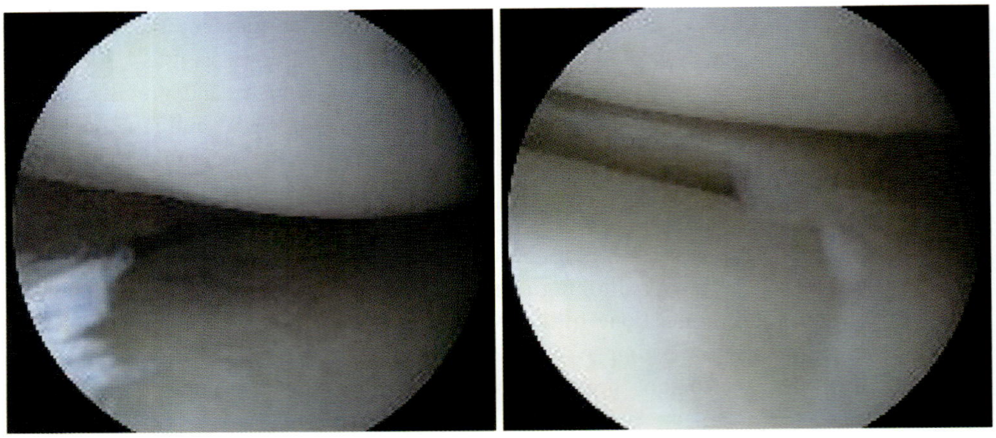

Fig. 4.30 The medial and lateral compartments were explored through the anteromedial and anterolateral portals respectively; the medial compartment shows arthritic changes and a degenerated meniscus with previous partial meniscectomy

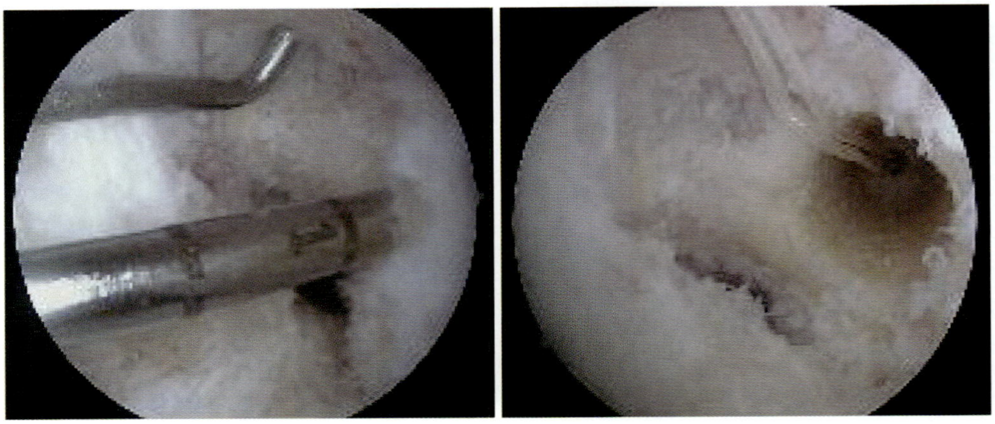

Fig. 4.31 The new femoral tunnel was drilled in the anatomic footprint through the anteromedial portal; the current position is lower and is surrounded by a sufficient bone bridge (seen here from the anteromedial portal)

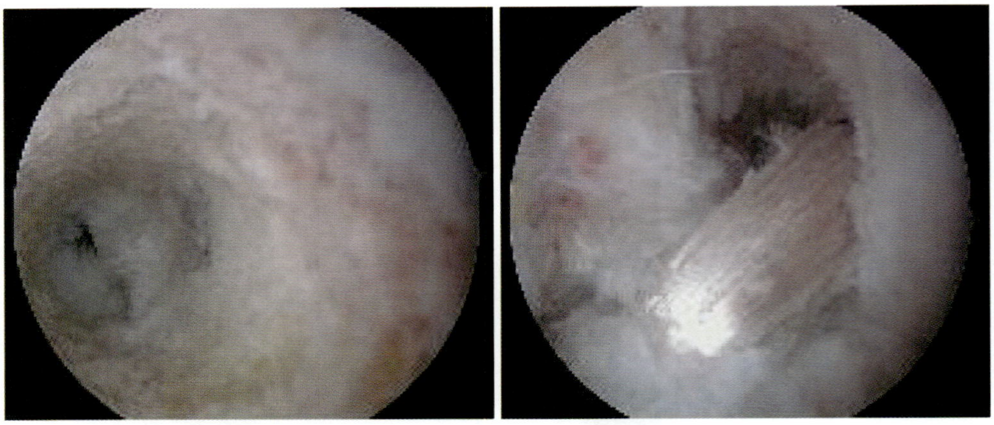

Fig. 4.32 We then drilled a new tibial tunnel converging towards the same aperture. Seen here from inside the distal tunnel; proper placement of the new ligament seen here through the anterolateral portal

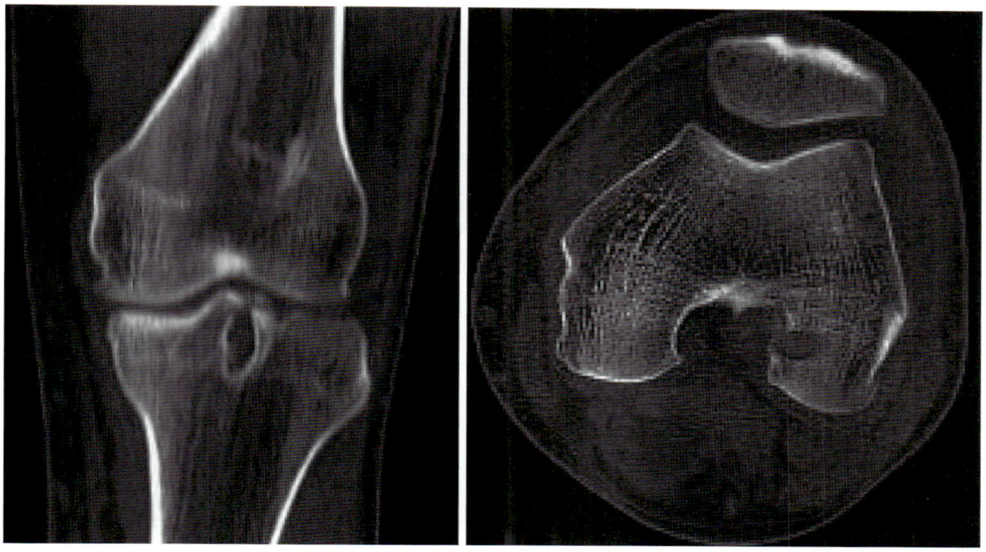

Fig. 4.33 Tunnel convergence towards the apertures can be seen on the postoperative coronal and axial CT

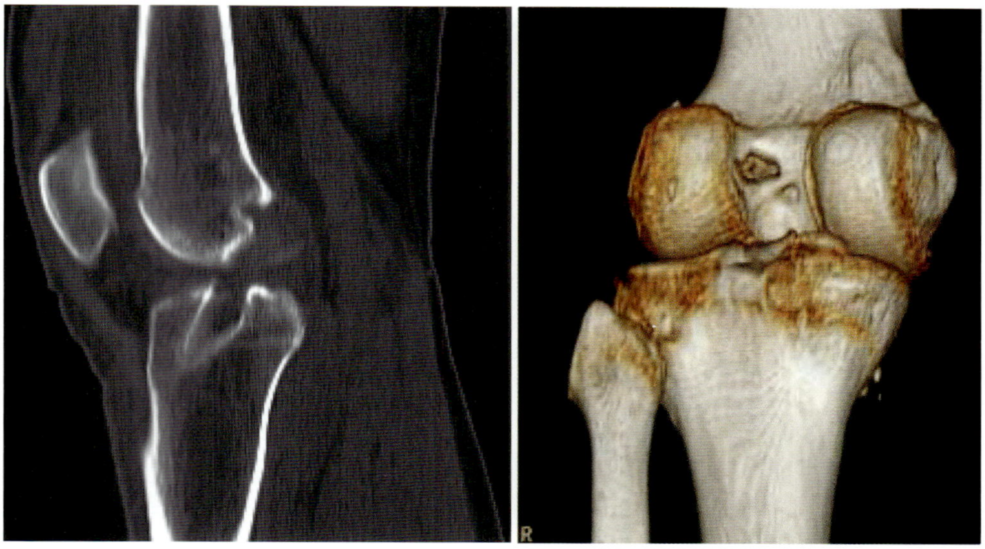

Fig. 4.34 Sagittal CT and 3D volume rendering (posteromedial oblique view) showing proper positioning of the new tunnels

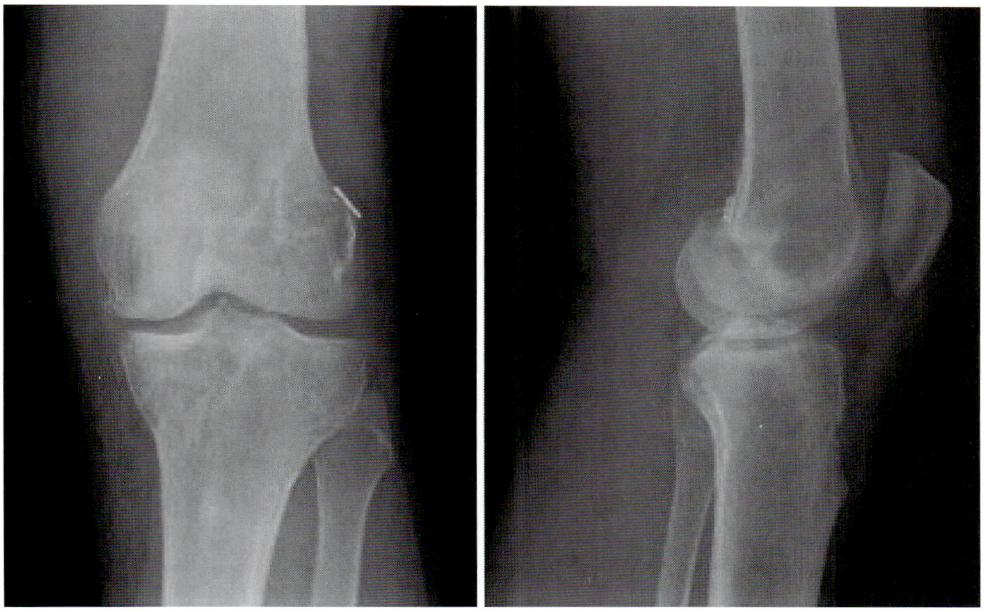

Fig. 4.35 AP and lateral postoperative X-rays showing adequate new tunnel positioning and arthritic degeneration of the medial compartment

4.7 Initial Anatomic Reconstruction

When the previous SB tunnels are in the anatomic location and there is only limited enlargement, they can be redrilled to a slightly larger size and reused [15]. When the initial and planned anatomic tunnels are partially overlapping or significant enlargement has occurred additional bone grafting is required. This is usually performed as staged arthroscopic procedures spaced 3 months apart [43].

Revision after failed DB reconstructions is more challenging. If the tunnels are well placed and not enlarged, they can also be redrilled and used as is. If significant enlargement has occurred, the options usually are staged procedures with bone grafting or an over the top procedure [45]. If any of the two index bundles overlap with the planned location for revision, a staged procedure or slightly over the top positioning of the (antero-medial) AM bundle can be accepted [44].

Case Example

A 34 years old male with bilateral ACL reconstructions using hamstrings grafts and trans AM femoral drilling. The right knee primary reconstruction was made 5 years ago. The patient had a new traumatic event 6 months before he decided to undergo revision. The patient had a history of giving way and the clinical exam found antero-posterior instability (anterior drawer, and Lachman 3+). The sagittal MRI T2 of the left knee was suggestive for a proximal torn graft (Fig. 4.36). CT exam showed proper tunnels (Fig. 4.37). We performed one stage anatomic SB revision. Arthroscopic exploration confirmed the torn graft (Fig. 4.38). After debridement (Fig. 4.39) the medial and lateral compartments were explored and found the medial compartment had grade II chondral lesions and a damaged meniscus (Fig. 4.39). Ipsilateral B-PT-B was harvested and prepared into a size 8 neoligament. The new femoral tunnel was drilled in the center of the old one to a size 9 in depth and 11 at the aperture through the anteromedial portal (Fig. 4.40). We then drilled the tibial tunnel converging towards the same aperture (Fig. 4.41). For fixation we used absorbable (PLLA) interference screw on the femur (10.28) and tibia (10.30) in 20° of flexion. Proper fixation of the new ligament can be seen through the anterolateral portal (Fig. 4.42).

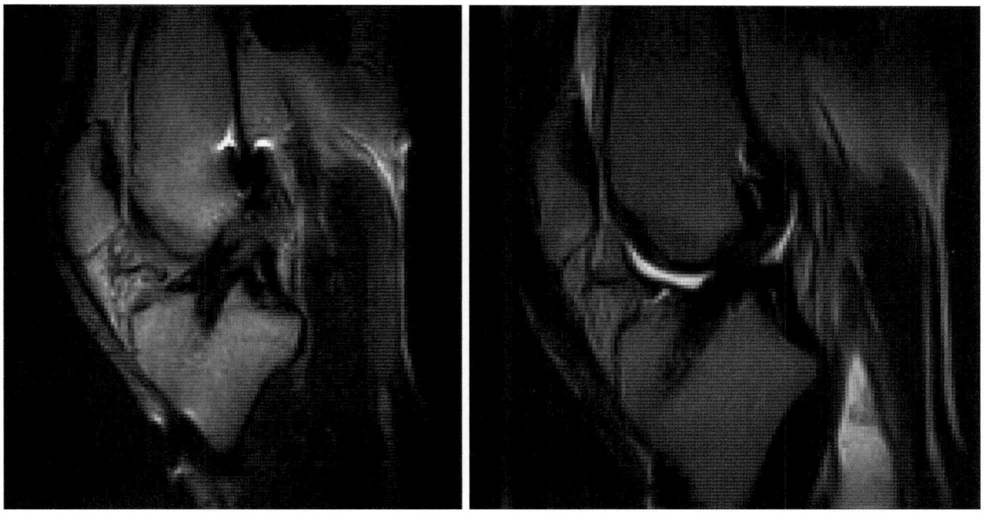

Fig. 4.36 The sagittal MRI T2 of the left knee was suggestive for a proximal torn graft. On the right, the 9 moths follow-up with a healing graft and thickened patellar tendon

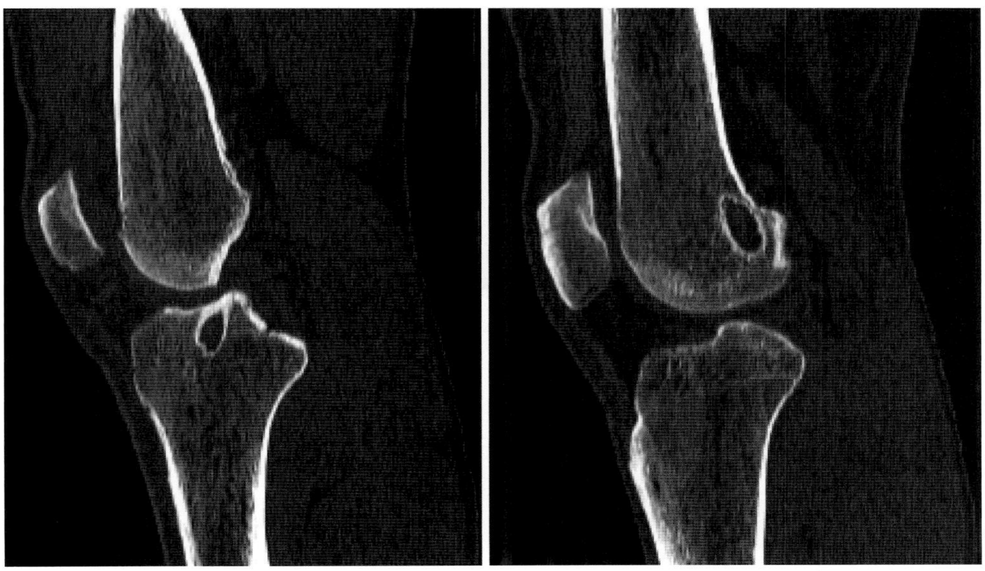

Fig. 4.37 CT exam showed proper tunnels

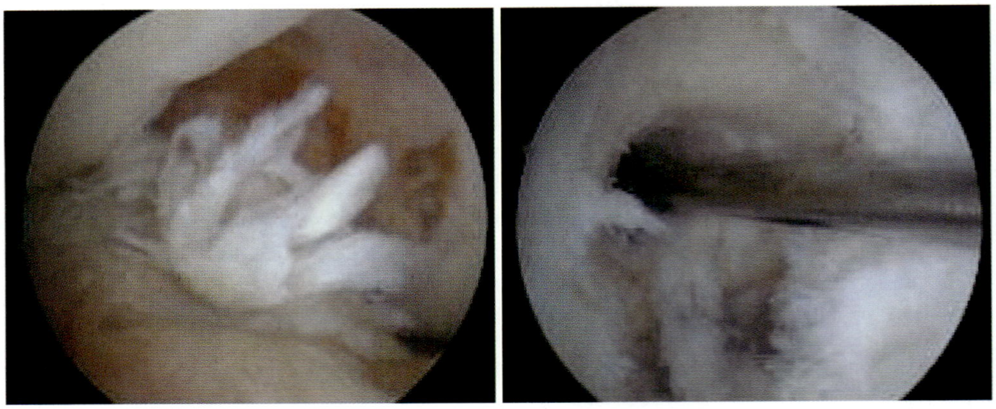

Fig. 4.38 Arthroscopic exploration confirmed the torn graft (anterolateral portal) and the new femoral tunnel was drilled in the center of the old one

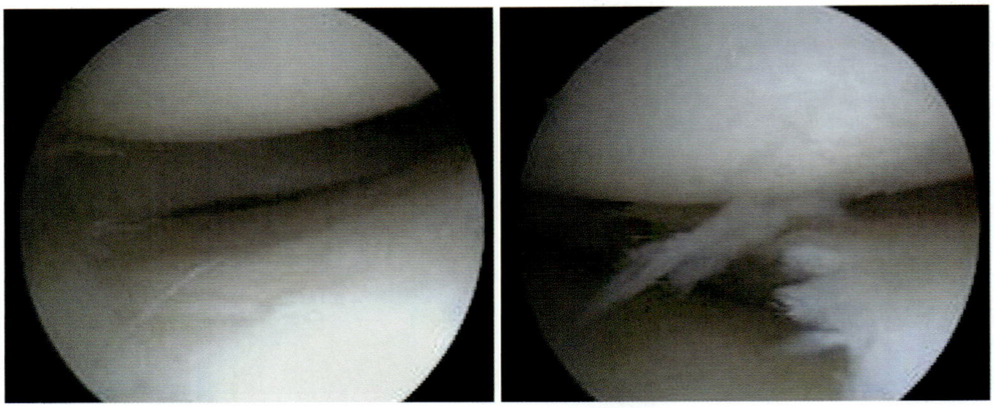

Fig. 4.39 The lateral and medial compartments were explored and found the medial compartment had grade II chondral lesions and a damaged meniscus

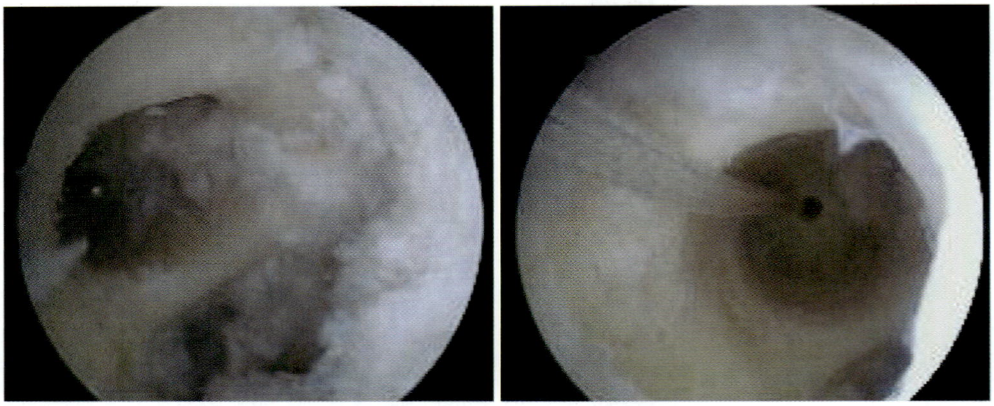

Fig. 4.40 The new femoral tunnel was drilled to a size 8 in depth and 10 at the aperture, through the anteromedial portal

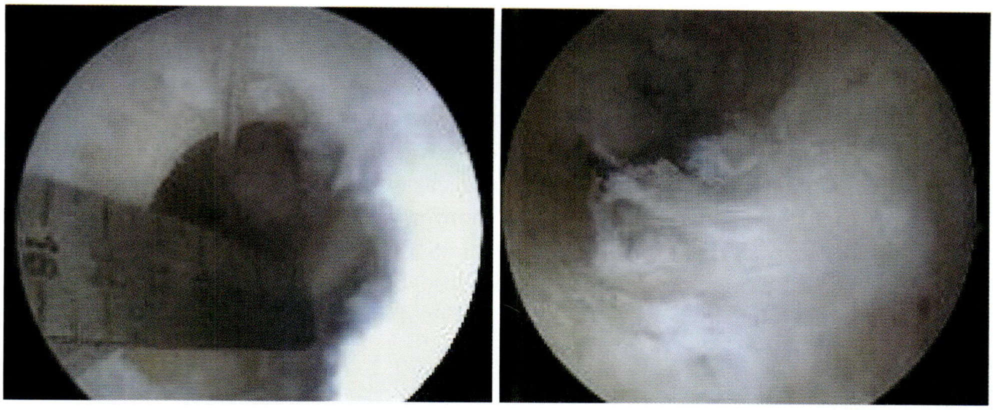

Fig. 4.41 The new femoral tunnel was drilled in the anatomic footprint. We then drilled the tibial tunnel converging towards the same aperture. Seen here from inside the distal tunnel

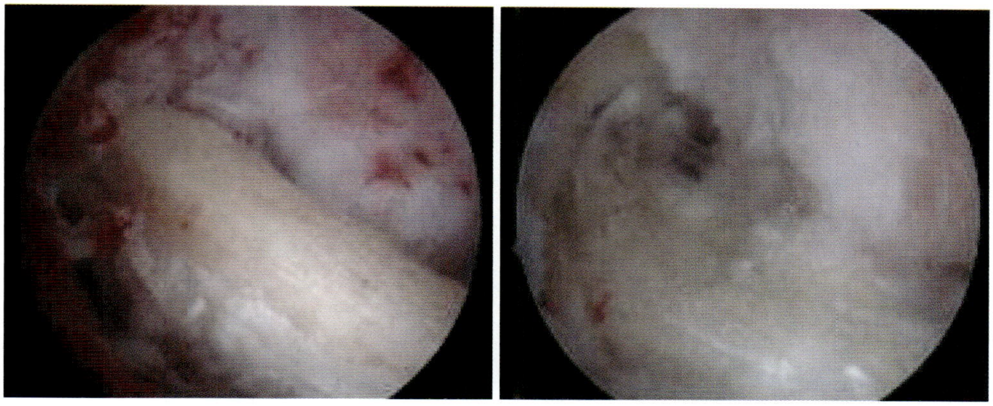

Fig. 4.42 Proper fixation of the new ligament seen here through the anterolateral portal

Case Example

A 28 years old male with right knee ACL reconstruction using hamstrings grafts and anatomic SB technique. The sagittal MRI T2 was suggestive for a completely torn neoligament (Fig. 4.43). The patient had a history of giving way and locking after a recent trauma. The clinical exam found antero-posterior instability (anterior drawer, and Lachman 3+). We performed one stage anatomic SB revision. Arthroscopic exploration confirmed the absence of the graft, with the remnant attached to the PCL (Fig. 4.44). After debridement we performed medial meniscectomy. Ipsilateral B-PT-B was harvested and prepared into a size 8 neoligament. The new femoral tunnel was drilled in the center of the old one to a size 9 at the aperture through the anteromedial portal. We then drilled the tibial tunnel converging towards the same aperture. For fixation we used absorbable (composite) interference screw on the femur (8.28) and tibia (10.30) in 20° of flexion. Fixation of the new ligament can be seen through the anterolateral portal (Fig. 4.45).

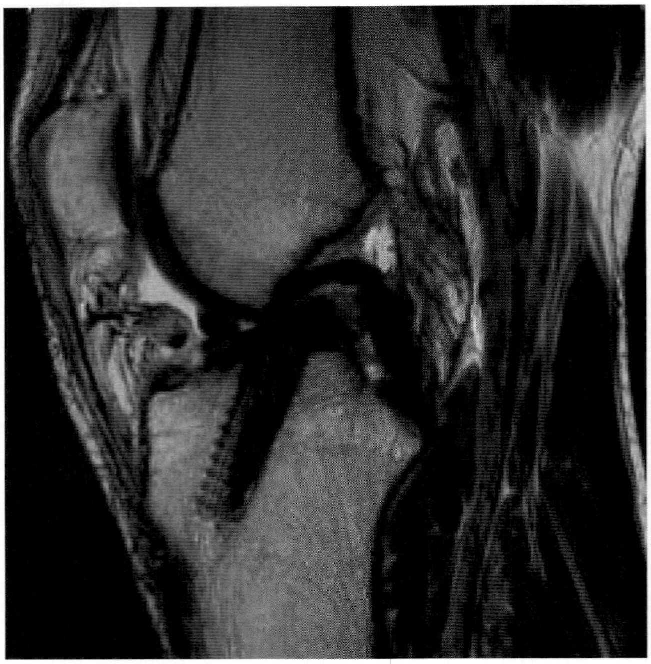

Fig. 4.43 Sagittal MRI T2 suggestive for a completely torn neoligament and a bucket handle medial meniscus tear with the internal border in the intercondylar space

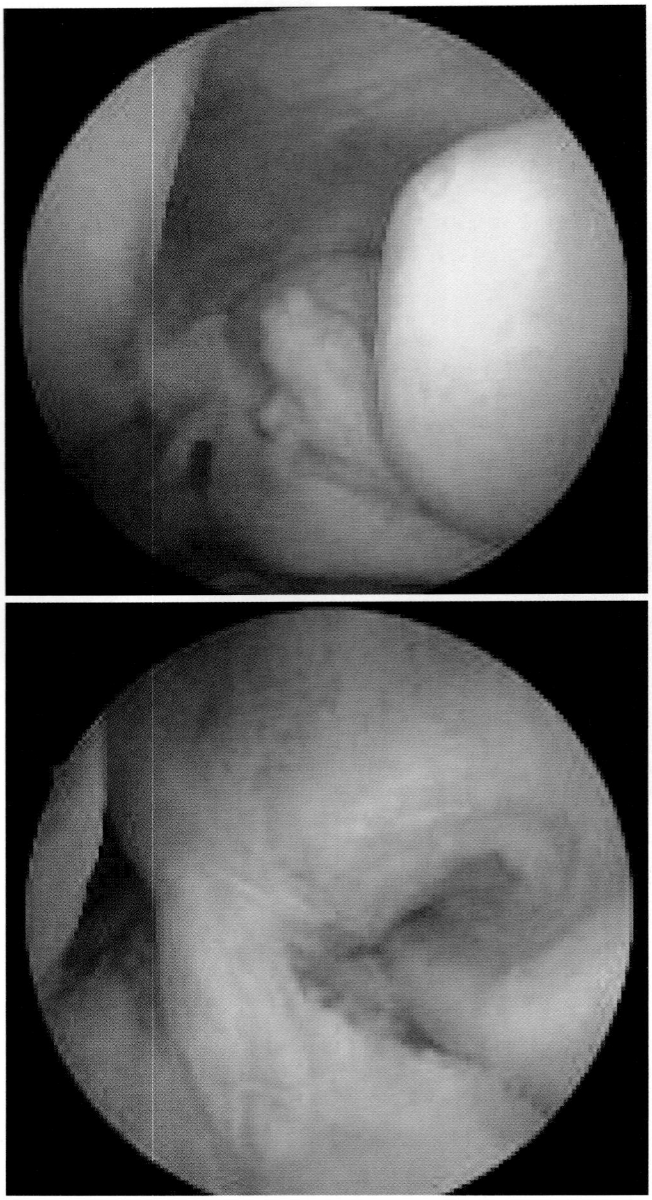

Fig. 4.44 Arthroscopic exploration (anterolateral portal) confirmed the absence of the graft, with the remnant attached to the PCL

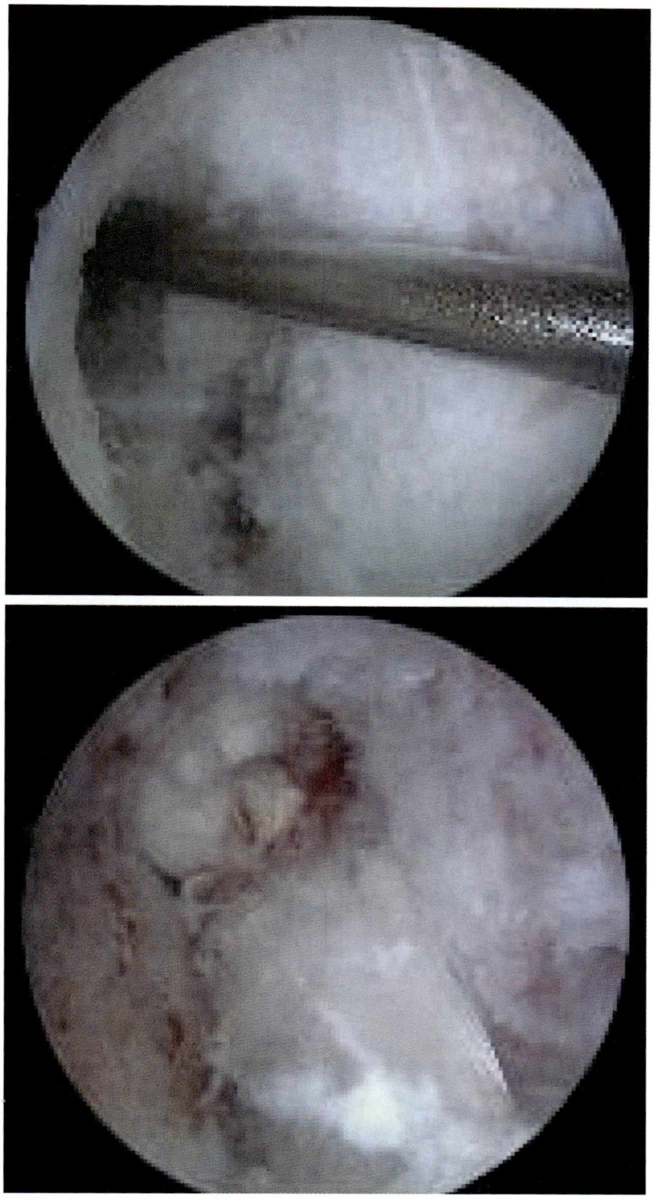

Fig. 4.45 The new femoral tunnel was drilled in the center of the old one through the anteromedial portal. For fixation we used absorbable (composite) interference screws. Proper placement of the new ligament

4.8 Outcomes After Revision ACL

Overall, the results after revision reconstructions are satisfactory [13] but poorer compared to primary procedures [36, 47]. Repeat surgery, associated lesions and greater heterogeneity of the cases might explain why these knees are stable but less clinically satisfied [46]. This aspect should be clarified with the patients prior to surgery [3, 22, 53].

The postoperative outcomes are evaluated in the same manner after primary and revision ACL reconstructions. Pain and patient perceived stability, range of motion and antero-posterior laxity are mostly reported using IKDC (International Knee Documentation Committee), KOOS (Knee injury and Osteoarthritis Outcome Score) and Tegner Lysholm scores, anterior drawer, Lachman and pivot shift or KT-1000 arthrometer (MEDmetric, San Diego, CA) testing. No relation was found between clinical or stability results and MRI findings [19].

Weiler et al. reported worse Lysholm but similar IKDC scores and objective knee stability for revision reconstructions compared to primary procedures [47]. Another study also reported decreased KOOS scores and more degenerative changes in revision patients but comparable IKDC functional outcome and stability [54]. For revision patients, Denti et al. reported that of patients most patients had good or excellent clinical scores (82 % for IKDC and 70 % for Lysholm), 68 % of patients had negative Lachman tests and 90 % had KT-1000 side-to-side difference of maximum 5 mm [49]. For DB reconstructions, only the positive pivot-shift test appears to be more prevalent after revision procedures [50].

The Nordic registries have the advantage of presenting data from very high volumes of patients. The KOOS scores for ACL revisions in the Danish report are 73 for symptoms, 78 for pain, 84 for activities of daily living, 52 for sports and 48 for quality of life [22]. These values are lower than for primary procedures but better than what is expected after multiligament reconstructions [25]. Especially sports and quality of life KOOS scores are decreased in the setting of revision ACL procedures. These values rose from 42 and 39 preoperatively to only 50 at follow-up while KT-1000 increased from 6.2 to 2.5 respectively. The Swedish registry also reported lower KOOS values for revisions at all examinations [4]. The French multicenter ACL revision evaluation found lower IKDC values and pivot-shift results, but the outcomes were better if the menisci were preserved and the cause was femoral malposition [23]. In general, mean Lysholm and IKDC scores after revision ACL should be expected at 82.1 and 74.8 respectively [8].

Osteoarthritic changes appear to be an important outcome factor after revision reconstruction [19]. One measure that could potentially prevent degeneration is reducing the time until the secondary procedure [48]. In the MOON and MARS groups, a previous meniscectomy increased the likelihood of articular cartilage damage [51]. Meniscal repair exhibits protective chondral properties even in revision surgery, which underlines the importance of meniscal preservation [52].

Failure rates for revision reconstructions are three to four times higher than for primary procedures [8, 36]. They vary from 6 % at 6 years [3, 22], to 11 % [14] and even 13.7 % [8]. Isolated ACL revision can have twice as high revision rated compared to reconstructions associated with extra-articular tenodesis [14].

When even the revision ACL fails, the question can sometimes be whether or not further surgery is advisable. Patients might predominantly choose to decline a re-revision [14]. Lysholm and IKDC scores can improve postoperatively to 82 and 80 respectively in the absence of grade 3 to 4 chondral damage, which leads to less favorable clinical outcomes and return to prior activity levels [55].

References

1. Maletis GB, Granan LP, Inacio MC, Funahashi TT, Engebretsen L. Comparison of community-based ACL reconstruction registries in the U.S. and Norway. J Bone Joint Surg Am. 2011;93 Suppl 3:31–6.
2. Maletis GB, Inacio MC, Funahashi TT. Analysis of 16,192 anterior cruciate ligament reconstructions from a community-based registry. Am J Sports Med. 2013;41(9):2090–8.
3. Lind M, Menhert F, Pedersen AB. Incidence and outcome after revision anterior cruciate ligament reconstruction: results from the Danish registry for knee ligament reconstructions. Am J Sports Med. 2012;40(7):1551–7.
4. Ahldén M, Samuelsson K, Sernert N, Forssblad M, Karlsson J, Kartus J. The Swedish National Anterior Cruciate Ligament Register: a report on baseline variables and outcomes of surgery for almost 18,000 patients. Am J Sports Med. 2012;40(10):2230–5.
5. Wright RW, Dunn WR, Amendola A, Andrish JT, Bergfeld J, Kaeding CC, Marx RG, McCarty EC, Parker RD, Wolcott M, Wolf BR, Spindler KP. Risk of tearing the intact anterior cruciate ligament in the contralateral knee and rupturing the anterior cruciate ligament graft during the first 2 years after anterior cruciate ligament reconstruction: a prospective MOON cohort study. Am J Sports Med. 2007;35(7):1131–4.
6. Hettrich CM, Dunn WR, Reinke EK; MOON Group, Spindler KP. The rate of subsequent surgery and predictors after anterior cruciate ligament reconstruction: two- and 6-year follow-up results from a multicenter cohort. Am J Sports Med. 2013;41(7):1534–40.
7. Wright RW, Huston LJ, Spindler KP, Dunn WR, Haas AK, Allen CR, Cooper DE, DeBerardino TM, Lantz BB, Mann BJ, Stuart MJ. Descriptive epidemiology of the Multicenter ACL Revision Study (MARS) cohort. Am J Sports Med. 2010;38(10):1979–86.
8. Wright RW, Gill CS, Chen L, Brophy RH, Matava MJ, Smith MV, Mall NA. Outcome of revision anterior cruciate ligament reconstruction: a systematic review. J Bone Joint Surg Am. 2012;94(6):531–6.
9. Mayr R, Rosenberger R, Agraharam D, Smekal V, El Attal R. Revision anterior cruciate ligament reconstruction: an update. Arch Orthop Trauma Surg. 2012;132:1299–313.
10. Middleton KK, Hamilton T, Irrgang JJ, Karlsson J, Harner CD, Fu FH. Anatomic anterior cruciate ligament (ACL) reconstruction: a global perspective. Part 1. Knee Surg Sports Traumatol Arthrosc. 2014;22(7):1467–82.
11. Wasserstein D, Khoshbin A, Dwyer T, Chahal J, Gandhi R, Mahomed N, Ogilvie-Harris D. Risk factors for recurrent anterior cruciate ligament reconstruction: a population study in Ontario, Canada, with 5-year follow-up. Am J Sports Med. 2013;41(9):2099–107.
12. Shelbourne KD, Gray T, Haro M. Incidence of subsequent injury to either knee within 5 years after anterior cruciate ligament reconstruction with patellar tendon autograft. Am J Sports Med. 2009;37(2):246–51.
13. Ferretti A, Conteduca F, Monaco E, De Carli A, D'Arrigo C. Revision anterior cruciate ligament reconstruction with doubled semitendinosus and gracilis tendons and lateral extra-articular reconstruction. J Bone Joint Surg Am. 2006;88(11):2373–9.
14. Trojani C, Beaufils P, Burdin G, Bussière C, Chassaing V, Djian P, Dubrana F, Ehkirch FP, Franceschi JP, Hulet C, Jouve F, Potel JF, Sbihi A, Neyret P, Colombet P. Revision ACL reconstruction: influence of a lateral tenodesis. Knee Surg Sports Traumatol Arthrosc. 2012;20(8):1565–70.
15. van Eck CF, Schreiber VM, Liu TT, Fu FH. The anatomic approach to primary, revision and augmentation anterior cruciate ligament reconstruction. Knee Surg Sports Traumatol Arthrosc. 2010;18(9):1154–63.
16. Shino K, Mae T, Nakamura N. Surgical technique: revision ACL reconstruction with a rectangular tunnel technique. Clin Orthop Relat Res. 2012;470(3):843–52.
17. Miyawaki M, Hensler D, Illingworth KD, Irrgang JJ, Fu FH. Signal intensity on magnetic resonance imaging after allograft double-bundle anterior cruciate ligament reconstruction. Knee Surg Sports Traumatol Arthrosc. 2014;22(5):1002–8.
18. Hosseini A, Lodhia P, Van de Velde SK, Asnis PD, Zarins B, Gill TJ, Li G. Tunnel position and graft orientation in failed anterior cruciate ligament reconstruction: a clinical and imaging analysis. Int Orthop. 2012;36(4):845–52.
19. Ahn JH, Lee YS, Chang MJ, Yim HS. Analysis of revision anterior cruciate ligament reconstruction according to the combined injury, degenerative change, and MRI findings. Knee. 2010. doi:10.1016/j.knee.2010.11.001.
20. Marchant BG, Noyes FR, Barber-Westin SD, Fleckenstein C. Prevalence of nonanatomical graft placement in a series of failed anterior cruciate ligament reconstructions. Am J Sports Med. 2010;38(10):1987–96.
21. Morgan JA, Dahm D, Levy B, Stuart MJ, MARS Study Group. Femoral tunnel malposition in ACL revision reconstruction. J Knee Surg. 2012;25(5):361–8.
22. Lind M, Lund B, Faunø P, Said S, Miller LL, Christiansen SE. Medium to long-term follow-up after ACL revision. Knee Surg Sports Traumatol Arthrosc. 2012;20(1):166–72.
23. Trojani C, Sbihi A, Djian P, Potel JF, Hulet C, Jouve F, Bussiere C, Ehkirch FP, Burdin G, Dubrana F, Beaufils P, Franceschi JP, Chassaing V, Colombet P, Neyret P. Causes for failure of ACL reconstruction and influence of meniscectomies after revision. Knee Surg Sports Traumatol Arthrosc. 2011;19(2):196–201.
24. Magnussen RA, Lawrence JT, West RL, Toth AP, Taylor DC, Garrett WE. Graft size and patient age are predictors of early revision after anterior cruciate ligament reconstruction with hamstring autograft. Arthroscopy. 2012;28(4):526–31.
25. Lind M, Menhert F, Pedersen AB. The first results from the Danish ACL reconstruction registry: epidemiologic and 2 year follow-up results from 5,818 knee ligament reconstructions. Knee Surg Sports Traumatol Arthrosc. 2009;17(2):117–24.
26. van Eck CF, Kropf EJ, Romanowski JR, Lesniak BP, Tranovich MJ, van Dijk CN, Fu FH. Factors that influence the intraarticular rupture pattern of the ACL graft following singlebundle reconstruction. Knee Surg Sports Traumatol Arthrosc. 2011;19(8):1243–8.
27. van Eck CF, Kropf EJ, Romanowski JR, Lesniak BP, Tranovich MJ, van Dijk CN, Fu FH. ACL graft re-rupture after double-bundle reconstruction: factors that influence the intra-articular pattern of injury. Knee Surg Sports Traumatol Arthrosc. 2011;19:340–6.

28. Suomalainen P, Järvelä T, Paakkala A, Kannus P, Järvinen M. Double-bundle versus single-bundle anterior cruciate ligament reconstruction: a prospective randomized study with 5-year results. Am J Sports Med. 2012;40(7):1511–8.
29. Rahr-Wagner L, Thillemann TM, Pedersen AB, Lind MC. Increased risk of revision after anteromedial compared with transtibial drilling of the femoral tunnel during primary anterior cruciate ligament reconstruction: results from the Danish Knee Ligament Reconstruction Register. Arthroscopy. 2013;29(1):98–105.
30. Hoser C, Tecklenburg K, Kuenzel KH, Fink C. Postoperative evaluation of femoral tunnel position in ACL reconstruction: plain radiography versus computed tomography. Knee Surg Sports Traumatol Arthrosc. 2005;13(4):256–62.
31. Marchant Jr MH, Willimon SC, Vinson E, Pietrobon R, Garrett WE, Higgins LD. Comparison of plain radiography, computed tomography, and magnetic resonance imaging in the evaluation of bone tunnel widening after anterior cruciate ligament reconstruction. Knee Surg Sports Traumatol Arthrosc. 2010;18(8):1059–64.
32. Webster KE, Feller JA, Elliott J, Hutchison A, Payne R. A comparison of bone tunnel measurements using computed tomography and digital plain radiography after anterior cruciate ligament reconstruction. Arthroscopy. 2004;20:946–50.
33. Lehmann AK, Osada N, Zantop T, Raschke MJ, Petersen W. Femoral bridge stability in double-bundle ACL reconstruction: impact of bridge width and different fixation techniques on the structural properties of the graft/femur complex. Arch Orthop Trauma Surg. 2009;129(8):1127–32.
34. Kopf S, Forsythe B, Wong AK, Tashman S, Anderst W, Irrgang JJ, Fu FH. Nonanatomic tunnel position in traditional transtibial single-bundle anterior cruciate ligament reconstruction evaluated by 3-D computed tomography. J Bone Joint Surg Am. 2010;92:1427–31.
35. Magnussen RA, Debieux P, Benjamin B, Lustig S, Demey G, Servien E, Neyret P. A CT-based classification of prior ACL femoral tunnel location for planning revision ACL surgery. Knee Surg Sports Traumatol Arthrosc. 2012;20(7):1298–306.
36. Noyes FR, Barber-Westin SD. Revision anterior cruciate surgery with use of bone-patellar tendon-bone autogenous grafts. J Bone Joint Surg Am. 2001;83-A(8):1131–43.
37. Ahn JH, Lee YS, Ha HC. Comparison of revision surgery with primary anterior cruciate ligament reconstruction and outcome of revision surgery between different graft materials. Am J Sports Med. 2008;36(10):1889–95.
38. Mayr HO, Willkomm D, Stoehr A, Schettle M, Suedkamp NP, Bernstein A, Hube R. Revision of anterior cruciate ligament reconstruction with patellar tendon allograft and autograft: 2- and 5-year results. Arch Orthop Trauma Surg. 2012;132:867–74.
39. Ferretti A, Monaco E, Caperna L, Palma T, Conteduca F. Revision ACL reconstruction using contralateral hamstrings. Knee Surg Sports Traumatol Arthrosc. 2013;21(3):690–5.
40. Mariscalco MW, Flanigan DC, Mitchell J, Pedroza AD, Jones MH, Andrish JT, Parker RD, Kaeding CC, Magnussen RA. The influence of hamstring autograft size on patient-reported outcomes and risk of revision after anterior cruciate ligament reconstruction: a Multicenter Orthopaedic Outcomes Network (MOON) Cohort Study. Arthroscopy. 2013;29(12):1948–53.
41. Forkel P, Petersen W. Anatomic reconstruction of the anterior cruciate ligament with the autologous quadriceps tendon: primary and revision surgery. Oper Orthop Traumatol. 2014;26(1):30–42.
42. Zantop T, Petersen W. Double bundle revision of a malplaced single bundle vertical ACL reconstruction: ACL revision surgery using a two femoral tunnel technique. Arch Orthop Trauma Surg. 2008;128(11):1287–94.
43. Franceschi F, Papalia R, Del Buono A, Zampogna B, Diaz Balzani L, Maffulli N, Denaro V. Two-stage procedure in anterior cruciate ligament revision surgery: a five-year follow-up prospective study. Int Orthop. 2013;37(7):1369–74.
44. Hofbauer M, Muller B, Murawski CD, Baraga M, van Eck CF, Fu FH. Strategies for revision surgery after primary double-bundle anterior cruciate ligament (ACL) reconstruction. Knee Surg Sports Traumatol Arthrosc. 2013;21(9):2072–80.
45. Marcacci M, Zaffagnini S, Bonanzinga T, Marcheggiani Muccioli GM, Bruni D, Iacono F. Over-the-top double-bundle revision ACL reconstruction. Knee Surg Sports Traumatol Arthrosc. 2012;20:1404–8.
46. Thomas NP, Kankate R, Wandless F, Pandit H. Revision anterior cruciate ligament reconstruction using a 2-stage technique with bone grafting of the tibial tunnel. Am J Sports Med. 2005;33(11):1701–9.
47. Weiler A, Schmeling A, Stöhr I, Kääb MJ, Wagner M. Primary versus single-stage revision anterior cruciate ligament reconstruction using autologous hamstring tendon grafts: a prospective matched-group analysis. Am J Sports Med. 2007;35(10):1643–52.
48. Ohly NE, Murray IR, Keating JF. Revision anterior cruciate ligament reconstruction: timing of surgery and the incidence of meniscal tears and degenerative change. J Bone Joint Surg Br. 2007;89(8):1051–4.
49. Denti M, Lo Vetere D, Bait C, Schonhuber H, Melegati G, Volpi P. Revision anterior cruciate ligament reconstruction: causes of failure, surgical technique, and clinical results. Am J Sports Med. 2008;36(10):1896–902.
50. Muneta T, Hara K, Ju YJ, Mochizuki T, Morito T, Yagishita K, Sekiya I. Revision anterior cruciate ligament reconstruction by double-bundle technique using multi-strand semitendinosus tendon. Arthroscopy. 2010;26(6):769–81.
51. Borchers JR, Kaeding CC, Pedroza AD, Huston LJ, Spindler KP, Wright RW, MOON Consortium and the MARS Group. Intra-articular findings in primary and revision anterior cruciate ligament reconstruction surgery: a comparison of the MOON and MARS study groups. Am J Sports Med. 2011;39(9):1889–93.
52. Brophy RH, Wright RW, David TS, McCormack RG, Sekiya JK, Svoboda SJ, Huston LJ, Haas AK, Steger-May K, Multicenter ACL Revision Study (MARS) Group. Association between previous meniscal surgery and the incidence of chondral lesions at revision anterior cruciate ligament reconstruction. Am J Sports Med. 2012;40(4):808–14.
53. Gifstad T, Drogset JO, Viset A, Grøntvedt T, Hortemo GS. Inferior results after revision ACL reconstructions: a comparison with primary ACL reconstructions. Knee Surg Sports Traumatol Arthrosc. 2013;21(9):2011–8.
54. Kievit AJ, Jonkers FJ, Barentsz JH, Blankevoort L. A cross-sectional study comparing the rates of osteoarthritis, laxity, and quality of life in primary and revision anterior cruciate ligament reconstructions. Arthroscopy. 2013;29(5):898–905.
55. Griffith TB, Allen BJ, Levy BA, Stuart MJ, Dahm DL. Outcomes of repeat revision anterior cruciate ligament reconstruction. Am J Sports Med. 2013;41(6):1296–301.

Multiligamentary Knee Injury

5

Dinu Vermesan and Florin Ramadani

Multiligamentary knee lesions are complex injuries, often associated with knee dislocations. They are the result of high force trauma and usually involve tears of the ACL, PCL and at least one of the collateral ligaments. Knee dislocations are serious injuries, and great care must be taken while providing emergency treatment, regarding the vascular structures that pass through the posterior aspect of the knee. In the unfortunate case that the dislocation was not spontaneously reduced, the doctor must immediately proceed in doing so, as prolonged interruption of vascular flux can lead to thrombosis and serious ischemia of the leg.

D. Vermesan, MD, PhD (✉)
Department of Orthopedics and Trauma,
University of Medicine and Pharmacy 'Victor Babes' Timisoara,
2 Eftimie Murgu Square, Timisoara 300041, Romania

I-st Clinic of Orthopedics and Trauma,
Emergency Clinical County Hospital Timisoara,
10 Iosif Bulbuca Blvd, Timisoara 300736, Romania
e-mail: vermesan@gmail.com

F. Ramadani, MD, PhD
Unfallchirurgie, Klinikum Wels-Grieskirchen,
42 Grieskirchner St, Wels A-4600, Austria

University of Medicine and Pharmacy 'Victor Babes' Timisoara,
Timisoara, Romania
e-mail: florin.ramadani@liwest.at

R. Prejbeanu (ed.), *Atlas of Knee Arthroscopy*,
DOI 10.1007/978-1-4471-6593-4_5, © Springer-Verlag London 2015

5.1 Knee Dislocation

The types of knee dislocations are described based on the direction of the tibia's translation in relation with the femur, resulting in five main types: anterior, posterior, lateral, medial and rotator [1, 2]. They are usually the result of high traumatic accidents, but can appear in certain situations due to low energy trauma. Even though the dislocation may not be clinically evident, a knee is considered to have had a self-reduced dislocation, if three or more ligaments are injured [3–5].

A study conducted by Frassica et al. on a series of patients, found posterior dislocations to have the highest incidence (70 %), followed by anterior (25 %) and rotational dislocations (5 %) [6]. Also, the posterior dislocations are known to have the highest incidence of vascular complications, due to the direction of the force that produces it (hyperextension). It is very important to correctly distinguish between the types of dislocation and perform a correct assessment of the patient in order to have a proper case management further on (Fig. 5.1).

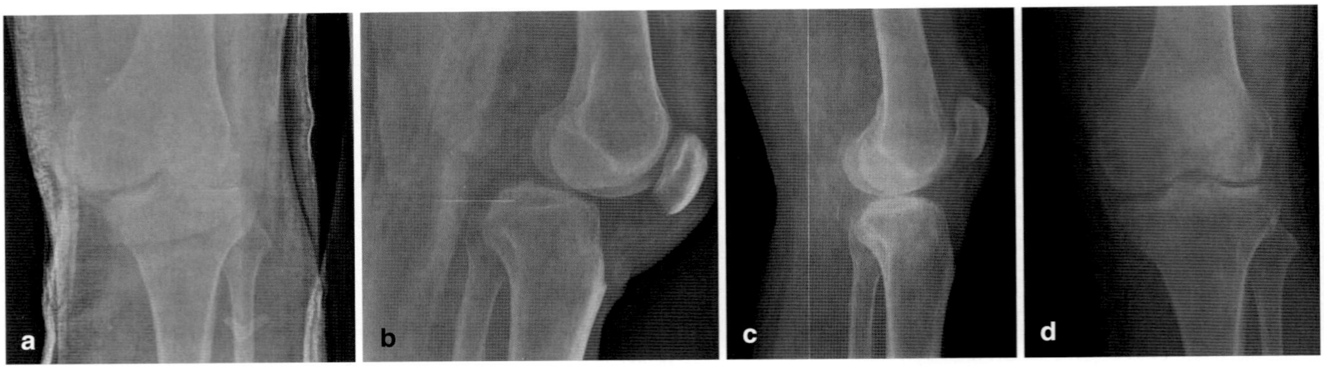

Fig. 5.1 Irreducible posterior dislocation of the left knee in an elderly male: AP and lateral X-rays from emergency presentation (**a**, **b**) and 8 weeks after open reduction and conservative management (orthosis immobilization and physical therapy) (**c**, **d**)

5.1.1 Clinical Signs and Emergency Procedures

The initial clinical evaluation of the patient is of utmost importance and must be carried out as soon as possible, depending on the overall status of the patient. The patient is usually in great pain, the knee is swollen (hemarthrosis) and very often deformed (if the dislocation has not been reduced prior to his arrival). The pulse must be checked distal to the knee, and the reduction procedures must be carried out immediately after observing the x-rays. It is important to mention that normal pulses, capillary refill or Doppler signal does not rule out eventual vascular injury [7].

The reduction is obtained by applying an axial (traction) force on the ankle while another doctor manipulates the proximal tibia in the appropriate direction. X-ray confirmation is mandatory, and immobilization in a long leg splint or trans-calcaneal extension is strongly advised.

Irreducible dislocations, open dislocations and prolonged ischemia are strong indicators for an emergency surgical procedure. Otherwise, MRI and clinical evaluation after 3–6 weeks from the trauma are needed in order to establish the surgical treatment. After the patient has overcome the acute phase, a proper clinical examination can be done which includes the Lachmann, anterior and posterior drawer and dial tests. These tests are specific to ligament injuries and can clearly demonstrate the grade of laxity and instability the knee has.

5.1.2 Patient Management

Multiple associated soft tissue injuries of the knee following dislocations are very hard to manage surgically and require a great deal of surgical skill and clinical experience. Depending on the structures that are affected, multiligamentary knee lesions can be resolved in different ways.

The ACL rupture is a definite indication for reconstruction, especially when associated with other instability issues of the knee. The reconstruction of the ACL was thoroughly discussed earlier on. The PCL is known to have intrinsic healing capabilities if properly managed. Thus, the bracing must include a method of pushing the tibia slightly anterior in order to allow for optimal healing parameters. If conservative PCL management is what we desire, an MRI investigation must be performed 4–6 weeks after immobilization in order to evaluate its condition.

The MCL ligament usually heals by itself after 4–6 weeks of stiff bracing. In certain ACL/PCL/MCL injuries, it is recommended to delay the surgical procedure of ACL and/or PCL reconstruction until after the eventual healing of the MCL. In unfortunate cases, the MCL must require reconstruction procedures to be carried out alongside with the other injured ligaments. Injuries that associate ACL and PCL with posterolateral corner tears must be surgically addressed and repaired between the 2nd and 3rd week after the trauma. This allows for optimal capsular closure and arthroscopic repair for the other affected structures as well as the posterolateral corner (Fig. 5.2).

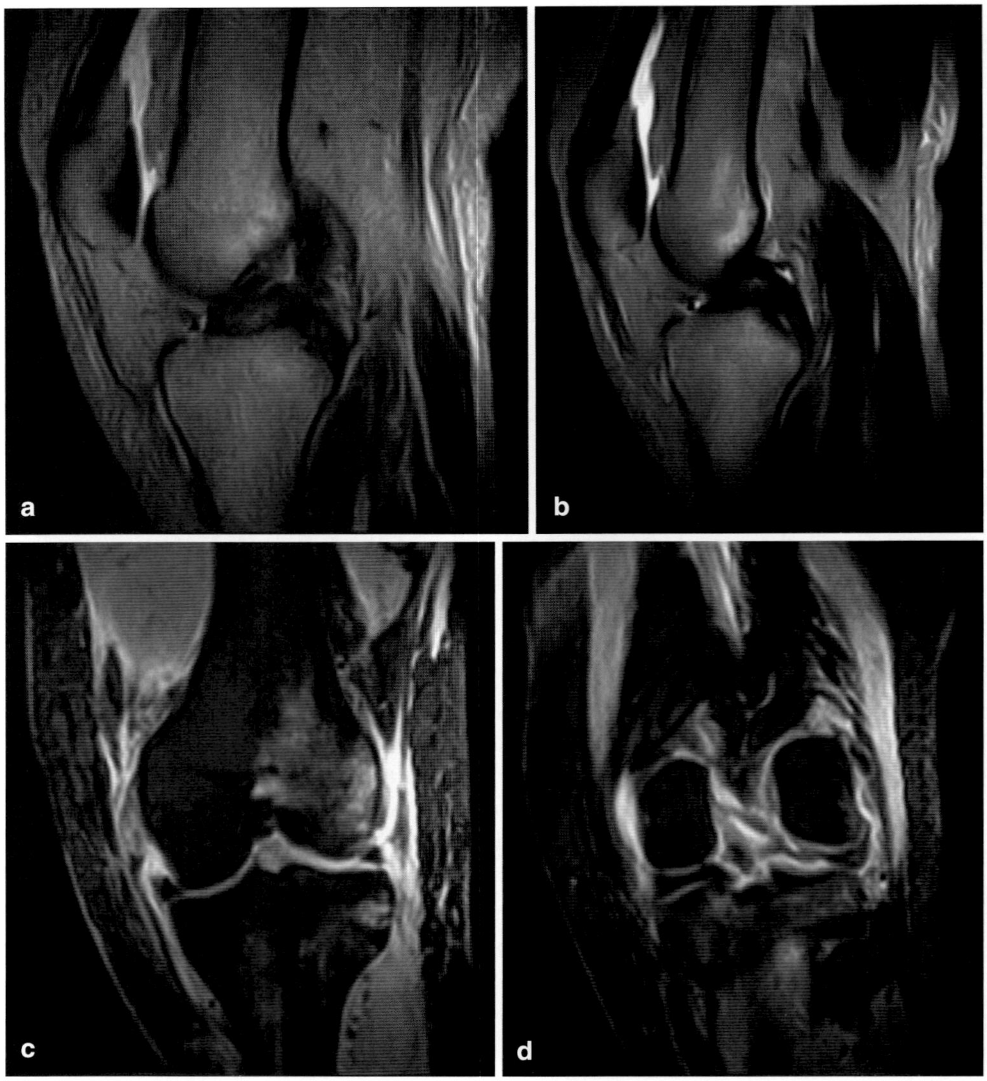

Fig. 5.2 Left knee MRI of a young male patient with multiligamentary injury: sagittal T2 with torn ACL at the femoral insertion (**a**) and PCL at the tibial insertion (**b**); coronal views showing complete (grade III) MCL rupture from the femoral insertion, bone edema on the lateral femoral condyle (**c**) and tibial plateau and ruptured PCL (**d**)

5.2 Posterior Cruciate Ligament (PCL) Tears

PCL tears represent 5–37 % of all ligament injuries, being less frequent than ACL tears but more difficult to handle with. The incidence in a general population was measured at 3 % [8]. They can occur in multiligamentary knee trauma [9, 10] or in athletes frequently in a hyperflexion movement [11, 12]. There has been great controversy regarding the treatment of PCL tears. Some author suggest that in case of multiligamentary association, the PCL should be treated surgically [13–17] and others believe that conservative treatment leads to acceptable results [14].

5.2.1 Examination

PCL tears lead to posterior knee laxity, sensation of uncontrolled hyperflexion and sometimes anterior knee pain. This type of injury translates into a highly positive posterior drawer test in knee flexion [3, 5, 7, 33]. According to the posterior laxity the knee has during the posterior drawer test, Harner and Hoher have established a classification for PCL tears. Grade I tears correspond to 0–5 mm of laxity, grade II tears present 5–10 mm of posterior tibial translation and grade III have more than 10 mm of posterior stress laxity [18]. Of course MRI and bilateral knee stress x-rays still carry a very important role in the imaging diagnosis of PCL rupture. For a good treatment to be offered, all of the other possibly associated ligament tears should be identified.

5.2.2 Treatment

Conservative treatment is considered a good option for PCL tears if they are not associated with other ruptured ligaments, whether the rupture is acute or chronic, exception being only grade III isolated ruptures in young athletes. Surgical treatment is an indication for combined ligamentary lesions that include PCL tears.

The PCL can be reconstructed using either a single bundle (SB) or double bundle (DB) technique. There have been many studies that compared the outcomes of both procedures, but there has been insufficient strong proof to confirm that DB technique is a clear advantage regarding rehabilitation and knee kinematics over the SB technique [19–23].

Most of the authors that use the SB technique use the footprint of the antero-lateral bundle to place the femoral insertion of the reconstructed PCL [24]. This footprint is located between the 9 and 12 o'clock positions looking at the notch [25]. Fifty articles on PCL reconstruction were reviewed and the reported positions for femoral insertion were between 10:00 and 11:00 o'clock, and from 2.5 to 13 mm depth regarding the edge of the articular cartilage [24].

The main advantage of the DB technique is that it decreases posterior tibial translation and laxity, unlike the SB that has had somewhat low results regarding this issue [20, 26–28]. The femoral footprint is usually left in place in order to allow for a proper fixation of the neoligament. A posteromedial portal is usually established under arthroscopic guidance and the PCL guide is placed on the tibial footprint of the PCL. With the aid of the guide, the two tunnels (AL and PM) are drilled, paying absolute caution to the neurovascular structures. The proper position of the tunnels is confirmed with an AP fluoroscopic view. The AL (1 o'clock) and PM (4 o'clock) femoral tunnels are drilled with the knee in 130° and 110° flexion. Graft positioning is done for the AL bundle first and then for the PM bundle taking note that proper tension should be performed before fixation.

5.2.3 Conclusion

Although the results of PCL reconstruction using the SB and DB techniques are still very controversial, it is safe to say that both can be used and give good results, given that the patient is chosen carefully and the procedure is performed with no complications. Another influencing factor is the postoperative rehabilitation which must be carried out by a specialized physiotherapist while taking into account for the case particularities and eventual other morbidities.

Even if PCL reconstruction is achieved, the patient must be aware that it cannot eliminate the posterior laxity that was once offered by the original ligament. Associated instabilities must be addressed before the PCL reconstruction in order to ensure good functional outcomes (Figs. 5.3 and 5.4).

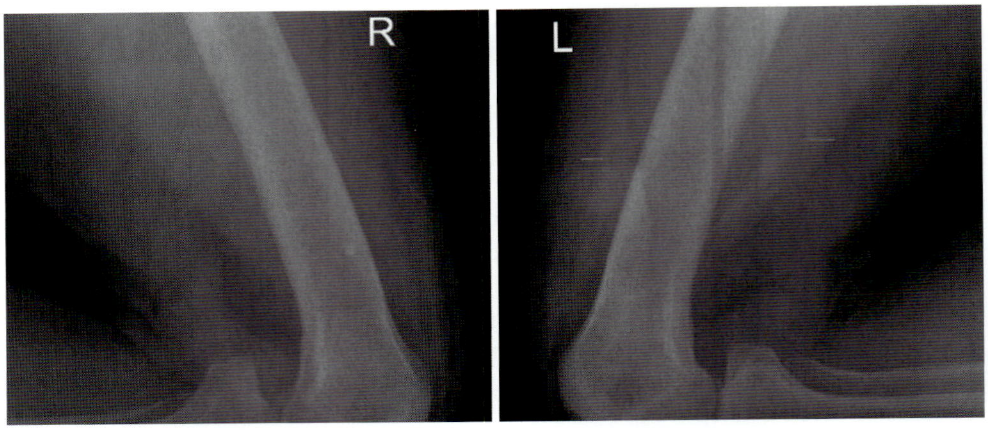

Fig. 5.3 An adult male patient with positive posterior drawer – stress X-ray of the right knee, suggestive of PCL injury

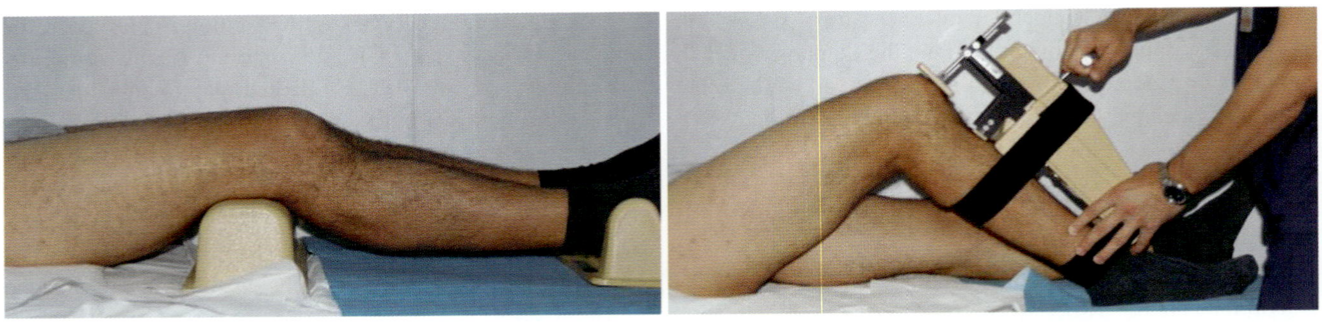

Fig. 5.4 A middle aged male patient with residual laxity and a history of distal femoral fracture. Positive posterior drawer – stress X-ray of the right knee suggestive of PCL insufficiency. KT-1,000 examination

5.3 Multiligamentary Surgical Repair

5.3.1 Posteromedial Corner

The posteromedial corner is made up of three ligaments that provide this portion of the knee with static and dynamic stability. These three ligaments are: the superficial medial collateral ligament, the posterior oblique ligament and the deep medial collateral ligament.

LaPrade et al. described an anatomic reconstruction technique of the proximal and distal avulsions of the superficial medial collateral ligament and the posterior oblique ligament using two separate grafts. Their approach was through an incision that expands from the medial side of the patella and continues 7–8 cm distal to the joint line, down the tibia. Once they found the attachment and insertion points of these two structures tunnel were drilled with the aid of guiding pins. Graft sizes should be 16 cm for the superficial MCL and 12 cm for the posterior oblique ligament. Femoral fixation was obtained through bioabsorbable screws. Then the posterior oblique ligament is fixed on the tibia with the knee in full extension and the superficial MCL with the knee in 20° of flexion.

Preoperative IKDC increased after postoperative rehabilitation from 43.5 (14–65) to 76.2 (54–88). Valgus stress gap decreased from 6.2 mm (3.5–14) to 1.3 mm (1.0–2) [29]. This model of reconstruction is anatomic and it is based upon careful dissection and identifying the origins and insertion of the two affected structures in order to ensure optimum results.

5.3.2 Posterolateral Corner

The posterolateral corner has three main stabilizing ligaments. The fibular collateral ligament (FCL), popliteofibular ligament (PFL) and popliteus tendon (PLT) ensure the knee has stability, external rotation and varus laxity resistance. A proper MRI and varus stress x-rays are very important in assessing the patient status both preoperatively and after the surgery.

In an attempt to find the proper treatment algorithm, especially surgical-wise, LaPrade et al. conducted quantitative studies in order to better define the anatomy of the region and establish anatomical landmarks of the involved ligaments [30, 31]. The authors established average lengths on all of the three ligaments, and came to a conclusion on the best surgical approach for the reconstruction of the posterolateral corner. The popliteus tendon was found to have an important role in not only dynamic stabilization of the knee, but also in providing static alignment and stability, calling it the "fifth ligament" of the knee [32].

For their reconstruction technique, Laprade et al. used multiple combinations of graft selections and surgical approaches in order to establish the best option in dealing with the pathology. For FCL reconstruction which had a native length of 71 mm, they preferred a semitendinosus autograft, due to its average long length compared to the patellar tendon graft (48 mm). Insertion points of the graft were placed at the femoral end (1.4 mm proximal and 3.1 mm posterior to the lateral epicondyle) and on the fibular head with interference screws and 20° knee flexion. The PLT reconstruction technique was also described using a semitendinosus autograft. The femoral insertion of the PLT was determined to be 18.5 mm anterior and distally from the FCL insertion. Its tibial insertion is common with the PFL and it is placed under the lateral tibial plateau, near the tibio-fibular joint line. Both tendons entering the tunnel are pulled through it towards the anterior exit where they are secured with an interference screw inserted from anterior [29].

In a study conducted to evaluate this method of treatment for acute grade 3 PLC injuries, IKDC mean values reached 81.5 (more than 2 year follow-up) from their initial mean value of 29.1 (preoperatively). Cincinnati values also increased from a mean value of 21.9–81.4. Varus stress x-rays showed a very good improvement as well. Preoperatively the side-to-side was 6.2 mm and at follow-up visits it decreased to a value of 0.1 mm. One single patient required a revision surgery [33].

5.3.3 Conclusions

Multiligamentary knee lesions are complex injuries that require an experienced approach and correct systematization. The clinical context of having a multiple traumatized patient with other additional pathologies, the risk of neurovascular affection and the need for interdisciplinary treatment makes these types of knee injuries the target of high skilled specialists.

Great caution must be taken at the initial clinical examination, the follow-up visits, the surgical planning including graft management and the postoperative treatment. Surgical timing must be chosen carefully and according to the healing progress of the injured ligaments. Some surgeons may also prefer using allografts during these reconstructions due to patient morbidity and high demand for ligament repair.

The progress that has be made up until now in treating multiligamentary knee lesions, makes us believe that the future directions are very good. Having advanced from treating ligament injuries conservatively, the reconstructing them (single bundle and double bundle) and even associating multiple ligament reconstructions on the same knee, places a strong believe that many big steps will be achieved in this field. The new trend of associating autologous platelet rich fibrin matrix with the grafts seems to have favorable results as reported by various specialist [34] (Figs. 5.5, 5.6 and 5.7).

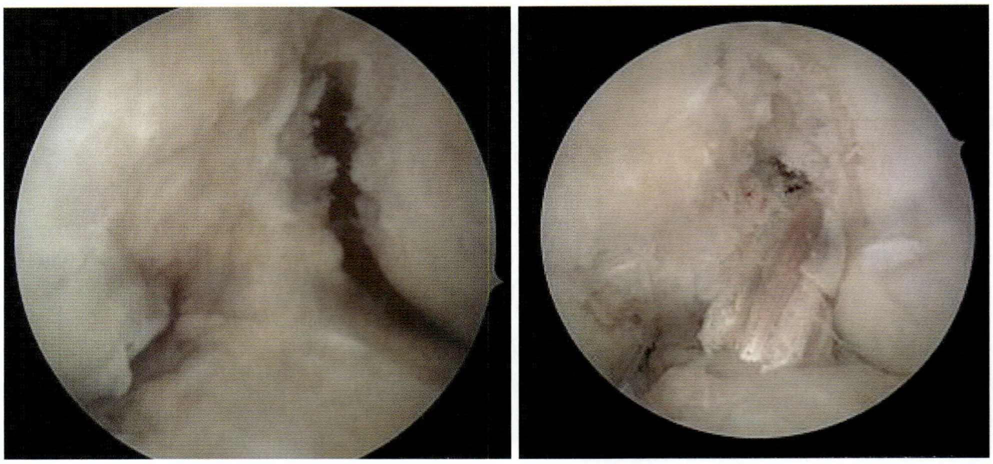

Fig. 5.5 Arthroscopic views from the anterolateral portal before and after SB ACL reconstruction in an obese adult patient, 6 months after knee dislocation and conservative treatment of the PCL and MCL

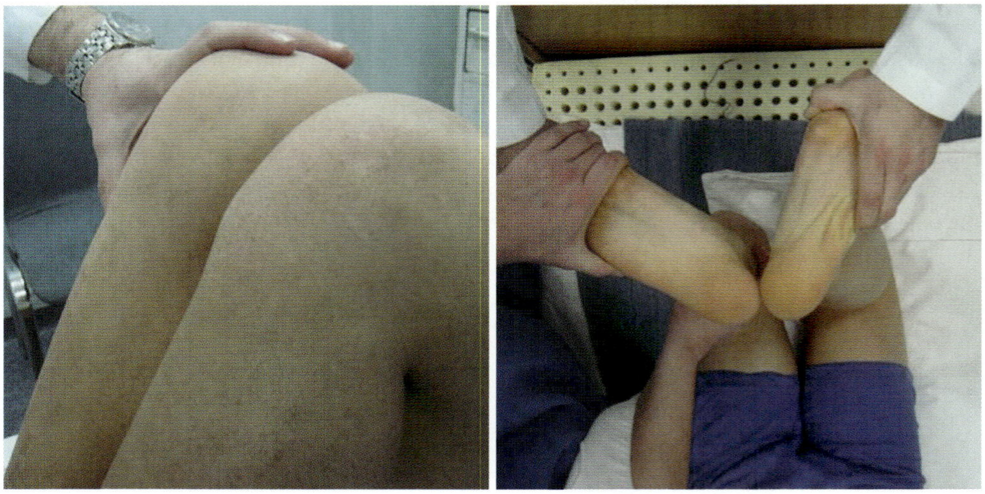

Fig. 5.6 Posterior slack of the right knee and positive dial test of the right knee in a young soccer player with old PCL – PLC injury

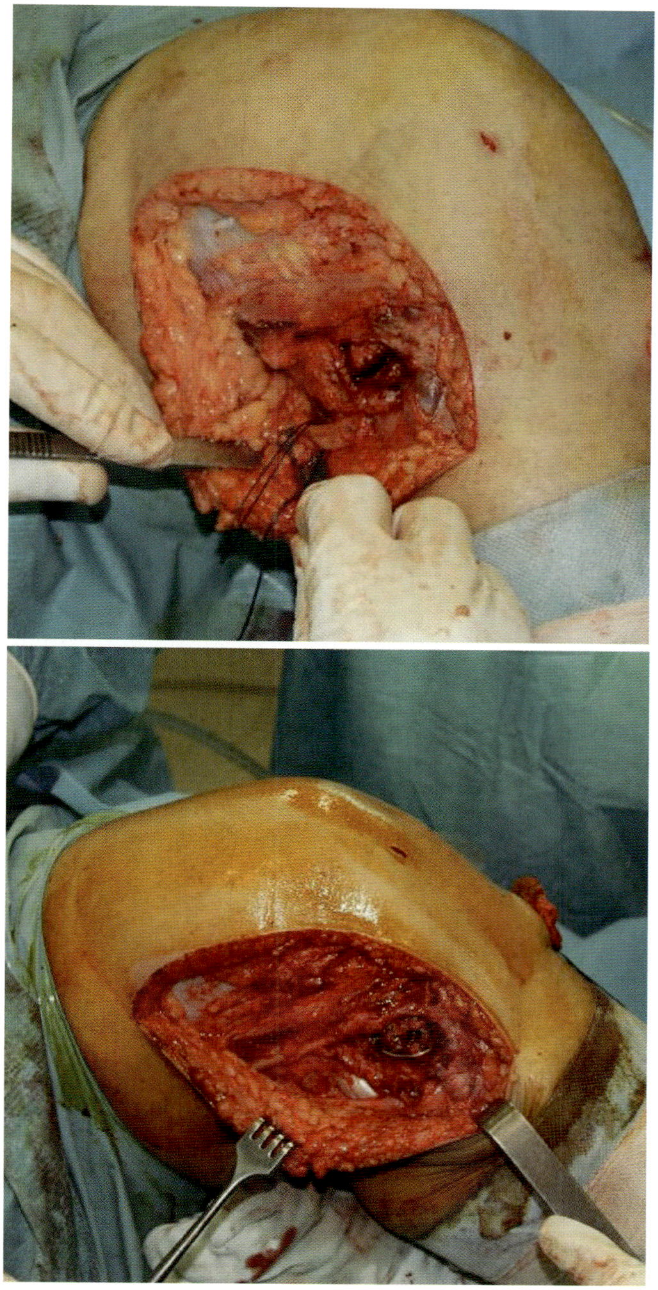

Fig. 5.7 Osteosynthesis for avulsion fracture of the peroneal head with LCL and biceps femoris insertions in an elderly female

References

1. Ghalambor N, Vangsness CT. Traumatic dislocation of the knee: a review of the literature. Bull Hosp Joint Dis. 1995;54(1):19–24.
2. Good L, Johnson RJ. The dislocated knee. J Am Acad Orthop Surg. 1995;3(5):284–92.
3. Fanelli GC, Gianotti BF, Edson CJ. Arthroscopically assisted combined posterior cruciate ligament/posterior lateral complex reconstruction. Arthroscopy. 1996;12(5):521–30.
4. Shelbourne KD, Porter DA, Clingman JA, et al. Low-velocity knee dislocation. Orthop Rev. 1991;20:995–1004.
5. Wascher DC, Dvirnak PC, Decoster TA. Knee dislocation: initial assessment and implications for treatment. J Orthop Trauma. 1997;11(7):525–9.
6. Frassica FJ, Sim FH, Staeheli JW, et al. Dislocation of the knee. Clin Orthop Relat Res. 1991;263:200–5.
7. Cone JC. Vascular injury associated with fracture dislocations of the lower extremity. Clin Orthop Relat Res. 1989;243:30–5.
8. Miyasaka K, Daniel D. The incidence of knee ligament injuries in the general population. Am J Knee Surg. 1991;4:3–8.
9. Fanelli GC. Posterior cruciate ligament injuries in trauma patients: part II. Arthroscopy. 1995;11:526–9.
10. Janousek AT, Jones DG, Clatworthy M, et al. Posterior cruciate ligament injuries of the knee joint. Sports Med. 1999;28:429–41.
11. Fowler PJ, Messieh SS. Isolated posterior cruciate ligament injuries in athletes. Am J Sports Med. 1987;15:553–7.
12. Parolie JM, Bergfeld JA. Long-term results of nonoperative treatment of isolated posterior cruciate ligament injuries in the athlete. Am J Sports Med. 1986;14:35–8.
13. Schulte KR, Chu ET, Fu FH. Arthroscopic posterior cruciate ligament reconstruction. Clin Sports Med. 1997;16:145–56.
14. Boynton MD, Tietjens BR. Long term follow-up of the untreated isolated posterior cruciate ligament-deficient knee. Am J Sports Med. 1996;24:306–10.
15. Cooper DE. Treatment of combined posterior cruciate ligament and posterolateral injuries of the knee. Oper Tech Sports Med. 1999;7:135–42.
16. Harner CD, Höher J. Evaluation and treatment of posterior cruciate ligament injuries. Am J Sports Med. 1998;26(3):471–82.
17. Veltri DM, Deng XH, Torzilli PA, et al. The role of the cruciate and posterolateral ligaments in stability of the knee. A biomechanical study. Am J Sports Med. 1995;23:436–43.
18. Grood ES, Stowers SF, Noyes FR. Limits of movement in the human knee. Effect of sectioning the posterior cruciate ligament and posterolateral structures. J Bone Joint Surg. 1988;70:88–97.
19. Race A, Amis AA. PCL reconstruction. In vitro biomechanical comparison of "isometric" versus single and double bundled "anatomic" grafts. J Bone Joint Surg. 1998;80-B:173–9.
20. Harner CD, Janaushek MA, Kanamori A, et al. Biomechanical analysis of a double-bundle posterior cruciate ligament reconstruction. Am J Sports Med. 2000;28:144–51.
21. Bergfeld JA, et al. A biomechanical comparison of posterior cruciate ligament reconstructions using single and double-bundle tibial inlay techniques. Am J Sports Med. 2005;33(7):976–81.
22. Markolf KL, Zemanovic JR, McAllister DR. Cyclic loading of posterior cruciate ligament replacements fixed with tibial tunnel and inlay methods. J Bone Joint Surg Am. 2002;84-A(4):518–24.
23. Wiley WB, et al. Kinematics of the posterior cruciate ligament/posterolateral corner-injured knee after reconstruction by single- and double-bundle intra-articular grafts. Am J Sports Med. 2006;34(5):741–8.
24. Apsingi S1, Bull AM, Deehan DJ, et al. Femoral tunnel placement for PCL reconstruction in relation to the PCL fibre bundle attachments. Knee Surg Sports Traumatol Arth. 2009;17(6):652–9.
25. Edwards A, Bull AMJ, Amis AA. The attachments of the fiber bundles of the posterior cruciate ligament: an anatomic study. Arthroscopy. 2007;23:284–90.
26. Amis AA. Posterior cruciate ligament reconstruction: the double-bundle method is most effective for restoring posterior tibiofemoral laxity. In: Johnson DP, Williams RJ, editors. Controversies in knee surgery. Oxford/New York: Oxford University Press; 2004. p. 375–83.

27. Mannor DA, Shearn JT, Grood ES, et al. Two bundle posterior cruciate ligament reconstruction. An in vitro analysis of graft placement and tension. Am J Sports Med. 2000;28:833–45.
28. Race A, Amis AA. PCL reconstruction – in vitro biomechanical comparison of "isometric" versus single and double bundled "anatomic" grafts. J Bone Joint Surg [Br]. 1998;80:173–9.
29. LaPrade RF, Wijdicks CA. Surgical technique: development of an anatomic medial knee reconstruction. Clin Orthop Relat Res. 2012;470:806–14.
30. LaPrade RF, Hamilton CD. The fibular collateral ligament-biceps femoris bursa. An anatomic study. Am J Sports Med. 1997;15:439–43.
31. LaPrade RF, Ly TV, Wentorf FA, Engebretsen L. The posterolateral attachments of the knee: a qualitative and quantitative morphologic analysis of the fibular collateral ligament, popliteus tendon, popliteofibular ligament, and lateral gastrocnemius tendon. Am J Sports Med. 2003;31:854–60.
32. LaPrade RF, Wozniczka JK, Stellmaker MP, Wijdicks CA. Analysis of the static function of the popliteus tendon and evaluation of an anatomic reconstruction: the fifth ligament of the knee. Am J Sports Med. 2010;38:543–9.
33. Geeslin AG, LaPrade RF. Outcomes of treatment of acute grade-III isolated and combined posterolateral knee injuries: a prospective case series and surgical technique. J Bone Joint Surg Am. 2011;93(18):1672–83.
34. Weiler A, Forster C, Hunt P, et al. The influence of locally applied platelet derived growth factor BB on free tendon graft remodeling after anterior cruciate ligament reconstruction. Am J Sports Med. 2004;4:881–91.

6 Arthroscopic Treatment of Intraarticular Fractures Around the Knee

Radu Prejbeanu and Dan Crisan

The knee joint is comprised of three bones, the femur, the patella and the tibia, all of which can have intraarticular fractures. However, not all of these fractures can be addressed arthroscopically and not all will be described in this chapter. Displaced patellar fractures are usually treated by open fashion as are the intraarticular fractures of the distal femur that are regularly high-energy fractures and so comminuted that they make open reduction a necessity.

Arthroscopy for proximal tibial fracture (ARIF) is not a new addition to the therapeutic arsenal. It has been tempted for almost as long as arthroscopy was introduced into the mainstream of orthopedic practice as it has been believed to be of great value to directly visualize the reduction of the articular surface and create a smooth anatomic reduction with no steps or gaps. This has proved to be rather difficult in clinical practice as comminuted tibial plateau fractures tend to associate bone loss in the metaphyseal area often with fragments of tibial cartilage missing or unfit for a anatomic reduction. Comminuted fractures of the tibial plateau pose extreme technical challenges to the treating surgeon and represent a challenge even to the senior orthopedic surgeon. Restoration of the articular surface, anatomical reduction, rigid fixation, early rage of movement are the guiding principles when treating such a complex, intraarticular fracture. A remarkable evolution of recommended treatment options has occurred over the past 50 years, as techniques of surgical stabilization of fractures and implants available have developed. Clearly, each fracture requires individualized decision-making regarding the choice of internal or external fixation, type of approach, and there are a large number of variables that can dictate what the ideal implant should be for an individual fracture. However, there is a general consensus that external fixators both planar and circular and both knee spanning and knee sparing have a lower risk of infection than conventional compression plating techniques [1–3]. On the other hand modern locking plates have allowed the development of minimally invasive approaches with great consideration for the soft tissues. They also allow for unilateral plating, even for complex fracture patterns thus further minimizing the added soft tissue trauma and lowering the risk of infection compared to conventional plating techniques. Furthermore, adding a plate, either lateral or medial, or two plates in case of a severely comminuted fracture can augment external fixation techniques.

Schatzker et al. proposed a classification system (Fig. 6.1) of tibial condyle fractures based on the fracture pattern and fragment anatomy divided into six types. The first three types (I, II, and III) are typically the result of low-energy injury. The second three types (IV, V, and VI) are typically the result of high-energy injury. However, relatively low-energy trauma to osteoporotic bones may produce fracture patterns similar to those of high-velocity injuries. The magnitude of the force determines both the degree of fragmentation and the degree of displacement [4, 5]. Although not a perfect or complete system this is the most widely used classification for fractures of the proximal tibia. Other useful classification system is the AO/ASIF.

The Schatzker classification of tibial plateau fractures [6]:

Type I is a split fracture of the lateral condyle usually as a result of valgus and axial force. This pattern usually appears in young patients so there is no compression of the fractured fragment because of the strong cancelous bone.

R. Prejbeanu, MD, PhD • D. Crisan, MD (✉)
Department of Orthopedics and Trauma,
University of Medicine and Pharmacy 'Victor Babes' Timisoara,
2 Eftimie Murgu Square, Timisoara 300041, Romania

I-st Clinic of Orthopedics and Trauma,
Emergency Clinical County Hospital Timisoara,
10 Iosif Bulbuca Blvd, Timisoara 300736, Romania
e-mail: raduprejbeanu@gmail.com; crisan.dan@gmail.com

R. Prejbeanu (ed.), *Atlas of Knee Arthroscopy*,
DOI 10.1007/978-1-4471-6593-4_6, © Springer-Verlag London 2015

Type II is a split-compression fracture of the lateral condyle, also a result of combined valgus-axial forces but the more porotic bone of older patients produces a collapse of the cancelous structure under the articular surface.

Type III is a pure compression fracture of the lateral condyle, it can be localized anywhere on the articular surface, the result of an axial force.

Type IV is a fracture of the medial plateau, with a of split or split-compression pattern. It is the result of either a varus or an axial compression force, usually greater than the force that produces a lateral condyle fracture.

Type V is a fracture of both condyles, split and split-compression. An axial force produces it with the knee in full extension.

Type VI is a complex bicondylar fracture with diaphyseal extension. The result of high-energy trauma, usually the fragments are depressed and impacted, separated from the diaphysis.

In the AO/OTA classification, the proximal tibia is denoted as segment 43 and is divided into three main categories. Type A fractures are extraarticular. Type B fractures are partial articular and are subdivided into three main categories: B1 are pure splits, B2 are pure depression and B3 are split-depression. Type C fractures are complete articular fractures and are also subdivided into three subtypes: Type C1 is articular and metaphyseal simple, Type C2 is articular simple, Type C2 is articular simple and metaphyseal multifragmentary and Type C3 is articular multifragmentary. The AO classification separates fractures of the tibial plateau based on their articular involvement in:

These classification systems were all initially based on the radiographic appearance of the fracture and are all subject to intra- and interobserver variability. Traditionally, tibial plateau fractures are classified based on plain anteroposterior (AP) and lateral plain radiographs but it is well known that several fracture patterns exist that are not well represented in existing two-dimensional (2D) fracture classifications. For example, recognition of a posteromedial fragment is important in preoperative planning as it may require an additional surgical approach and/or supplementary fixation methods. It is well recognized that posteromedial shear fractures, as well as fractures in the coronal plane, are easily overlooked on plain AP radiographs.

As CT scanning provides better imaging of bone tissue it should make for a more accurate assessment of the tibial plateau fractures. However, there is conflicting evidence in literature regarding the improvement in the intra- and interobserver variability in classifying tibial plateau fractures using both plain radiographs and CT scanning. Intra- and inter-observer reliability and/or diagnostic accuracy of the most common classification systems for tibial plateau fractures – the AO and Schatzker classifications – are widely studied in orthopedic literature based on plain radiographs [7]. Better, more detailed, imaging form CT scans means that fracture patterns that are not visible on plain X-Rays can be visualized and assessed. This is especially true for fracture patterns that are not very well represented on traditional biplane imaging, such as pure depression patterns and posteromedial shear fractures. Recently, Gardner et al. disagreed that Schatzker III fractures exist, stating that a shear pattern existed in all of the cases that they have investigated [8]. Although Schatzker III fractures are cited to represent up to 30 % of the fracture patterns [5, 9, 10], we found a much lower rate of Schatzker III fractures in our practice of around 7 %. CT and MRI imaging are more accurate than plain radiography for classification of tibial plateau fractures, and the use of cross-sectional imaging can improve surgical planning. MRI is especially useful for determining the association and extent of associated lesions (collateral ligaments, menisci, anterior cruciate ligament, posterior cruciate ligament). While its value cannot be undermined, its costs prohibit the routine use of MRI in fractures of the tibial plateau. Kode et al. compared MR imaging with CT for evaluation of tibial plateau fractures and found that MR imaging was equivalent or better in determining the degree of fracture displacement [11]. In many cases, CT findings mirror those of conventional radiography.

Classically the intraoperative evaluation of the articular surface was be done under direct visualization, something that can be difficult in certain combinations of fracture patterns and approaches (especially a lateral approach for a fracture with a medial component), but some authors favor the use of arthroscopy for its lower rate of infectious complications [12, 13]. Taking all this into the account we agree that the therapeutic indication for arthroscopically assisted fixation of proximal tibia fractures is limited to simple split fractures, split depression and pure depression fractures (Schatzker type I, II, III and simple type IV) as well as avulsion fractures of the ACL insertion and osteochondral fractures this being supported by the opinion of other authors [6, 14],

The use of arthroscopy is according to Musahl et al. better suited for Schatzker III pure depression fractures, one of the uncommon forms of tibial plateau fractures, but while this obviously varies from surgeon to surgeon not all tibial plateau fractures is amenable to arthroscopic aided reduction and fixation techniques. The arthroscopic treatment of proximal tibial fractures is reserved to those fracture patterns where the direct visualization of the fracture can add a definite value to the fracture reduction process. Another factor to be accounted for is the positive liquid pressure that is necessary to perform a knee arthroscopy. It should not hinder the fracture reduction process nor create extensive swelling in an already swollen knee and further increasing the risk for compartment syndrome. Also there is at least one case cited in literature where embolism form arthroscopy fluid occurred in a patient with a tibial plateau fracture that was treated by arthroscopy [15]. Other early complications for ARIF techniques such as DVT and knee effusions maintain the same trend being fewer and less serious than those for standard ORIF techniques but they may have the selection bias of simpler cases fracture patterns that receive the arthroscopic treatment in their favor [16]. Arthroscopy with an articular fracture of the tibial plateau is a technically challenging surgery for the less experienced surgeon but it will also be of great help in identifying and treating associated meniscal injuries or other articular lesions. A fluid pump will control bleeding but low pressure should be maintained to decrease the risks associated with excessive fluid extravasation [17].

Another type of intraarticular injuries that can be addressed arthroscopically is the fractures of the tibial eminence that are synonymous with intercondylar eminence avulsion fractures. Displaced avulsions of the tibial spine are equivalent to ruptures of the anterior cruciate ligament. They present to general orthopedists as well as a wide variety of orthopedic subspecialty surgeons including sports medicine and pediatrics. Restoration of normal knee kinematics is dependent on anatomic reduction and fixation of the avulsed fragment. Because this injury is typically sustained by the skeletally immature patient, epiphyseal fixation is ideal to avoid physeal injury, which can lead to angular limb deformity [18]. Lafrance et al. consider that although most fractures heal successfully, residual laxity usually persists because of prefracture anterior cruciate ligament midsubstance attenuation. This does not typically manifest in subjective instability, and reconstruction of the anterior cruciate ligament is rarely required [19].

Prince et al. found that ACL injuries in skeletally immature patients are seen more often in boys. In addition, tibial avulsion fractures and partial tears are more common in younger, less rigid skeletons that can absorb the forces of trauma. As children mature, complete ACL tears and associated injuries occur in frequencies approaching those patterns seen in adults [20].

Sometimes when close reduction of the fragment is attempted this is obtained incompletely due to soft tissue interposition. Kocher et al. found that 65 % of type III fractures and 26 % of type II fractures had entrapment of the anterior horn of the meniscus, most commonly medial [21]. Other authors have confirmed this as well, particularly in type III fractures. This is why most authors such as Accousti et al. consider the treatment algorithm for tibial eminence fracture management with regard to displaced and irreducible fractures to require arthroscopic or open treatment, based on surgeon preference [22, 23]. Objective sagittal plane laxity does not translate into long-term clinical or subjective instability. However, every effort should be made to obtain the best possible reduction with stable fixation, when needed, to maximize function.

The classification system of Meyers and McKeever (Fig. 6.2) is the current standard used to classify these fractures and to guide treatment [24]. It is based on the degree of displacement, mainly on the lateral x-ray. Zaricznyj modified this classification [25] to include a fourth type – comminuted fractures of the tibial spine, which applies mostly to adults:

The Mayer and Mc Keevers classification, modified by Zariczynj:

Type I: minimal displacement of the tibial spine fragment

Type II: displacement of the anterior third to half of the avulsed fragment, which is lifted upward but remains hinged on its posterior border

Type III: complete separation of the avulsed fragment from the proximal tibial epiphysis, usually associated with upward displacement and rotation

Type III A involves only ACL insertion

Type III B involves entire intercondylar eminence.

Type IV comminuted fractures of tibial spine.

Song et al. reviewed their cohort of patients with displaced tibial spine avulsions and identified eight cases of type II and ten of type III in children and two cases of type II, 15 of type III, and five of type IV in adults. A higher incidence of type IV fractures was encountered in the adult group. Adults had higher incidences of accompanied meniscal injuries and type IV fractures than children. Significant differences were found in mean Lysholm scores, 99.3 points in children and 89.5 in adults. However, no significant differences were found between adults and children in terms of range of motion, the Lachman test and the Pivot-shift test, and instrumented anterior laxity. Lysholm scores of ACL avulsion fractures were better in children than in adults. Possible causes of these results are higher incidences of accompanying meniscal injury and type IV fracture in adults. However, no intergroup differences were found in terms of stabilities [26].

Arthroscopic treatment is advocated by the majority of authors as the best current option [27–31]. This allows for a complete evaluation and treatment of associated lesions, optimal reduction with removal of any possible soft tissue entrapment, accurate estimate of the size of the fragment (the chondral part is not visualized on x-rays and thus the fragment is usually undersized) and adequate internal fixation using suture, wire or screws. Reynders et al. presented a series of 26 cases of displaced fractures of the intercondylar eminence of the tibia treated with an arthroscopically placed, intrafocal screw with washer. Sixteen patients had a type II tibial eminence fracture according to Meyers and McKeever (mean age, 15 years; male/female ratio, 11:5) and ten patients had a type III tibia eminence fracture (mean age, 17 years; male/female ratio, 1:1). They encountered neither stiffness nor iatrogenic chondral abrasion. All but three patients with type II had some degree of residual laxity, without apparent impact on the clinical result. In four patients with a type III lesion, a residual laxity without functional deficit was noticed. In two cases with a type III lesion, a reconstruction of the anterior cruciate ligament was necessary 3 years after trauma. In four patients with a type III fracture, the fragment remained elevated, with minor impairment of the mobility (extension lag). No mechanical failure or infection was seen in this series. The authors found the intrafocal screw fixation for displaced fracture of the intercondylar eminence to be a reliable and safe technique, although complete restoration of the anteroposterior knee stability was seldom seen [32]. Lubowitz et al. recommend arthroscopic reduction and internal fixation for all displaced (type III) fractures and believe this should also be considered for all cases of displaced type II fractures. Fractures without displacement after closed reduction require careful evaluation to rule out meniscal entrapment. Subjective results are found to be uniformly excellent, despite reports of objective anteroposterior laxity [29].

Kocher et al. reviewed their results in six patients at minimal 2-year follow-up. They found mean postoperative Lysholm and Tegner scores of 99.5 and 8.7, respectively. One patient had a grade A Lachman (normal) test, three had grade B (nearly normal), and two had grade C (abnormal). Instrumented knee laxity showed side-to-side differences of greater than 3 mm in 4 of 6 patients [33].

In contrast, Wilfinger et al. performed a retrospective clinical analysis in a single department and identified 43 patients. Twenty-three were female and 20 male. The mean age at trauma was 11.5 years (6–16 years). Only 1 patient required a change of therapy and needed open reduction. Thirty-eight patients were available for follow-up at an interval of 1–7.5 years after trauma (mean 3.5 years). None of the patients reported pain, swelling, disability or giving-way, or was handicapped in their daily life. Of 26 magnetic resonance imaging examinations, we found a missing anterior cruciate ligament in 1 and a partial rupture in another patient. Based on these results, the authors recommend nonoperative management as the primary treatment for tibial spine fractures in children [34].

Rademakers et al. included 44 displaced tibial spine fractures in a study. The mean age at time of accident was 24 years (range 9–57 years). Out of these, 16 patients had an open physis at the time of trauma. After a mean follow-up of 16 years (range 5–27 years), the median knee ROM was 130° (range 115–140°). As measured with an objective testing device, no statistically significant difference of anteroposterior stability between the injured and uninjured legs was found, with a mean difference of 1 mm (range −3.9 to 6.9 mm). The Lysholm score showed good to excellent results in 86 % of the patients. The patients with open physis at the time of index surgery did not develop axial misalignment in the long term [35] (Fig. 6.3).

Early range-of-motion exercises are essential to prevent loss of extension. Repair using nonabsorbable suture fixation, when of adequate strength to allow early range-of-motion, has the advantages of eliminating the risks of comminuting of the fracture fragment, posterior neurovascular injury, and need for hardware removal, compared with screws.

Osteochondral fractures are a type of traumatic injury that can benefit fully from the advantages of arthroscopic treatment. Articular cartilage is a avascular, aneural and alymphatic tissue that covers the articular ends of bones. It serves as al low friction high wear resistance surface to ideal provide mobility and strength. However due to its poor vascularization it has rather limited regenerative capabilities. Cartilage lesions of the knee are rather common in children and adolescents representing a more difficult pathological entity due to the young age of the patients and the risk of secondary degenerative disease in case of a poor management. Ostehochondral fractures (OCF) are most prevalent in this age group due to a higher risk of direct knee trauma, skeletal immaturity in girls predisposing them to lateral patellar dislocation with secondary OCF and a more elastic ligamentary apparatus. The mechanism of OCF is believed to be the shear stress forces that appear during a lateral patellar dislocation. Their frequency in the pediatric and adolescent population is 43/100,000 with an incidence varying from 5 to 39 % after dislocation [36]. Association with intercondylar eminence fractures, a rare event, has been reported in literature [37] as well as ACL lesions and Segond fractures [38].

Positive diagnosis can be made on plain radiographs, usually on the lateral view, for OCFs that have a large enough bony fragment (Fig. 6.4). MRI is the imaging investigation of choice for these lesions as it is able to detect smaller, chondral fragments and can also asses the status of the MPFL and detect other articular. The gold standard for the detection of these lesions remains the arthroscopic evaluation of the joint [39, 40].

Treatment of these injuries can be conservative for nondisplaced fractures. Surgical treatment includes arthroscopic removal of the articular loose bodies if they are old or too small to be fixed with marrow stimulating techniques for defects smaller than 2 cm^2 and mosaicplasty or osteochondral autograft transplantation system (OATS), autologous chondrocyte implantation (ACI) and the matrix induced chondrocyte implantation (MACI). Large fragments in an acute setting should be fixed with screws, K wires, pull out sutures, biological glue or resorbable pins [41–43] (Fig. 6.5). As far as the reconstructive techniques of the articular cartilage are concerned Benthien et al. concluded that all operative procedures yielded comparable improvements, none being superior to the other and that the majority of studies evaluated by this review is insufficient for EBM purposes more coherent studies with LOE of I or II are needed [44]. Postoperative protocols vary with some authors allowing weight bearing as tolerated in extension for the first 6 weeks [41].

In conclusion arthroscopy is widely used in treating various types of fractures around the knee. It provides a minimally invasive, reduced risk surgery, an increased benefit for an already injured joint, with excellent postoperative results providing a correct surgical indication combined with an impeccable technique.

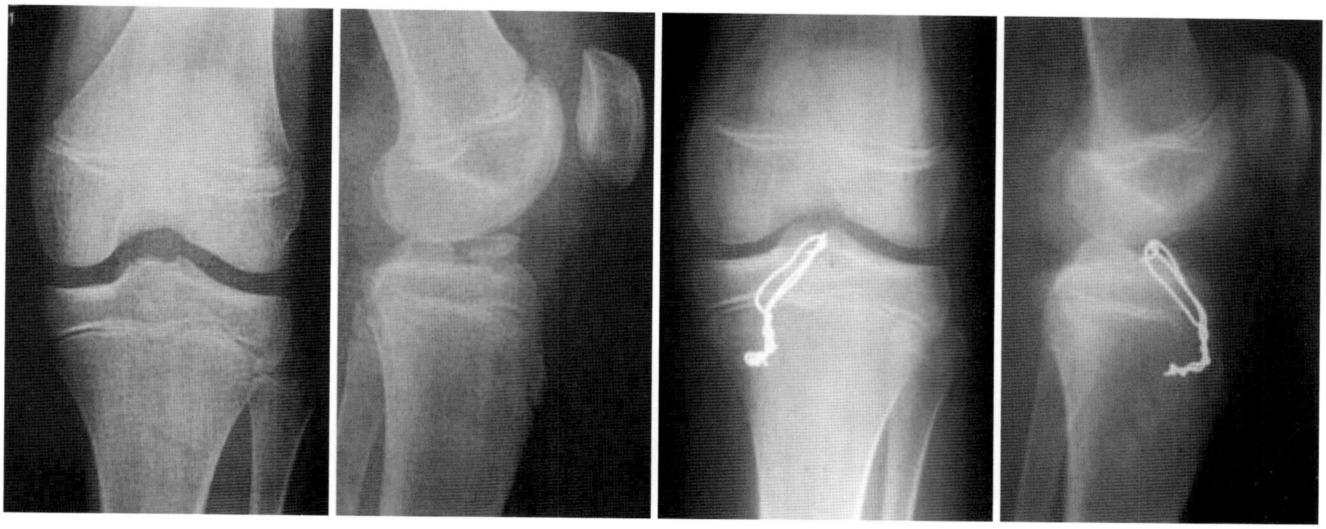

Fig. 6.1 AP and lateral X-ray views of a 12 years old girl with a type IIIA tibial spine avulsion. AP and lateral X-rays after arthroscopic reduction and internal fixation with wire (postoperative and 6 months follow-up)

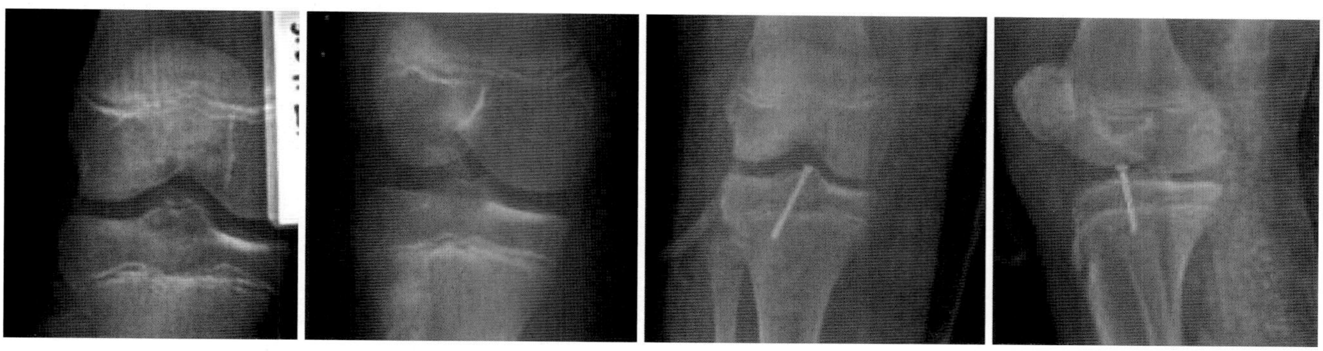

Fig. 6.2 AP and lateral emergency X-ray views of a 11 years old girl with a type IIIA tibial spine avulsion. AP and lateral X-rays after arthroscopic reduction and internal fixation with a cannulated screw

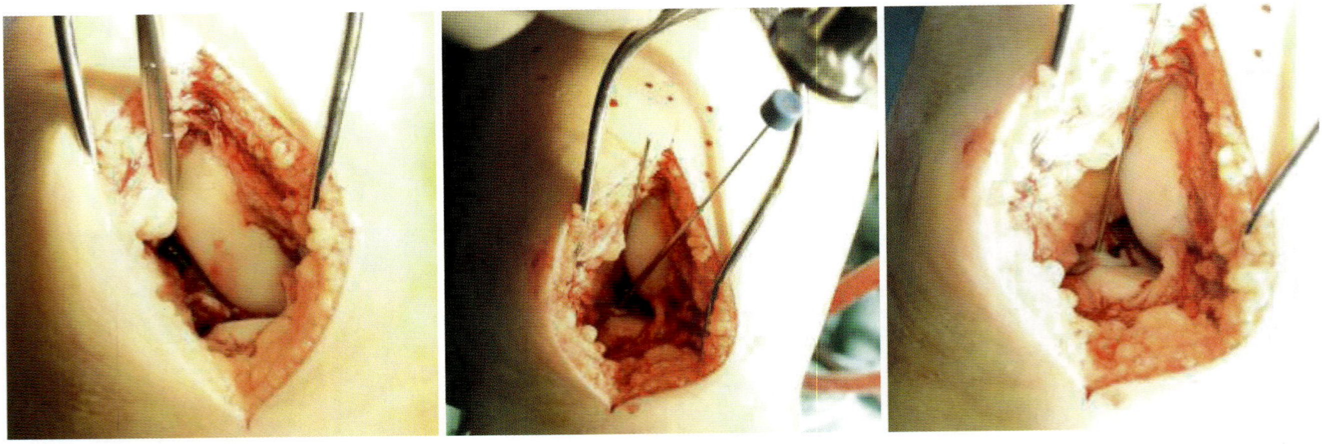

Fig. 6.3 Tibial spine avulsion: mini open medial arthrotomy, open reduction and internal fixation with absorbable pins (EthiPin, Ethicon Johnson & Johnson, Livingston, Scotland, UK)

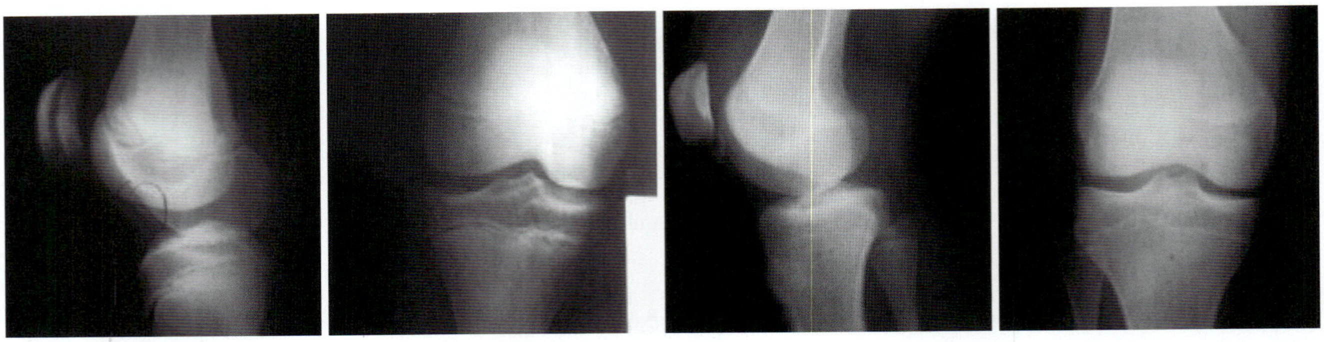

Fig. 6.4 Lateral and AP X-Ray showing a small articular bony fragment pertaining to a acute OCF after a spontaneously reduced patellar dislocation in a skeletally immature patient

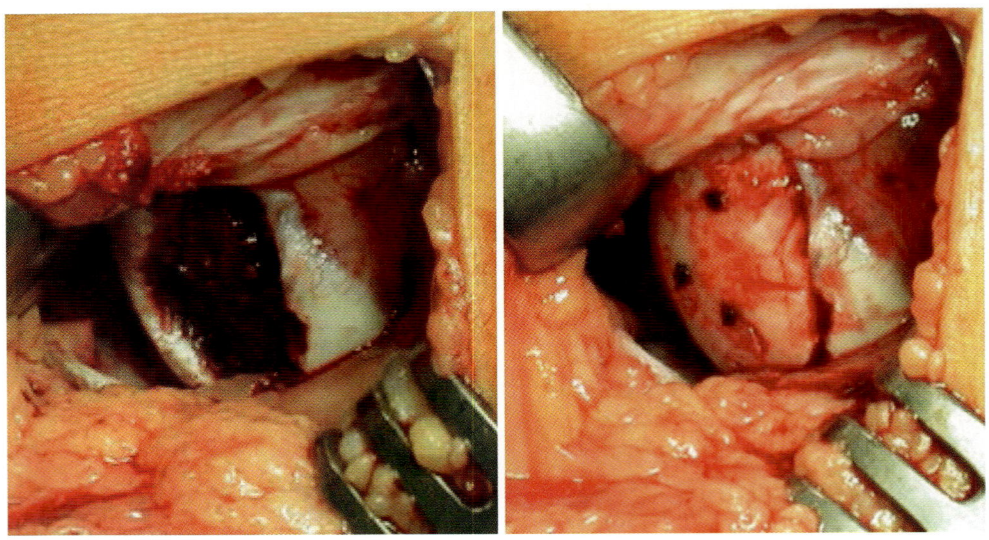

Fig. 6.5 Large (3 cm^2) acute osteochondral defect on the weight bearing surface of the lateral femoral condyle: lateral mini arthrotomy, open reduction and internal fixation with absorbable pins (EthiPin, Ethicon Johnson & Johnson, Livingston, Scotland, UK)

References

1. Mankar SH, Golhar AV, Shukla M, Badwaik PS, Faizan M, Kalkotwar S. Outcome of complex tibial plateau fractures treated with external fixator. Indian J Orthop. 2012;46(5):570–4.
2. Babis GC, Evangelopoulos DS, Kontovazenitis P, Nikolopoulos K, Soucacos PN. High energy tibial plateau fractures treated with hybrid external fixation. J Orthop Surg Res. 2011;6(1):35.
3. Musahl V, Tarkin I, Kobbe P, Tzioupis C, Siska PA, Pape H-C. New trends and techniques in open reduction and internal fixation of fractures of the tibial plateau. J Bone Joint Surg Br. 2009;91(4):426–33.
4. Schatzker J, McBroom R, Bruce D. The tibial plateau fracture. The Toronto experience 1968–1975. Clin Orthop Relat Res. 1979;138:94–104.
5. Markhardt BK, Gross JM, Monu JUV. Schatzker classification of tibial plateau fractures: use of CT and MR imaging improves assessment. Radiographics. 2009;29(2):585–97.
6. Lubowitz JH, Elson WS, Guttmann D. Part I: arthroscopic management of tibial plateau fractures. Arthroscopy. 2004;20(10):1063–70.
7. Doornberg JN, Rademakers MV, Bekerom MPVD, Kerkhoffs GM, Ahn J, Steller EP, et al. Two-dimensional and three-dimensional computed tomography for the classification and characterisation of tibial plateau fractures. Injury. 2011;42(12):1416–25.
8. Gardner MJ, Yacoubian S, Geller D, Suk M, Mintz D, Potter H, et al. The incidence of soft tissue injury in operative tibial plateau fractures: a magnetic resonance imaging analysis of 103 patients. J Orthop Trauma. 2005;19(2):79–84.
9. Charalambous CP, Tryfonidis M, Alvi F, Moran M, Fang C, Samarji R, et al. Inter- and intra-observer variation of the Schatzker and AO/OTA classifications of tibial plateau fractures and a proposal of a new classification system. Ann R Coll Surg Engl [Internet]. 2007;89(4):400–4. Available from: http://www.ncbi.nlm.nih.gov/entrez/query.fcgi?db=pubmed&cmd=Retrieve&dopt=AbstractPlus&list_uids=17535620.
10. Wicky S, Blaser PF, Blanc CH, Leyvraz PF, Schnyder P, Meuli RA. Comparison between standard radiography and spiral CT with 3D reconstruction in the evaluation, classification and management of tibial plateau fractures. Eur Radiol. 2000; 10(8):1227–32.
11. Kode L, Lieberman JM, Motta AO, Wilber JH, Vasen A, Yagan R. Evaluation of tibial plateau fractures: efficacy of MR imaging compared with CT. AJR Am J Roentgenol. 1994;163(1):141–7.
12. Dall'oca C, Maluta T, Lavini F, Bondi M, Micheloni GM, Bartolozzi P. Tibial plateau fractures: compared outcomes between ARIF and ORIF. Strategies Trauma Limb Reconstr. 2012;7(3):163–75.
13. Chan Y-S. Arthroscopy- assisted surgery for tibial plateau fractures. Chang Gung Med J. 2011;34(3):239–47.
14. Kayali C, Oztürk H, Altay T, Reisoglu A, Agus H. Arthroscopically assisted percutaneous osteosynthesis of lateral tibial plateau fractures. Can J Surg. 2008;51(5):378–82.
15. Hunter RE, Sgaglione NA. AANA advanced arthroscopy: the knee. Philadelphia: Saunders/Elsevier, Philadelphia, PA; 2010.
16. Papagelopoulos PJ, Partsinevelos AA, Themistocleous GS, Mavrogenis AF, Korres DS, Soucacos PN. Complications after tibia plateau fracture surgery. Injury. 2006;37(6):475–84.
17. McKeon BP, Bono JV, Richmond JC. Knee arthroscopy. Springer Science+Business Media, LLC, New York; 2009.
18. Fabricant PD, Osbahr DC. Management of a rare complication after screw fixation of a pediatric tibial spine avulsion fracture: a case report with follow-up to skeletal maturity. J Orthop Trauma. 2011;25(12):e115–9.
19. Lafrance RM, Giordano B, Goldblatt J, Voloshin I, Maloney M. Pediatric tibial eminence fractures: evaluation and management. J Am Acad Orthop Surg. 2010;18(7):395–405.
20. Prince JS, Laor T, Bean JA. MRI of anterior cruciate ligament injuries and associated findings in the pediatric knee: changes with skeletal maturation. AJR Am J Roentgenol. 2005;185(3):756–62.
21. Kocher MS, Micheli LJ, Gerbino P, Hresko MT. Tibial eminence fractures in children: prevalence of meniscal entrapment. Am J Sports Med. 2003;31(3):404–7.
22. Accousti WK, Willis RB. Tibial eminence fractures. Orthop Clin North Am. 2003;34(3):365–75.
23. Hudgens JL, Dahm DL. Treatment of anterior cruciate ligament injury in skeletally immature patients. Int J Pediatr. 2012;2012(6):932702–6.
24. Sapre V, Bagari V. Tibial spine avulsion fractures: current concepts and technical note on arthroscopic techniques used in management of these injuries [Internet]. InTech. 2013; 16 p. Available from: http://cdn.intechopen.com/pdfs/43257/InTech-Tibial_spine_avulsion_fractures_current_concepts_and_technical_note_on_arthroscopic_techniques_used_in_management_of_these_injuries.pdf.
25. Zaricznyj B. Avulsion fracture of the tibial eminence: treatment by open reduction and pinning. J Bone Joint Surg Am. 1977;59(8):1111–4.
26. Song E-K, Seon J-K, Park S-J, Yoon T-R. Clinical outcome of avulsion fracture of the anterior cruciate ligament between children and adults. J Pediatr Orthop B. 2009;18(6):335–8.
27. Senekovič V, Veselko M. Anterograde arthroscopic fixation of avulsion fractures of the tibial eminence with a cannulated screw. Arthroscopy. 2003;19:54–61.
28. Binnet MS, Gürkan I, Yilmaz C, Karakas A, Cetin C. Arthroscopic fixation of intercondylar eminence fractures using a 4-portal technique. Arthroscopy. 2001;17(5):450–60.
29. Lubowitz JH, Elson WS, Guttmann D. Part II: arthroscopic treatment of tibial plateau fractures: intercondylar eminence avulsion fractures. Arthroscopy. 2005;21(1):86–92.
30. McKoy BE, Stanitski CL. Acute tibial tubercle avulsion fractures. Orthop Clin North Am. 2003;34(3):397–403.
31. Mosier SM, Stanitski CL. Acute tibial tubercle avulsion fractures. J Pediatr Orthop. 2004;24(2):181–4.
32. Reynders P, Reynders K, Broos P. Pediatric and adolescent tibial eminence fractures: arthroscopic cannulated screw fixation. J Trauma. 2002;53(1):49–54.
33. Kocher MS, Foreman ES, Micheli LJ. Laxity and functional outcome after arthroscopic reduction and internal fixation of displaced tibial spine fractures in children. Arthroscopy. 2003;19(10):1085–90.
34. Wilfinger C, Castellani C, Raith J, Pilhatsch A, Höllwarth ME, Weinberg A-M. Nonoperative treatment of tibial spine fractures in children-38 patients with a minimum follow-up of 1 year. J Orthop Trauma. 2009;23(7):519–24.
35. Rademakers MV, Kerkhoffs G, Kager J. Tibial spine fractures: a long-term follow-up study of open reduction and internal fixation. J Orthop Trauma. 2009;23(3):203–7.
36. Nietosvaara Y, Aalto K, Kallio PE. Acute patellar dislocation in children: incidence and associated osteochondral fractures. J Pediatr Orthop. 1994;14(4):513–5.
37. Sharma G, Naik VA, Pankaj A. Displaced osteochondral fracture of the lateral femoral condyle associated with an acute anterior cruciate ligament avulsion fracture: a corollary of "the lateral femoral notch sign". Knee Surg Sports Traumatol Arthrosc. 2012;20(8):1599–602.
38. Tei K, Kubo S, Matsumoto T, Matsushita T, Matsumoto A, Kurosaka M, et al. Combined osteochondral fracture of the posterolateral tibial plateau and Segond fracture with anterior cruciate ligament injury in a skeletally immature patient. Knee Surg Sports Traumatol Arthrosc. 2012;20(2):252–5.
39. Friemert B, Oberländer Y, Schwarz W, Häberle HJ, Bähren W, Gerngross H, et al. Diagnosis of chondral lesions of the knee joint: can MRI replace arthroscopy? A prospective study. Knee Surg Sports Traumatol Arthrosc. 2004;12(1):58–64.

40. Braune C, Rehart S, Kerschbaumer F, Jäger A. Resorbable pin refixation of an osteochondral fracture of the lateral femoral condyle due to traumatic patellar dislocation: case management, follow-up and strategy in adolescents. Z Orthop Ihre Grenzgeb. 2004;142(1):103–8.
41. Lee BJ, Christino MA, Daniels AH, Hulstyn MJ, Eberson CP. Adolescent patellar osteochondral fracture following patellar dislocation. Knee Surg Sports Traumatol Arthrosc. 2013;21:1856–61.
42. Gkiokas A, Morassi LG, Kohl S, Zampakides C, Megremis P, Evangelopoulos DS. Bioabsorbable pins for treatment of osteochondral fractures of the knee after acute patella dislocation in children and young adolescents. Adv Orthop. 2012;2012(4):1–4.
43. Chotel F, Knorr G, Simian E, Dubrana F, Versier G, Society FA. Knee osteochondral fractures in skeletally immature patients: French multicenter study. Orthop Traumatol Surg Res. 2011;97(8 Suppl):S154–9.
44. Benthien JP, Schwaninger M, Behrens P. We do not have evidence based methods for the treatment of cartilage defects in the knee. Knee Surg Sports Traumatol Arthrosc. 2010;19:543–52.

7 Chondral Pathology

Radu Prejbeanu and Dinu Vermesan

Cartilage damage is one of the most difficult preoperative diagnoses to make in knee arthroscopy and it has the potential to progress to osteoarthritis over time. Currently there is no concrete evidence to show that articular cartilage repair can prevent the progression of a defect to osteoarthritis (OA). Also the methods of treating chondral defects are limited in effectiveness or technically difficult and expensive with rather questionable long time effects, as mentioned above. This makes arthroscopic cartilage surgery a challenging field with plenty of room for improvement and innovation.

Chondropathy is defined as the degenerative disease of the articular cartilage of a joint. It is a progressive "wear and tear" degradation of the articular cartilage that ultimately leads to the total disappearance of the cartilage on the weightbearing surfaces of the femoral and tibial condyles of the lateral or the medial compartment or both in advanced cases of osteoarthritis. Cartilage lesions can occur in the femoropatellar compartment as well most of these lesions appearing on the femoral side in the trochlear groove.

We prefer to use the Outerbridge classification for grading joint cartilage breakdown [1]. This classification system is widely used in practice because it allows the surgeon to quantize cartilage lesions in a simple and accurate yet reproducible manner:

- Grade 0 – normal (Fig. 7.1)
- Grade I – cartilage with softening and swelling (Fig. 7.2)
- Grade II – a partial-thickness defect with fissures on the surface that do not reach subchondral bone or exceed 1.5 cm in diameter (Fig. 7.3)
- Grade III – fissuring to the level of subchondral bone in an area with a diameter more than 1.5 cm (Fig. 7.4)
- Grade IV – exposed subchondral bone (Fig. 7.5)

R. Prejbeanu, MD, PhD • D. Vermesan, MD, PhD (✉)
Department of Orthopedics and Trauma,
University of Medicine and Pharmacy 'Victor Babes' Timisoara,
2 Eftimie Murgu Square, 300041 Timisoara, Romania

I-st Clinic of Orthopedics and Trauma,
Emergency Clinical County Hospital Timisoara,
10 Iosif Bulbuca Blvd, 300736 Timisoara, Romania
e-mail: raduprejbeanu@gmail.com; vermesan@gmail.com

R. Prejbeanu (ed.), *Atlas of Knee Arthroscopy*,
DOI 10.1007/978-1-4471-6593-4_7, © Springer-Verlag London 2015

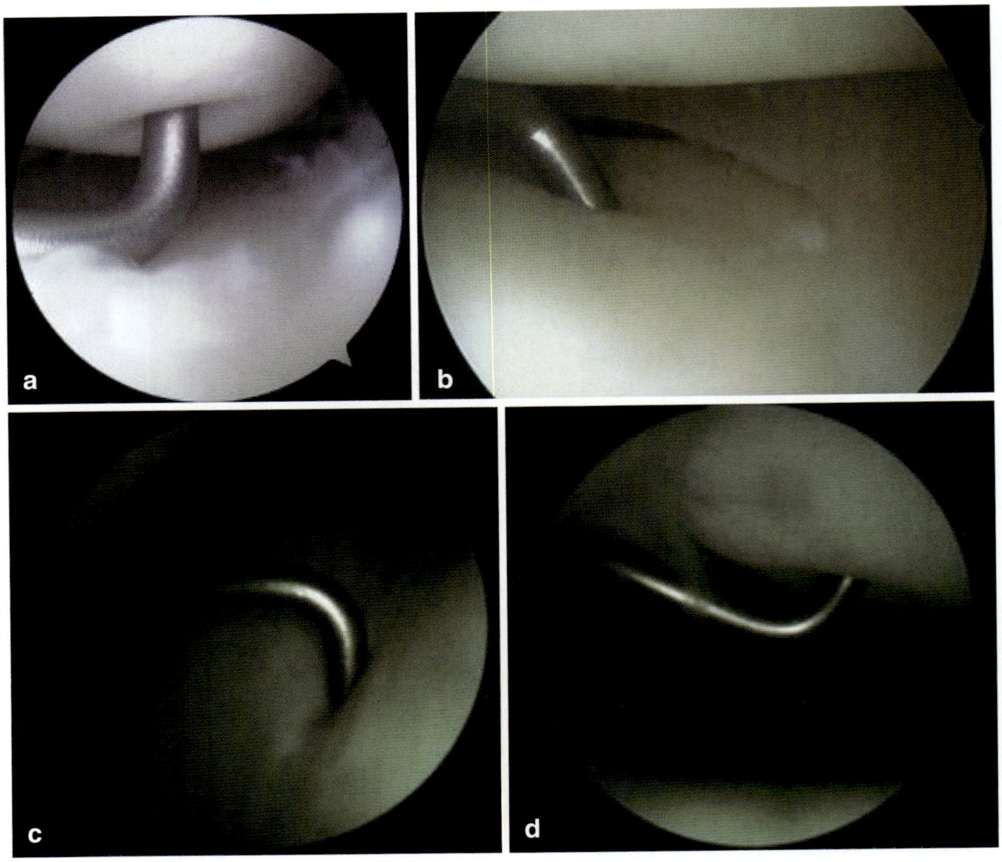

Fig. 7.1 Outerbridge I chondropathy of the internal femoral condyle (**a**), internal tibial plateau (**b**), trochlear groove (**c**) and of the patella (**d**)

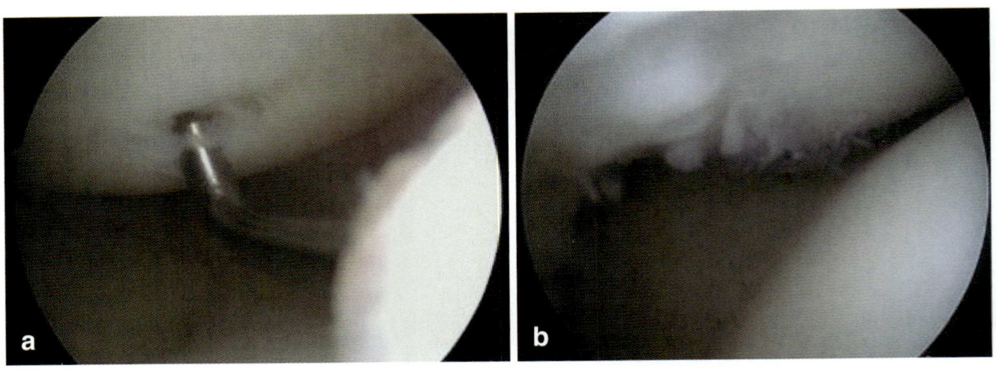

Fig. 7.2 Outerbridge II chondropathy of the internal femoral condyle (**a**) and trochlear groove (**b**)

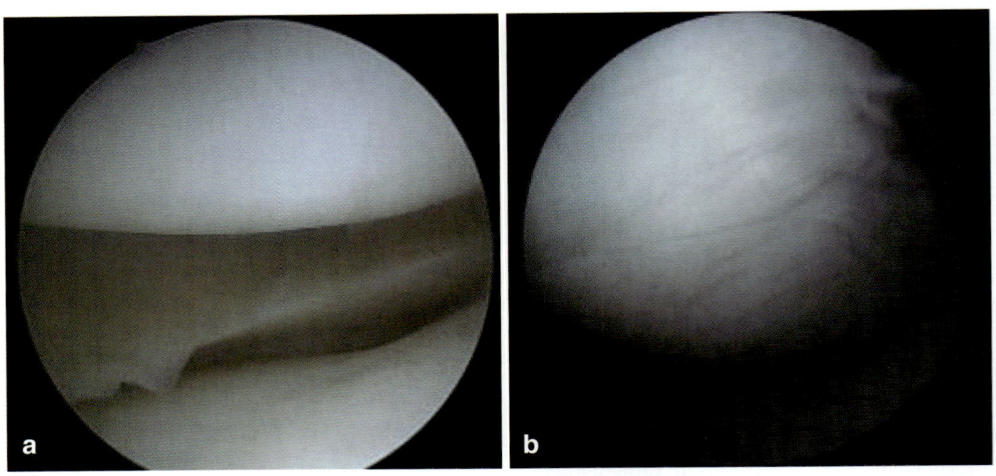

Fig. 7.3 Internal compartment with intact cartilage on the femoral and tibial condyles (**a**). Outerbridge II lesion of the internal femoral condyle. This is a lesion typical to chronic ACL deficient knees (**b**)

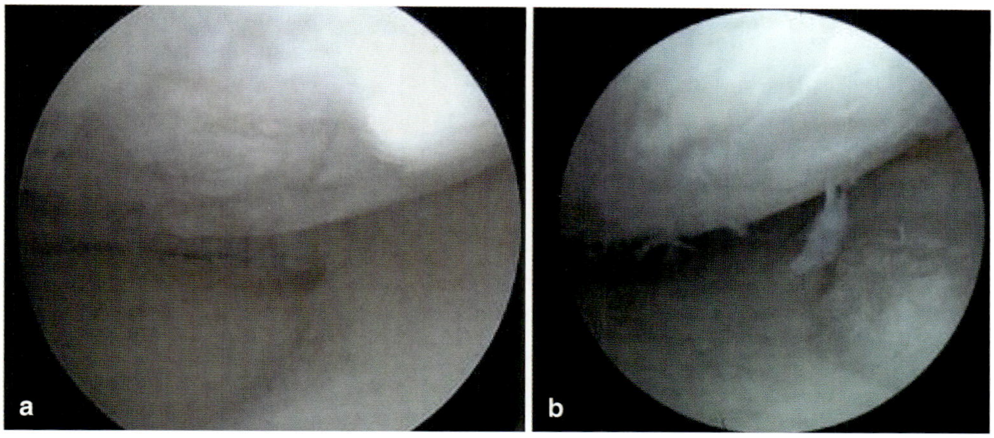

Fig. 7.4 Outerbridge III lesions of the internal femoral condyle. Note the meniscus has been partially removed, this goes to show that these are chronic lesions (**a**, **b**)

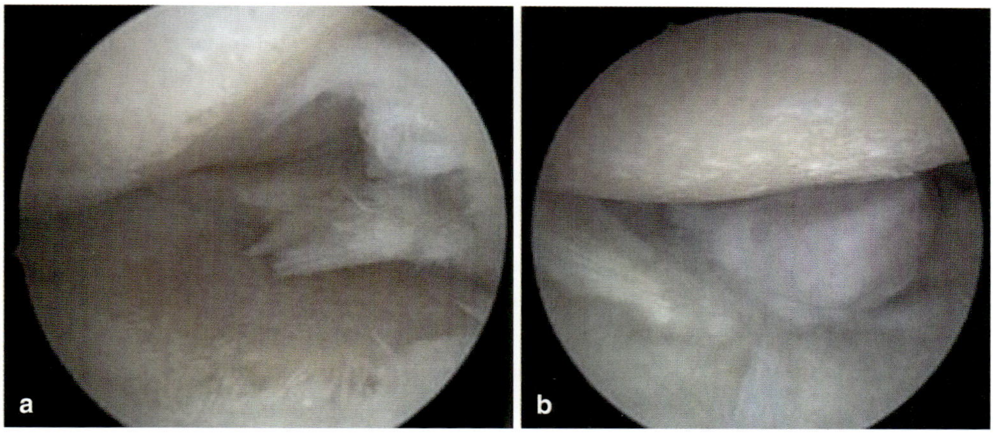

Fig. 7.5 Outerbridge IV lesions. *Left image* (**a**) shows mirrored lesions and in *right image* (**b**) we can see an articular loose body in the lateral recess

7.1 The Noyes Classification

- Grade 1: Cartilage surface intact
  - 1A = some remaining resilience;
  - 1B = deformation
- Grade 2A: Cartilage surface damaged (cracks, fibrillation, fissuring, or fragmentation); with less than half of cartilage thickness involved
- Grade 2B: Depth of involvement greater than half of cartilage thickness but without exposed bone
- Grade 3: Bone exposed
  - 3A = surface intact;
  - 3B = surface cavitation

The more recent ICRS (International Cartilage Repair Society) classification:

- Grade 0: Normal
- Grade 1: Nearly Normal (soft indentation and/or superficial fissures and cracks)
- Grade 2: Abnormal (lesions extending down to <50 % of cartilage depth)
- Grade 3: Severely Abnormal (cartilage defects >50 % of cartilage depth)
- Grade 4: Severely abnormal (through the subchondral bone)

The cartilage is an avascular and aneural tissue, thus its regenerative capacities are rather limited and this causes the progressive aspect of these degenerative lesions and the difficulty in treating these lesions. The classic therapeutic options of chondroplasty and microfractures can do only a little to resolve the actual pathology and do so only partially, the result being a fibrocartilage with mechanical proprieties that are not similar to that of the damaged hyaline cartilage and do not actually stop the overall degenerative process.

Calcium pyrophosphate dihydrate deposition (CPPD) or chondrocalcinosis (Fig. 7.6) is a rheumatologic condition caused by the accumulation of crystals of calcium pyrophosphate dihydrate in the connective tissues. It is sometimes used as a synonym for chondrocalcinosis, but the two pathologies, while similar, are not equal. Chondrocalcinosis represents the visible presence of calcification within tissues on an imaging study. According to Richette et al the correct definition would be: 'chondrocalcinosis' (CC)—radiographic calcification of articular fibro- or hyaline cartilage; 'pyrophosphate arthropathy'—structural abnormality of cartilage and bone associated with articular CPPD deposition; and 'pseudogout'—the clinical syndrome of acute synovitis associated with intraarticular CPPD deposition [2–4].

Cartilage lesions can also appear secondary to other joint pathologies such as ACL ruptures that cause secondary instability, synovial plicae, especially the mediopatellar plica causes cartilage damage, chronic synovitis or chronic, neglected meniscal tears. Another type of cartilage lesions are the ones caused by the operating surgeon – the iatrogenic injuries. Lack of experience, large instruments and vile maneuvers during joint exploration can cause cartilage lesions so an absolute delicacy is required to perform knee arthroscopic surgery. Another type of iatrogenic injures are those created by drills during the anatomic trans AM placement of the femoral tunnel during ACL reconstructions. To address this special, thinner, drills have been designed with only the diameter of the cutting surface (tip) of the drill changing, while the stem remains the same diameter (Fig. 7.7).

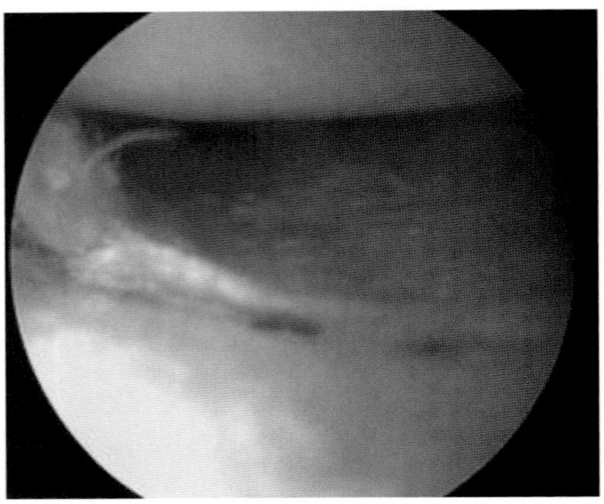

Fig. 7.6 Crystals of calcium deposited on the medial tibial plateau

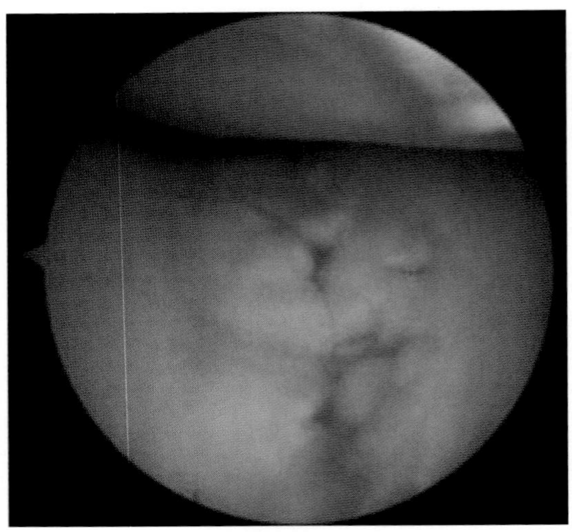

Fig. 7.7 This image shows a iatrogenic cartilage lesion of the trochlear groove made by the aggressive insertion of the canula or another instrument in the suprapatellar compartment of the knee joint

7.2 Articular Loose Bodies

A loose body is a free-floating piece of bone, cartilage or a foreign object in the knee joint, the most common joint for loose bodies. We will present in this chapter two types of articular loose bodies, the chondral and osteochondral types, different, iatrogenic, loose bodies will be presented in the complications chapter (Fig. 7.8).

Cartilaginous and bony intra-articular bodies float freely within the synovial fluid and can grow in dimension over time due to the nutritive proprieties of the synovial fluid. The most frequent cause of articular loose bodies is synovial osteochondromatosis, a cartilaginous metaplasia of the synovial membrane. It can also be caused by a fracture with avulsed fragment or detached, calcified meniscus, a detached bone spur, osteochondritis dissecans. Other, less frequent causes are synovial chondrosarcoma, pigmented villonodular synovitis, osteomyelitis and synovial chondrosarcoma.

Loose bodies can be found in knee joints years after the original traumatic event, moving from the suprapatellar compartment to the anterior, internal or external compartments and can cause reversible joint locking. Most often they tend to move in the lateral or medial recess and reside in the suprapatellar or, most often, in the posterior compartment of the knee because of the gravity effect, where they can become incarcerated. Because of the friction forces and the nutritional proprieties of the synovial fluid as the time passes they become rounded or oval in shape, as a more efficient way for them to travel trough the joint space with a minimal risk of creating secondary lesions.

Nevertheless in most of the cases they do create secondary lesions (Fig. 7.9), supplementary cartilage damage and meniscal injuries to name just a few. Chronic synovitis and secondary osteoarthritis both as a result of cartilage damage and synovial inflammation are a common end point, loose bodies are often found during TKA surgery.

Preoperative diagnosis of loose bodies can prove difficult at times, depending on the imaging method used for this. X-rays can detect osteochondral or calcified articular bodies, but fails to provide data for radiotransparent objects. CT and CT arthrography, while superior to plain X-rays do not provide the same amount of information as MRI does. But the imaging method of choice remains MR arthrography, superior to conventional MR in mapping out articular structures in joints with minimal fluid. No joint infiltration or fluoroscopic guidance is required. Removing articular loose bodies from the knee joint can be technically difficult (Fig. 7.10), especially for those trapped in the posterior compartment, where access is laborious with regular arthroscopic instruments.

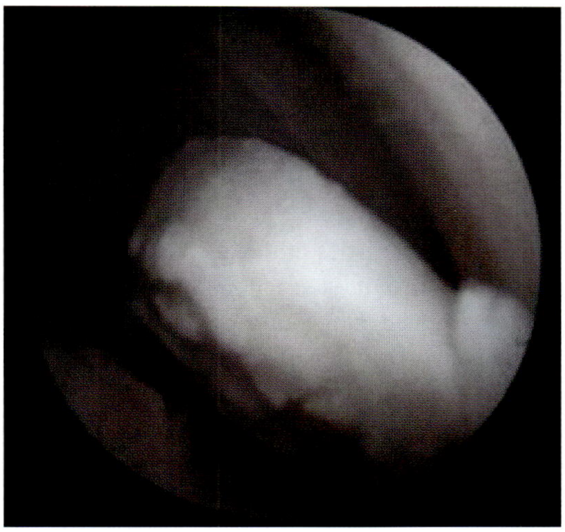

Fig. 7.8 This loose body in the lateral recess of the knee has started to have rounded edges, showing that some time has passed since the lesion was produced

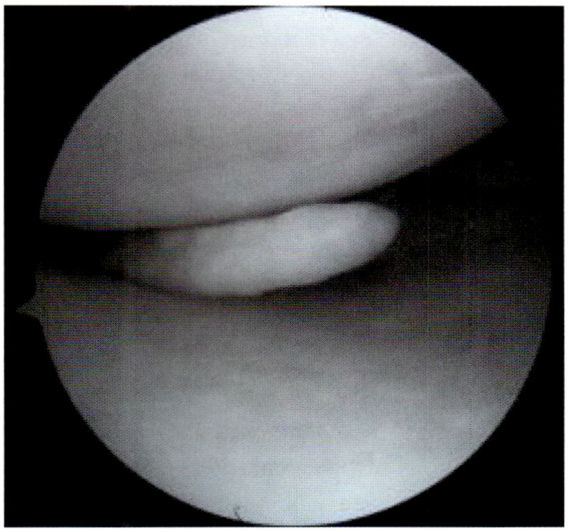

Fig. 7.9 Chronic chondral loose body in the internal compartment of the knee

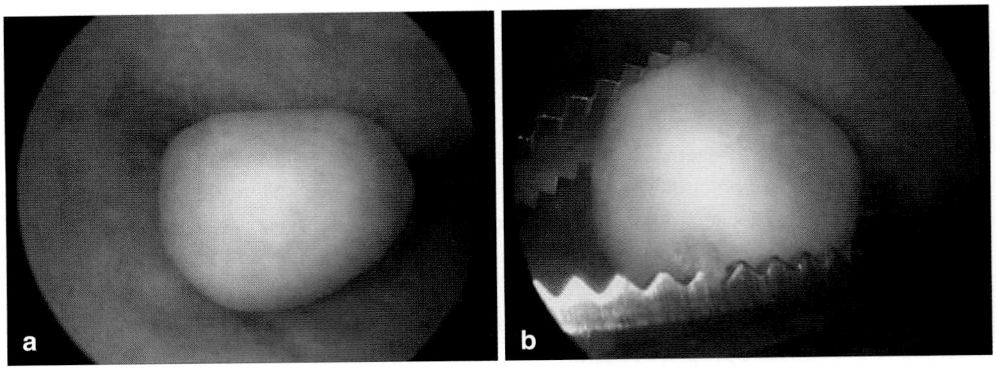

Fig. 7.10 Loose body associated with Outerbridge IV chondropathy (**a**) and the removal of the loose body (**b**)

7.3 Osteochondritis Dissecans

Osteochondritis dissecans (abbreviated OCD and OD) is a condition in which a fragment of bone in a joint is deprived of blood and separates from the rest of the bone, causing soreness and making the joint give way. While OCD may affect any joint, the most affected joint in the human body is the knee. Left untreated, it leads to secondary osteoarthritis caused by joint incongruity and aberrant wear patterns, especially in adult patients. OCD is classified as a juvenile (JOCD) or adult (AOCD) form based on the skeletal maturity of the patients, i.e. the presence or absence of open growth plates. OCD is one of the most common causes of knee pain in teenagers, with a peak in occurrence in the 10–15 years age group. JOCD has been recognised as a pathological entity for more than 100 years, but its pathogenesis is still widely debated, with no certain cause having been pinned down, it is believed to be caused by repetitive trauma [5–7] (Fig. 7.11).

Young people are involved in a wide array of sports that require intensive family support, thus early recognition of osteochondral lesions of the knee is easier to make [6, 8]. Osteochondritis dissecans OCD of the knee can be classified in an adult form and a juvenile form. However, these two forms of OCD have a different natural evolution in terms of the disease and the outcomes that they produce. JOCD has a better outcome under conservative treatment than the adult form with high degree of family involvement and commitment, the "compliance triad" of physician, parent, and child being the key element when a conservative treatment plan for JOCD is initiated. JOCD can be further subdivided in a adolescent form a juvenile form, depending on the status of the growth physis [5, 9, 10].

- Juvenile Osteochondritis Dissecans: wide open physis
- Adolescent Osteochondritis Dissecans: closing physis
- Adult Osteochondritis Dissecans: closed physis

Diagnosis and lesion location are made using standard AP and lateral radiographs and MRI. X-rays can determine the site of the lesion but magnetic resonance adds more detail to that information such as the state of the subchondral bone (bond edema, separation), cartilage condition and associated lesions. Radiographic grading is done with the Cahill classification but the most useful are the two classification systems are widely used for staging JOCD, the Hefti classification, based on MRI aspects and the arthroscopic Gühl classification.

The Hefti classification:

- Stage 1: Small change without clear margins of fragment
- Stage 2: Osteochondral fragment with clear margins but without fluid between the fragment and underlying bone
- Stage 3: Fluid is visible partially between fragment and underlying bone
- Stage 4: Fluid is completely surrounding the fragment, but the fragment is in situ.
- Stage 5: Fragment is completely detached and displaced (loose body).

The Gühl classification:

- Stage I: Intact Lesions
- Stage II: Lesions showing signs of early separation
- Stage III: Partially detached lesions
- Stage IV: Craters with loose bodies (Fig. 7.12)

Treatment algorithms have been developed for the treatment of OCD depending on the age of the patient, physeal maturity, the characteristics of the lesion (size location, grading) and symptoms. It is usual incomplete, stable JOCD lesions to be treated nonoperatively with good prognosis. Knee immobilization with partial weightbearing (4–6 weeks) is started after which, if the knee is pain free weightbearing progresses and rehab is started (knee ROM and strengthening exercises). No sports are allowed. A secondary clinical and X-ray evaluation is made at 3–4 months, if there are enough signs of healing return to sports is gradually permitted. Success rates have been reported to be of 50 % at 10–18 months.

Treatment of osteochondral lesions of the juvenile knee should be coordinated with the degree of articular cartilage impairment and the size of the lesion and most importantly the type of lesion. While conservative treatment for JOCD has a demonstrated success rate, with a secondary surgical indication, chronic lesions will benefit from arthroscopic treatment as well. For juvenile patients with OCD the first line of treatment is conservative therapy for which relatively good outcomes have been reported, Cahill reported a 56 % success rate on a series of 92 knees followed scintigraphically for an average of 4.2 years with no knee immobilization and a complete restriction of athletic activities. Other authors report similar success rates, with or without immobilization the higher number of stable lesions and healing under conservative treatment demonstrates that juvenile OCD has a much better prognosis than adult OCD. There is still debate over the role and length of immobilization but a general phased conservative treatment protocol has been produced [10–13].

Phase 1 (Weeks 0–6):

- Knee immobilisation (cast or brace)
- Partial weight bearing with crutches
- Pain free knee is a criteria for phase 2

Phase 2 (Weeks 6–12)

- No knee immobilization
- Weight bearing as tolerated
- Physical therapy: ROM and low impact strengthening (quads, hams).
- No sports
- X-ray – healing with clinical improvement – phase 3.

Phase 3 (from 3 to 4 months)

- A complete absence of symptoms allows for gradually loading the knee (running, jumping and eventually sports) with progressively increased intensity
- Follow-up MRI/scintigraphy shows the degree of lesion healing.

While conservative treatment is indicated for most patients with JOCD as the first line of treatment and surgical therapy is usually reserved for cases that failed to show signs of healing at follow-up, there are situations that imply surgery as the first line of treatment such as unstable lesions on MRI valuation and articular loose bodies from a lesion with a detached osteochondral fragment. The same cannot be said for AOCD, where because of the greater risk of instability the treatment of choice is early surgical intervention.

Surgical therapy for osteochondral lesions includes several options such as bone marrow stimulation techniques, subchondral drilling, loose fragment fixation, cartilage abrasion, loose body removal, allograft transplant, OATS and ACI. Treatment algorithms have been conceived to address these lesions, one of the most useful is the one described by Garrido et al., presented in Fig. 7.13 [13, 14].

Bone marrow stimulation include drilling the lesion for grade I and II stable JOCD and microfractures for chronic JOCD (Fig. 7.14). Microfractures represent the piercing of small holes in the area of the defect to allow for nutrient and growth factor rich blood to penetrate through to the joint space. This will allow the cartilaginous defect to be filled with fibrous cartilage. Subchondral drilling creates vascular channels in low grade stable OCD lesions or as a supplement to fragment fixation.

Antegrade drilling is done orthogonally under direct arthroscopic visualization using the standard portals or separate accessory portals. Retrograde drilling necessitates C-arm radioscopic control to avoid joint penetration or the secondary mobilisation of the osteochondral fragment or ACL tibial aiming device with or without sonography. Iliac crest bone graft supplementation has also been added to help in healing. Good and excellent results have been reported in literature. The healing rate was of 80 % in adolescent JOCD patients, with 70 % or more being able to return to sports.

Higher grade lesions (3 & 4) with unstable osteochondral fragments with a totally or partially detached fragment (trap door) and acute OCF's have an indication for fixation of the fragment. This can be achieved via metal screws (Herbert), metal or bioabsorbable pins or bio-screws (Fig. 7.14). Each have their advantages, some authors prefer the use of metal implants that need hardware removal surgeries to benefit from this second look arthroscopy to check the status of the cartilage [14–18].

Grafting the lesion is the most complex treatment method, reserved for the chronic, large size JOCD lesions. Autograft transplantation is a surgical option but availability is reduced to a small number of patients. It represents the harvesting of a osteochondral plugs from nonweightbearing areas of the joint and implanting them in the bed of the defect. One plug is sufficient for 2 cm^2 of lesion surface. Allografting is permitted in some countries by legislation, with instrumentation systems available to size and match the defect. NWB rehabilitations are started postoperatively. Good rates of survival have been reported for osteochondral grafts.

Autologus condhrocyte implantation allows the repair of defects up to 10 cm^2 and up to 8 mm in depth. Chondrocytes are harvested, grown in a cell culture in a lab and inserted in the defect in a pouch made by autologus periosteum or a synthetic collagen patch [7, 14, 18, 19].

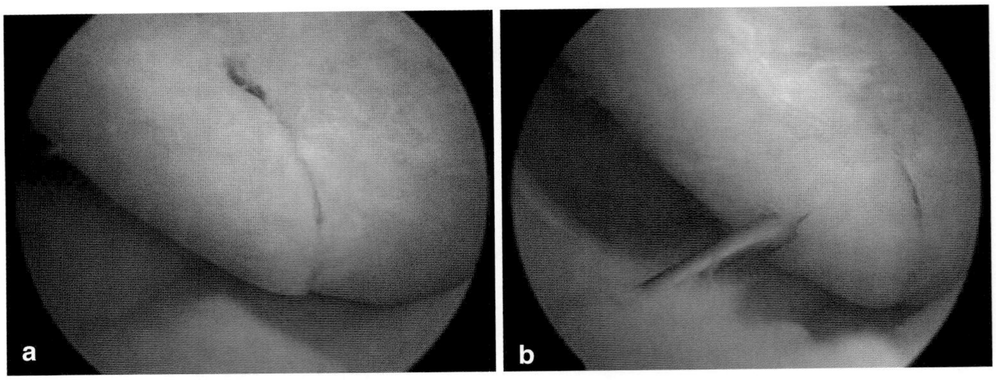

Fig. 7.11 The chronic cartilaginous lesion is seen with clear delimitation from the normal cartilage (**a**, **b**)

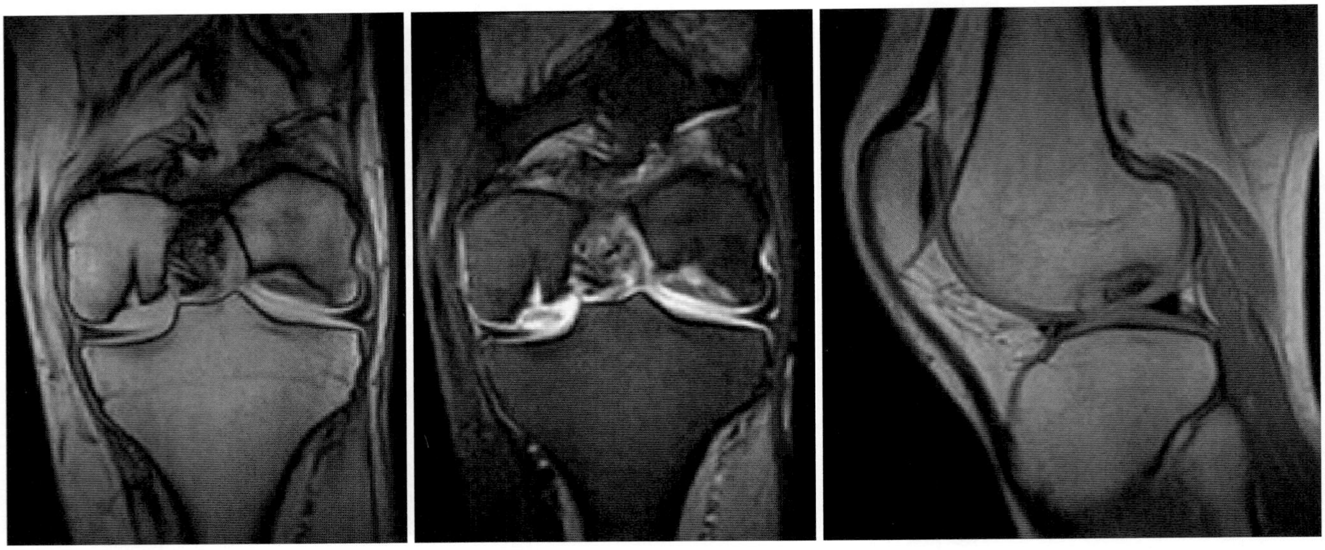

Fig. 7.12 MRI showing OCD Stage IV lesion on coronal T1 GFE, coronal STIR and sagital T1

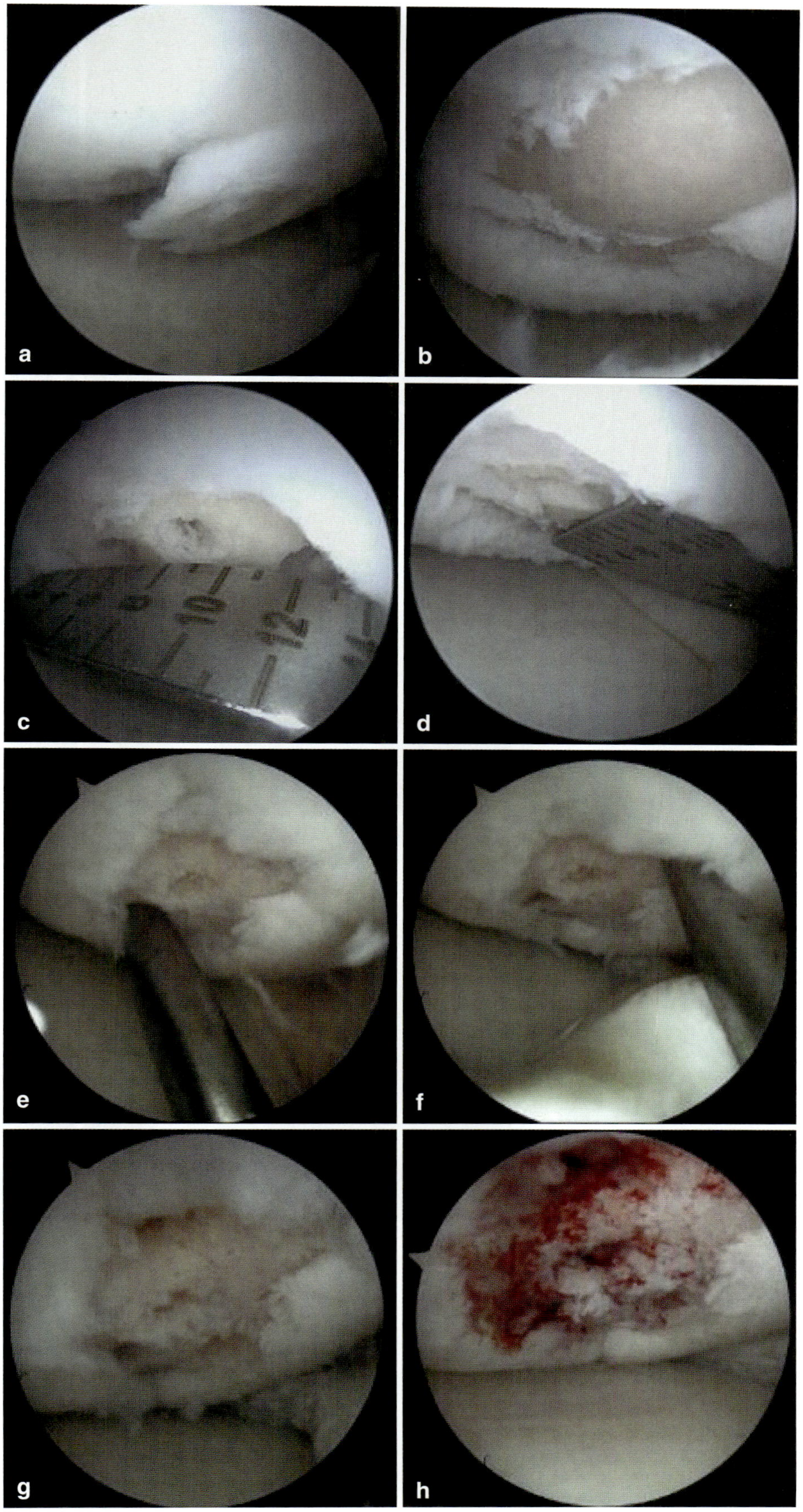

Fig. 7.13 The OCD lesion is visualized on the articular surface of the medial femoral condyle (**a**), the cartilage completely detached with a clear circumferential delimitation from the flat subchondral bone (**b**). Bone marrow stimulation – microfractures are seen (**c, e, f**), the ruler is used to size up the lesion (**d**). Chondroplasty was performed to help the fibrous cartilage blend with the normal unaltered cartilage. Microfracture technique: the subchondral bone is pierced with the perforator throughout the fracture bed, at a distance of 1 mm from the other, cartilage edges shaved; blood is seen coming out of the perforations (**g**, **h**)

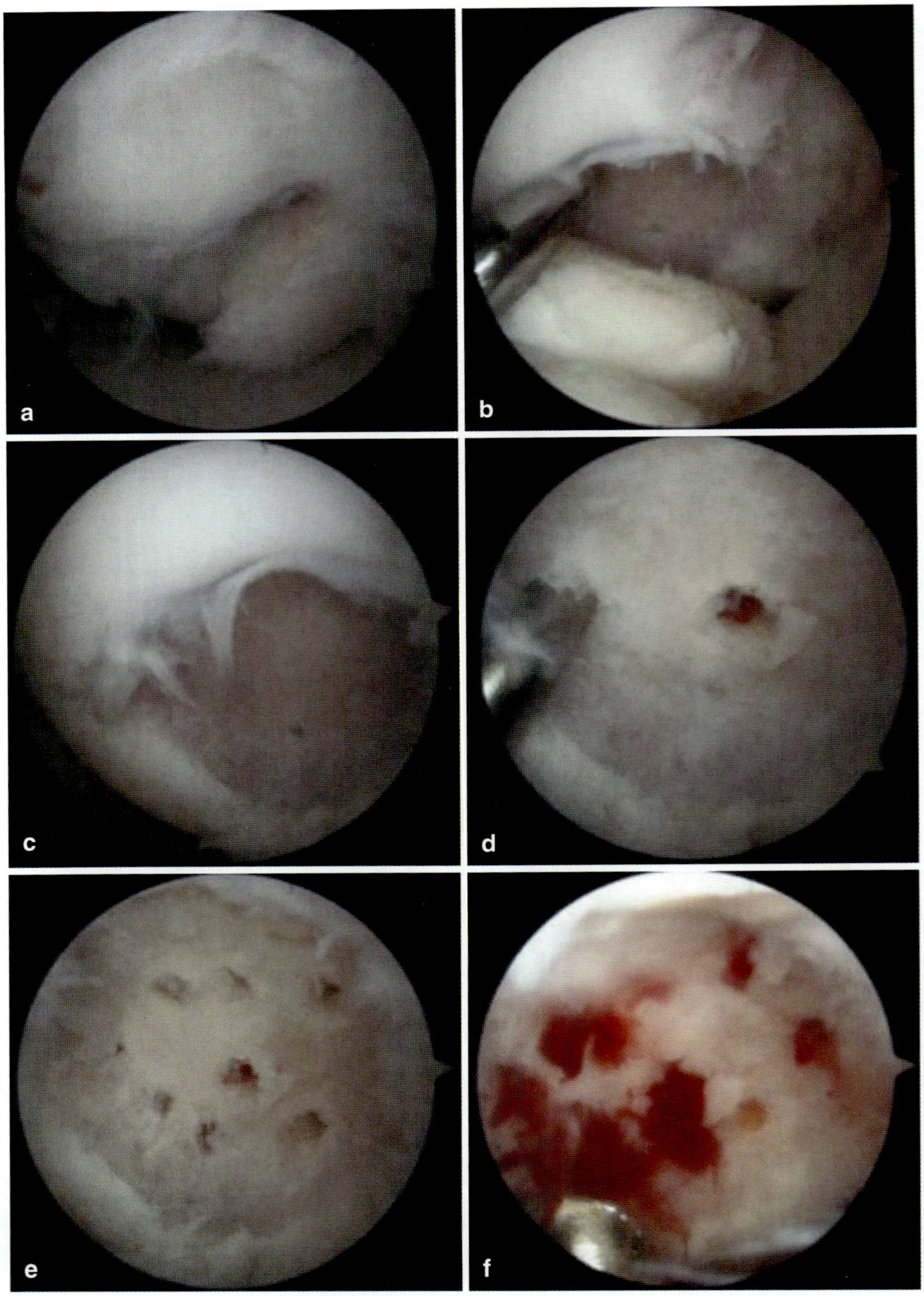

Fig. 7.14 AOCD lesion (**a**), the chondral fragment is removed (**b**, **c**, **d**), the subchondral bone bed is microfractured and the edges are shaved (**e**, **f**)

7.4 Cartilage Transplant

Cartilage is a avascular, aneural and alymphatic tissue that is comprised by a combination of water (67–80 %), matrix of proteoglycans, collagens and proteins that form a macromolecular framework for the rare cells of this cartilage, the chondrocytes. These take about 1–2 % of the tissue and are responsible for the production of the matrix. Because of the avascular nature of this tissue their nutrition is made by diffusion.

At the forefront of therapeutic options in treating cartilage lesions is the cartilage transplant. There are a few techniques available for the repair of the cartilage tissue, such as autologous transplant, allograft cartilage transplant and ACI (autologous chondrocyte implantation) a technique with several variations and the most difficult from a technical point of view. Still not a widely used method, mostly because of its high cost, not supported by insurance companies in every country, it requires two surgeries, one for harvesting the cartilage matrix and one for inserting the artificially grown cartilage in the knee. ACI has been demonstrated to be a good option for treating cartilage defects larger than 4 cm^2 resulting from osteochondritis dissecans or chronic osteochondral fracture. It is not, however, an option of treatment for degenerative cartilage loss (Fig. 7.15).

The initial surgery is a knee arthroscopy that serves for the debridement of the cartilage lesion, the sizing and preparation of its edges, the harvesting of a piece of unaffected cartilage from a non weightbearing region of the femoral condyles storing it in a special nutritive solution and sending it to the lab for chondrocyte multiplication. Associated lesions can be treated during this first, arthroscopic surgery stage. After sufficient cell multiplication that takes about 3–4 weeks the artificially grown cartilage base is returned from the lab and the second, implantation, surgery is scheduled. A medial parapatellar approach is selected with knee arthrothomy for better exposure of the articular surface. The chondrocyte matter is placed in the cleaned defect under a protective pouch made out of autologus periosteum or a synthetic mesh. The knee is immobilized in 20° of flexion, nonweightbearing for 4 weeks (Fig. 7.16).

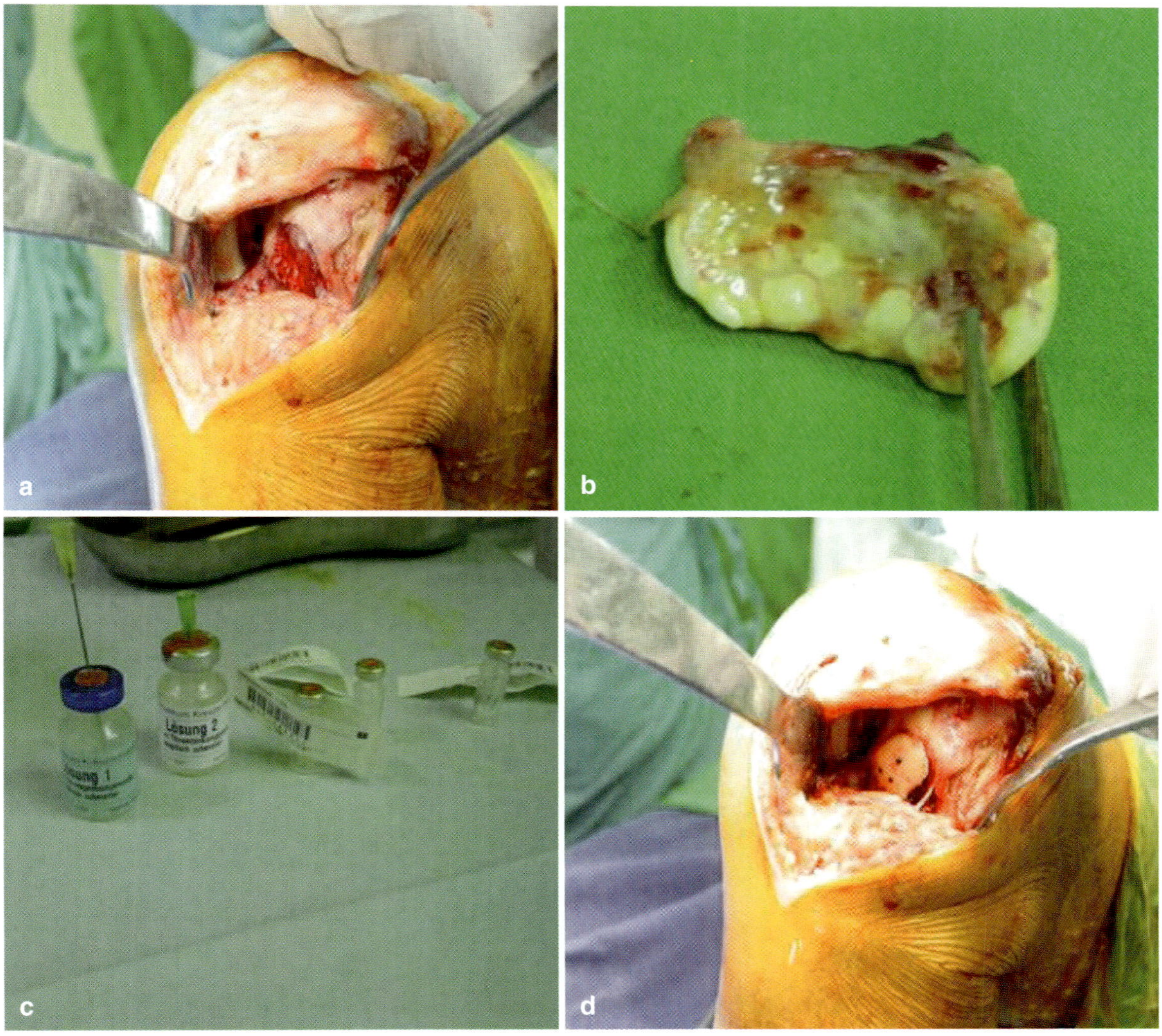

Fig. 7.15 The osteochondral defect of the medial femoral condyle is visualized trough the medial parapatellar arthrotomy (**a**) and the osteochondral fragment removed (**b**), artificially grown chondrocytes (**c**), that are applied in the lesion bed and the final aspect of repair after fixation of the OC fragment and insertion of the autologous chondrocytes (**d**)

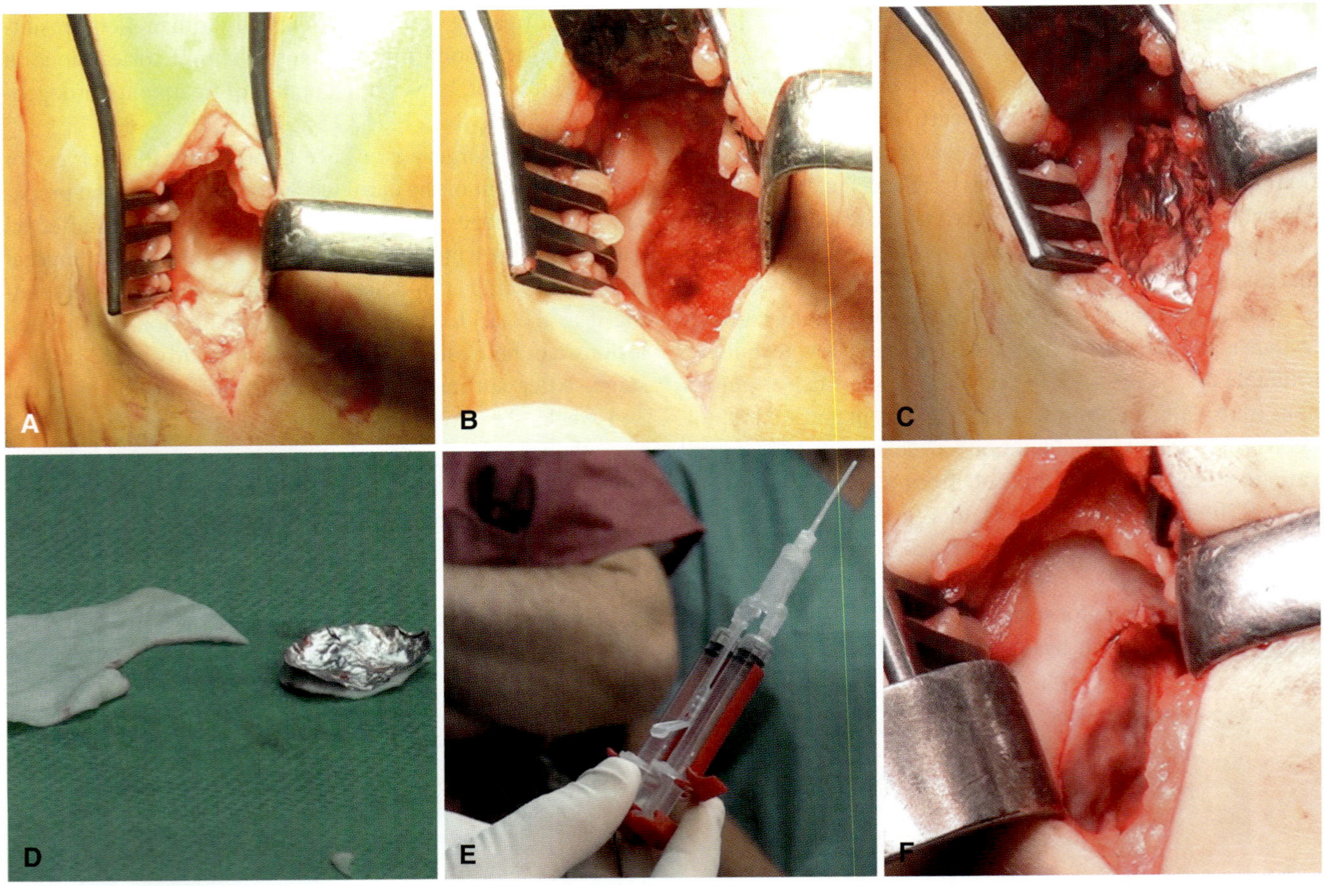

Fig. 7.16 Mini arthrotomy approach osteocondritis dissecans of the medial condyle, weight bearing area (**a**). After initial treatment the defect is filled with fibrous tissue (**b**). The area is debrided (**c**) and a mapping of the defect is performed to precisely cut the matrix (**d**). The fibrin glue is prepared (**e**) and the matrix is attached on site (**f**)

References

1. Cameron ML, Briggs KK, Steadman JR. Reproducibility and reliability of the outerbridge classification for grading chondral lesions of the knee arthroscopically. Am J Sports Med. 2003;31(1):83–6.
2. Richette P, Bardin T, Doherty M. An update on the epidemiology of calcium pyrophosphate dihydrate crystal deposition disease. Rheumatology (Oxford). 2009;48(7):711–5.
3. Ferrone C, Andracco R, Cimmino MA. Calcium pyrophosphate deposition disease: clinical manifestations. Reumatismo. 2011;63(4):246–52.
4. Zhang W, Doherty M, Bardin T, et al European League Against Rheumatism recommendations for calcium pyrophosphate deposition. Part I: terminology and diagnosis. Ann Rheum Dis. 2011;70(4):563–70.
5. Cahill B. Osteochondritis dissecans of the knee: treatment of juvenile and adult forms. J Am Acad Orthop Surg. 1995;3(4):237–47.
6. Polousky JD. Juvenile osteochondritis dissecans. Sports Med Arthrosc. 2011;19(1):56–63.
7. Kocher MS, Tucker R, Ganley TJ, Flynn JM. Management of osteochondritis dissecans of the knee: current concepts review. Am J Sports Med. 2006;34(7):1181–91.
8. Wall E, Stein Von D. Juvenile osteochondritis dissecans. Orthop Clin North Am. 2003;34(3):341–53.
9. Cahill BR, Ahten SM. The three critical components in the conservative treatment of juvenile osteochondritis dissecans (JOCD). Physician, parent, and child. Clin Sports Med. 2001;20(2):287–98, vi.
10. Cahill BR, Phillips MR, Navarro R. The results of conservative management of juvenile osteochondritis dissecans using joint scintigraphy. A prospective study. Am J Sports Med. 1989;17(5):601–5; discussion 605–6.
11. Kijowski R, Blankenbaker DG, Shinki K, Fine JP, Graf BK, De Smet AA. Juvenile versus adult osteochondritis dissecans of the knee: appropriate MR imaging criteria for instability. Radiology. 2008;248(2):571–8.
12. Shea KG, Jacobs JC, Grimm NL, Pfeiffer RP. Osteochondritis dissecans development after bone contusion of the knee in the skeletally immature: a case series. Knee Surg Sports Traumatol Arthrosc. 2013;21(2):403–7.
13. Samora WP, Chevillet J, Adler B, Young GS, Klingele KE. Juvenile osteochondritis dissecans of the knee: predictors of lesion stability. J Pediatr Orthop. 2012;32(1):1–4.
14. Pascual-Garrido C, Mcnickle AG, Cole BJ. Surgical treatment options for osteochondritis dissecans of the knee. Sports Health. 2009;1(4):326–34.
15. Wachowski MM, Floerkemeier T, Balcarek P, Walde TA, Schüttrumpf JP, Frosch S, et al. Mid-term clinical and MRI results after refixation of osteochondral fractures with resorbable implants. Z Orthop Unfall. 2011;149(1):61–7.
16. Trinh TQ, Harris JD, Flanigan DC. Surgical management of juvenile osteochondritis dissecans of the knee. Knee Surg Sports Traumatol Arthrosc. 2012;20(12):2419–29.
17. Lintz F, Pujol N, Pandeirada C, Boisrenoult P, Beaufils P. Hybrid fixation: evaluation of a novel technique in adult osteochondritis dissecans of the knee. Knee Surg Sports Traumatol Arthrosc. 2011;19(4):568–71.
18. Sasaki K, Matsumoto T, Matsushita T, Kubo S, Ishida K, Tei K, et al. Osteochondral autograft transplantation for juvenile osteochondritis dissecans of the knee: a series of twelve cases. Int Orthop. 2012;36(11):2243–8.
19. Cahill B. Treatment of juvenile osteochondritis dissecans and osteochondritis dissecans of the knee. Clin Sports Med. 1985;4(2):367–84.

Patellar Instability

8

Florin Ramadani and Horia Haragus

The symptomatic patello-femoral compartment can have a broad spectrum of causes and presentations. Anterior knee pain can be present without apparent pathological clinical findings. The etiology is ill-defined and patellar maltracking alone cannot explain all clinical presentations, especially the pain at rest. A history of trauma may lead to recurrent dislocations and instability if additional anatomical morphological abnormalities are present. Thus, numerous factors have to be evaluated in order to improve the accuracy of determining the cause of the symptoms.

The patella is the largest sesamoid bone in the human body. It serves as a connection between the large quadriceps muscles and the tibia, through the patellar tendon (Fig. 8.1).

F. Ramadani, MD, PhD
Unfallchirurgie, Klinikum Wels-Grieskirchen,
42 Grieskirchner St, Wels A-4600, Austria

University of Medicine and Pharmacy 'Victor Babes' Timisoara,
Timisoara, Romania
e-mail: florin.ramadani@liwest.at

H. Haragus, MD, PhD (✉)
Department of Orthopedics and Trauma,
University of Medicine and Pharmacy 'Victor Babes' Timisoara,
Timisoara, Romania

I-st Clinic of Orthopedics and Trauma,
Emergency Clinical County Hospital Timisoara,
10 Iosif Bulbuca Blvd, Timisoara 300736, Romania
e-mail: horia.haragus@yahoo.com

R. Prejbeanu (ed.), *Atlas of Knee Arthroscopy*,
DOI 10.1007/978-1-4471-6593-4_8, © Springer-Verlag London 2015

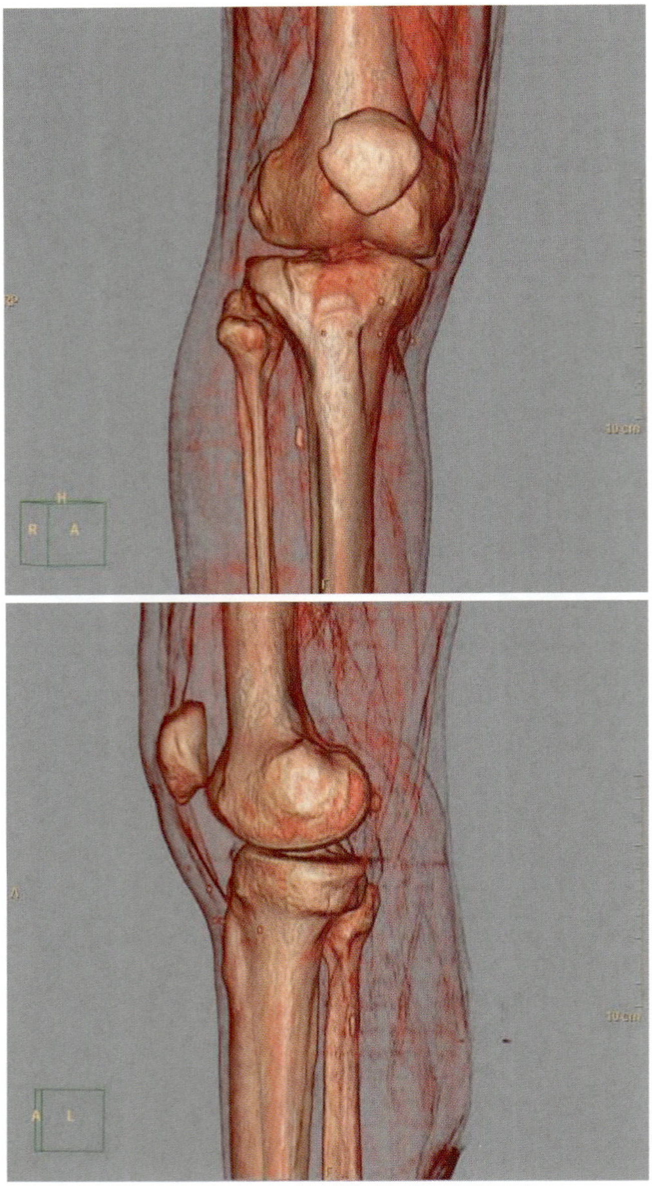

Fig. 8.1 anterior and medial views of the knee joint from volume rendered computed tomography depicting the normal anatomy and relations

8.1 Proximal Procedures

Patellar instability is a term that describes a multitude of causes that lead to chronic lateral patellar subluxation or recurrent episodes of dislocation. The clinical presentation is usually residual after an acute dislocation in patients with altered patello-femoral and extensor mechanism morphology.

The clinical exam findings are the most important when deciding for surgical treatment of patellar instability. The positive apprehension test is a very suggestive subjective measure of lateral instability. It is performed with the patient supine and the knee close to full extension. The examiner gently pushes lateral on the patella while the patient's intension is to apprehend and terminate the action. The lateral glide should have no firm endpoint and the translation should be greater than two quadrants (roughly patellar quarters) or 10 mm. The knee is put through flexion and the centration of the patella in the trochlea is observed. Permanent lateral dislocation will require more than MPFL reconstruction.

8.1.1 Lateral Release

Is commonly performed during arthroscopic procedures. However, the indications have reduced considerable and there is very little evidence to support isolated use. The main indication to performing lateral release, isolated or in association with proximal or distal procedures is excessive patellar tilt and lateral facet hyperpressure due to tightness of the lateral retinaculum or a dysplastic quadriceps. In other circumstances, lateral retinacular release may aggravate patellar instability in early flexion [2, 12].

The patellar tilt is the angle formed by the transverse axis of the patella to a line tangential to the posterior femoral condyles. 3D CT images visualize the abnormalities but are not able to quantify them (Fig. 8.2):

8.1.2 Medial Reefing

Medial plication can be done mini open or arthroscopic. Three to five sutures (PDS No.1) are started from the distal third of the patella. These are passed over the ruptured medial structures if visible, such as in acute cases. If not, a 2 cm bridging from the medial border of the patella can be selected. Simple or vertical mattress type sutures can be performed, with the later having a true plication effect. Stability during range of motion is verified and additional sutures may be added or cut if inappropriate patellar tracking is observed. For the arthroscopic technique, the sutures are passed similar to 'outside in' meniscal sutures: two needles are used to pass a No.1 PDS and looped No.2/0 PDS sutures respectively. The No.1 is then passed through the loop with the aid of the probe or a grasp. The procedure is repeated for each suture and all are tightened at the end, with the knee in 60° of flexion.

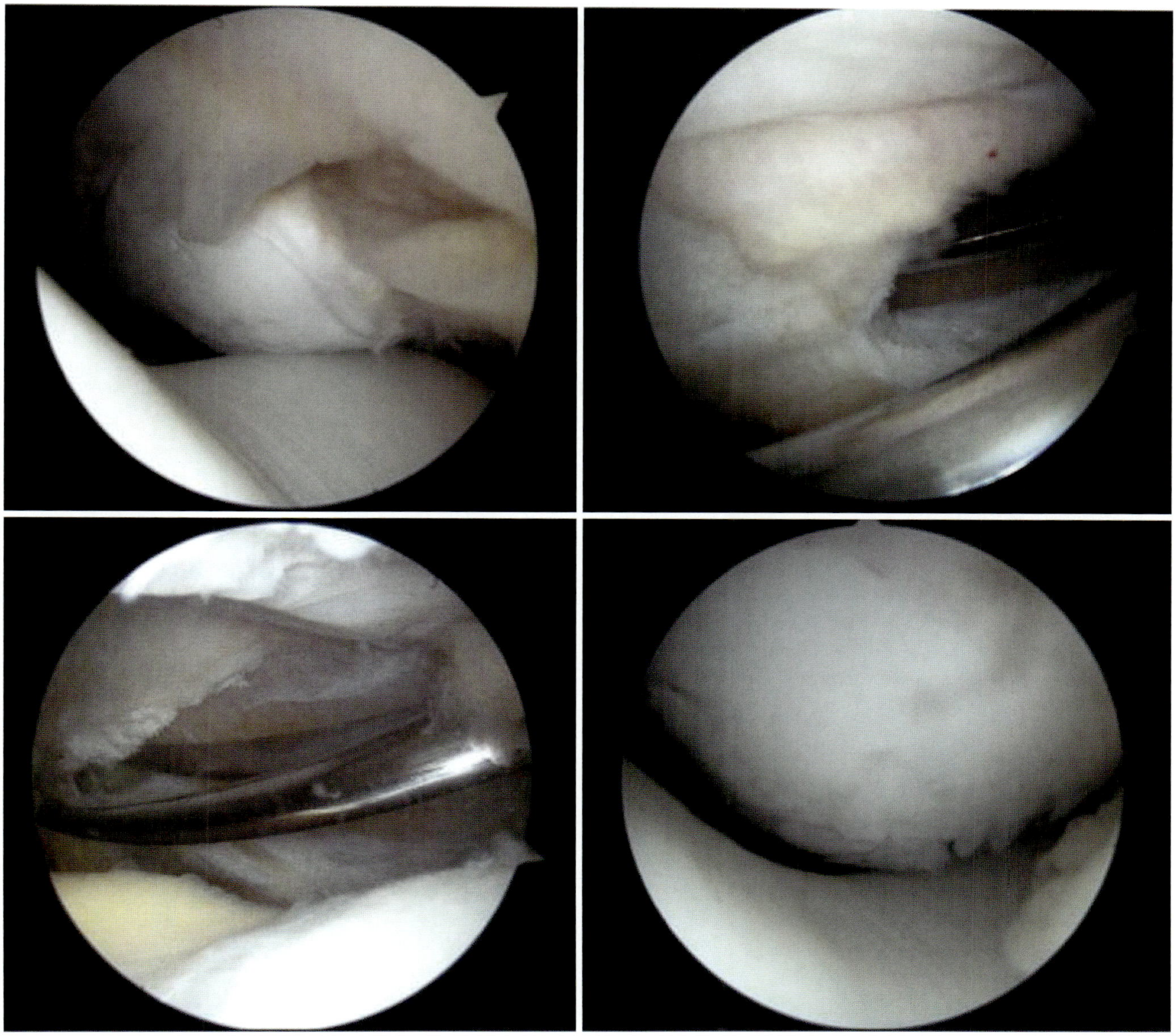

Fig. 8.2 Arthroscopic view through the anteromedial portal with the knee in extension; the patella is not centered in the trochlea. Lateral retinaculum release is performed with the scissors and this improves the tracking. The patellar cartilage is fragmented

8.2 MPFL Reconstruction

The acute lateral patella dislocation almost always tears the aponeurotic medial constraints and the medial patello-femoral ligament (MPFL). Nonsurgical approach is the recommended treatment for the initial episode, unless osteochondral fractures are loose in the joint. After reduction, the knee is immobilized in 20° of flexion. Gradual range of motion is started after two weeks with the orthosis on. Vastus medialis oblique (VMO) strengthening exercises are started after 6 weeks. This leads to 15–44 % recurrence rates, compared to 10–20 % after reconstruction of the MPFL, even in pediatric patients [19, 17].

The MPFL is the main passive medial restraint [1] and the VMO the main dynamic stabilizer, with obliquely oriented fibers. The MPFL is most taut with the quadriceps contracted and the knee in extension. During early flexion (20°), it resists lateral tensions and centers the patella in the trochlear groove [2]. The lateral trochlear facet becomes the main stabilizer in higher flexion (over 30°) [3]. It also resists lateral patellar tilt and rotation up to 90° of flexion.

Numerous variations for MPFL reconstruction have been described [14]. The procedure is suitable for a patient without significant anterior knee pain, with recurrent episodes of dislocation that are not permanent during flexion, a positive apprehension test and excessive lateral glide and mild patello-femoral arthritis at most. The MPFL reconstruction improves clinical symptoms and reduces the patellar tilt even in the presence of mild trochlear dysplasia or a TT-TG distance over 20 mm without tibial tuberosity medialization [15, 16] (Fig. 8.3).

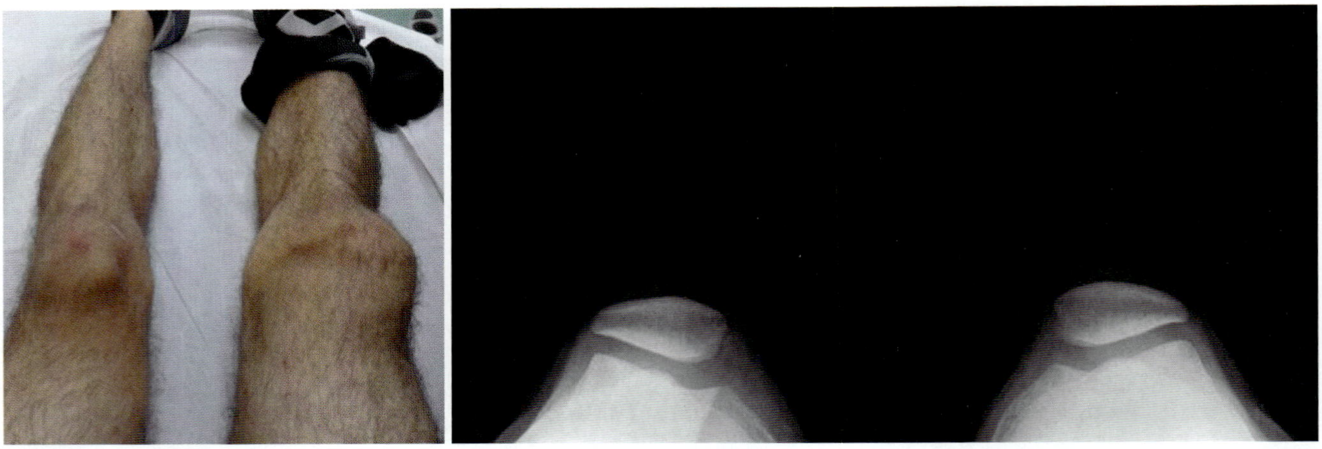

Fig. 8.3 Clinical aspect of recurrent (third) right patellar dislocation during sports. Merchant view shows a Wiberg type III patella, a wide trochlear groove angle and small bony avulsions on the right medial side

8.2.1 Surgical Technique

The patient is positioned supine with a Tourniquet cuff on the thigh and in the leg holder. The operating table can be complete or with the leg support dropped, leaving the knee flexed and the leg hanging down freely. The femoral tunnel is recommended to be checked intraoperatively with radioscopic imaging and thus a true lateral view of the distal femur should be possible when the patient is positioned and before sterile draping.

Standard arthroscopic anterolateral and anteromedial portals are used to confirm the inappropriate patellar tracking and explore the articulation. An accessory superolateral portal can facilitate examination of the patella in the trochlea as well as document postoperative reduction.

The most commonly used graft is the semitendinosus (semi T). The gracilis may not have sufficient length routinely but otherwise can also be used. The harvest is usually performed in the same fashion as for ACL reconstruction (see Sect. 3.7.1). Alternatively, the hamstrings can be harvested by slightly extending the incision made for the femoral fixation. A 24 mm long free semi T is cleaned of remaining muscle and 4 (2 cm) looped traction sutures (No.2 non- or absorbable) are saw on both free ends. It is than sized single and double (looped) for adequate tunnel accommodation.

A vertical incision is made on the medial side of the patella (3 cm). The dissection is advanced deeper but proud of the knee capsule (remains extraarticular). This vertically oriented ligament is found between layers 2 and 3, together with the medial collateral ligament. The patellar attachment of the MPFL is wider and located approximately at the junction of the upper and middle thirds of the patella, where the medial border becomes more vertical. The patellar bone is exposed and two tunnels are drilled 1 cm apart, close to the articular surface. These are used for the patellar attachment, which can be done either by transosseous tunnels or anchors. If the later is chosen, the 4.5 mm tunnels are advanced to a depth of 1 cm with exit holes on the anterior cortex of patella. This way the fracture risk is reduced, compared to drilling all the way through the lateral border. The graft is than attached to the patella at the middle of the loop using two anchors (Fig. 8.4);

A small (2 cm) incision is made between the adductor tubercle and the medial epicondyle. These structures usually can be palpated with the knee flexed to move the hamstrings posteriorly. The MPFL attaches to the femur in the saddle between the medial epicondyle and the adductor tubercle: 10 mm proximal and 2 mm posterior to the medial epicondyle or approximately 4 mm distal and 2 mm anterior to the adductor tubercle [13]. Dissection is carried deeper to expose the bone in the saddle created between these two structures. A pin with a loop for suture passage (from the ACL instrument set) is placed in the femoral insertion and the position is checked with intraoperative radioscopy (Fig. 8.5). For safer passage, it should be slightly angled proximal and anterior. This positioning is one of the most critical steps of the procedure. It should lie proximal to the intersection of the Blumensaat line and the posterior femoral cortex, along a line extending distal from the posterior cortex of the femoral shaft on a true lateral view (both condyles overlapping). Schöttle et al. found this radiographic location to be situated 1 mm anterior to the posterior cortex line, 2.5 mm distal to the posterior origin of the medial femoral condyle and proximal to the level of the posterior point of the Blumensaat line (Fig. 8.6) [20]. A forceps is passed from the femoral attachment between the layers and the sutures along with the graft are passed. By temporarily securing the graft to the pin a check of the reduction and the isometry can be performed.

The femoral positioning should allow for a relatively isometric behavior throughout the range of motion. The pin is then advanced through the lateral femoral cortex and an appropriately sized 20 mm tunnel is drilled. The graft's leader sutures are passed through. The tension is decided by pulling on the graft traction lines from the lateral side. It should not overload the patello-femoral compartment. Physiologic (less than 2 quadrants or 10 mm) lateral glide should be possible with the knee extended after reconstruction. The free ends are then secured in the femoral tunnel with the corresponding interference screw. Postoperatively, the patient is immobilized and weight-bearing is limited for the first 2 weeks. Range of motion exercises are started as soon as possible.

The isometric femoral fixation will pass near the open physes in skeletally immature patients. Alternative techniques have been described for pediatric patients, which use the adductor tendon. The graft is passed around the most distal portion, forming a sling. This way there is no interference with the growth physes. The position closely resembles the true isometric position of the native MPFL, although the result is a graft attached slightly more proximal.

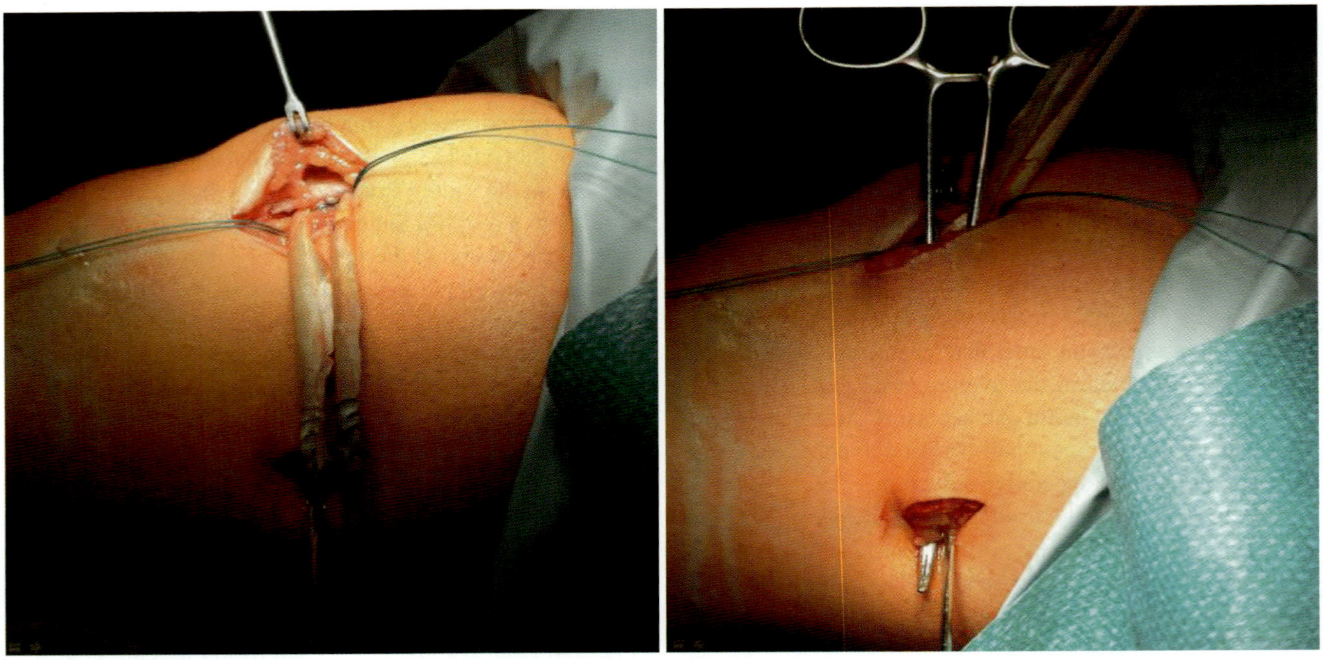

Fig. 8.4 The graft is attached to the patella using 2 anchors; leader sutures are than passed using a small forceps between layers 2 and 3

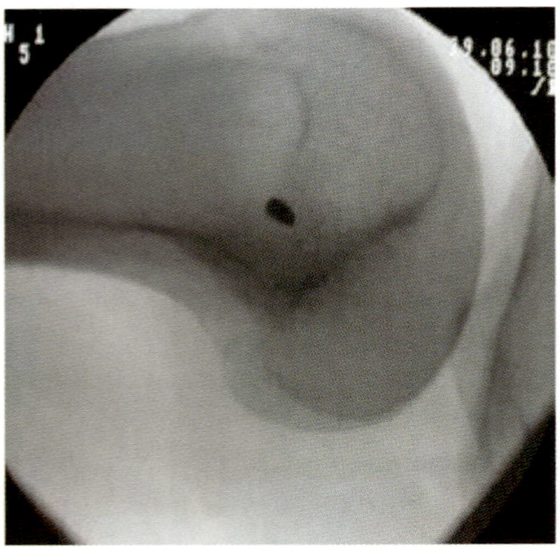

Fig. 8.5 The radiographic landmarks of the femoral insertion according to **Schöttle** et al.; a pin is placed in the femoral insertion and the position is checked with intraoperative radioscopy

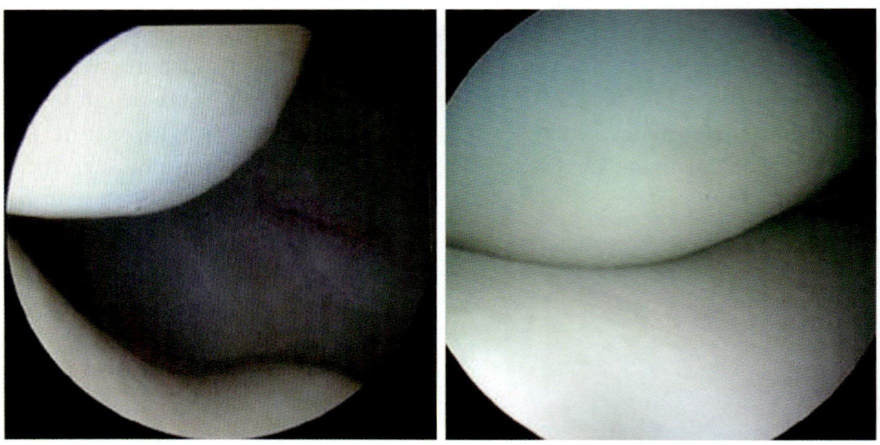

Fig. 8.6 Arthroscopic view through the anterolateral portal before and after MPFL reconstruction

8.3 Distal Realignment

8.3.1 Patellar Height

High riding patella is a cause of instability due to inappropriate entry in the trochlear groove during flexion initiation. There are three commonly used indexes to measure the position of the patella to the articular surface:

The Insall – Salvati ratio is defined by distracting the length of the patellar tendon from the maximum length of the patella in the sagittal plane. The normal value is between 0.8 and 1.2. The main drawback is that this ratio does not relate the height of the patella to the articular surface if the tibial tubercle insertion is abnormal.

Blackburne and Peel used [4] the ratio of the articular length of the patella to the height of the lower pole of the articular cartilage above the tibial plateau. Normal values were found between 0.54 and 1.06 [5].

Caton – Deschamps ratio measures the distance between the lower edge of the articular surface of the patella to the antero-superior angle of the tibia and the length of the articular surface of the patella. Normal values are between 0.6 and 1.2 [6].

To address the patella alta, a systematic review found tibial tubercle distalization was successful in normalizing patellar height and preventing recurrent patellar dislocation [18]. The procedure requires careful consideration of the amount of distalization required to set the patella in the normal range. The tibial tubercle is isolated and a generous sized tibial tubercle bone plug is removed using an osteotome. The lateral cut is performed in the coronal plane and the medial in almost a frontal plane. The depth of the cut should reach the subcortical spongia for a length of 5–7 cm. This improves healing and offers sufficient bone stock for reduction. The distal cut is repeated with the desired shortening and then stabilized with two bicortical screws from anterior to posterior (Fig. 8.7).

The 'Q angle' (quadriceps pull) was described by Brattstrom and represents the angle between the quadriceps pull and the patellar tendon with the knee in extension. It has not proved to be a reliable determinant of patellar tracking mainly since it is a static measure of a dynamic mechanism. Flexing the knee reduces the 'Q' angle due to internal tibial rotation. Increased femoral internal rotation and tibial external rotation can alter the 'Q' angle.

Torsional deformity such as increased femoral anteversion also leads to higher forces on the lateral patellar facet and is associated with symptomatic patello-femoral instability [10]. CT determination uses a proximal axial slice through the femoral head and a distal cut through the proximal trochleae. The angle between a line through the center of the femoral neck and the femoral epicondyles on superimposed images measures femoral anteversion (Fig. 8.8).

Patellar centration is most reliably evaluated by the TT-TG distance, which is a measure of the coronal alignment of the extensor mechanism. An axial slice is recorded through the proximal trochlea (the first cut with cartilage) and another through the tibial tuberosity. The distance between the middle of the tibial tubercle and the lowest point of the trochleae is measured, referenced perpendicular to the posterior condylar line. This distance can be dependent on the observer estimate of references as well as the size of the patient, since it is an absolute measure and tot a ratio.

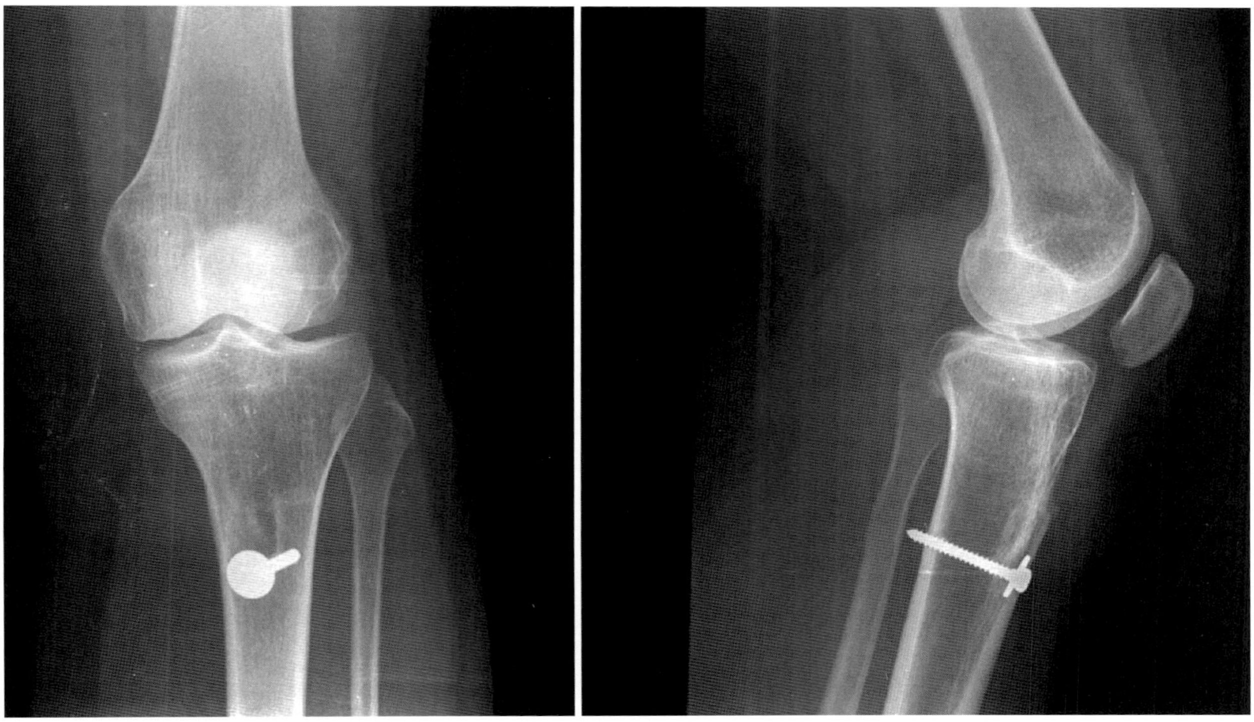

Fig. 8.7 Iatrogenic patella baha after excessive tibial tubercle distalization in an asymptomatic patient

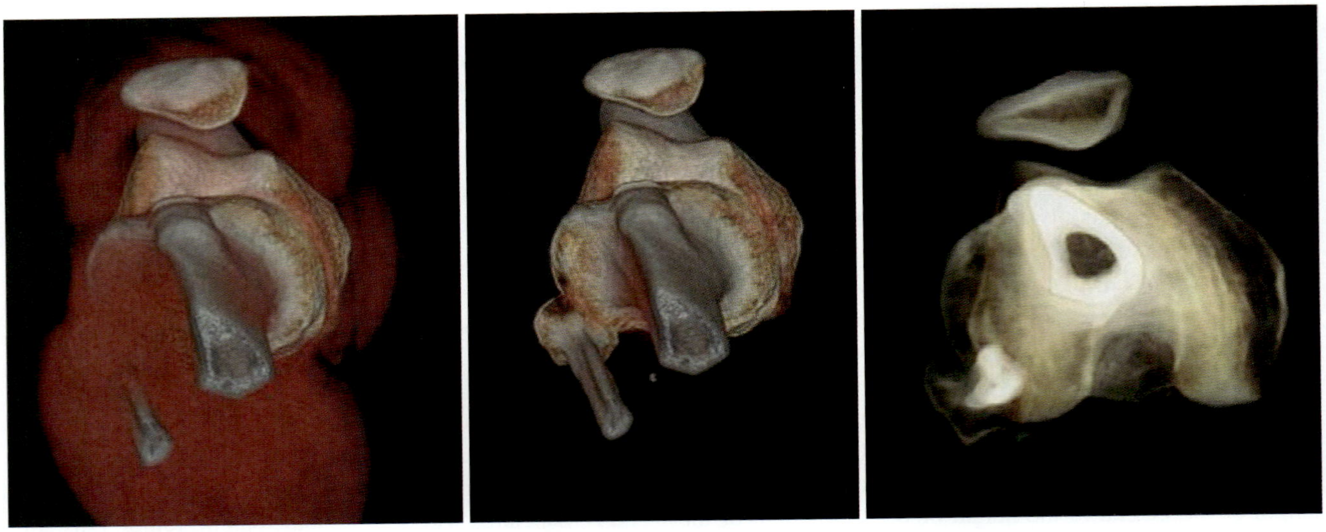

Fig. 8.8 3D CT volume rendering of the knee joint in extension showing the relationship of the patella to the trochleae and the tibial tuberosity; the physiologic external rotation of the tibial tubercle is apparent. 3D CT volume longitudinal axial transparent view shows the significance of the TT-TG measure in the extensor mechanism

8.3.2 Tibial Tubercle Medialization

The target is to normalize the TT-TG distance to less than 20, ideally 15 mm. This should provide a better function of the extensor mechanism with reduced lateral pull. Different techniques are described but they all involve dethatching the tibial tuberosity with a generous bone plug and reattaching it to a more biomechanically sound location.

The Elmslie-Trillat technique requires the tibial tuberosity to be removed and the proximal (tendon) end medialized while the distal is kept attached as much as possible. An osteotome is used to detach a tapered, shallow bone plug 5 cm long without a distal cut. Common associated additional procedures are lateral release, medial reefing or medial patellotibial ligament reconstruction by reattaching the medial third of the patellar tendon from the tibial tubercle to a more medial location [21]. Long term results are reported with controversial results [22].

The Fulkerson osteotomy is able to address medialization, anteriorization and distalization through a single tibial tuberosity relocation. By creating the osteotomy at an angle of approximately 30° from anterior to posterior and medial to distal, the medial translation will also provide some reduction in the patello-femoral contact pressures. This should foster any osteoarthritic changes from developing or aggravating [23].

8.3.3 Patello-Femoral Dysplasia

The axial radiographic examination proposed by Merchant is the most commonly accepted imaging modality of the patello-femoral space. The patient is placed supine on the table, with the knees [9] hanging off one side at 45° of flexion. The radiographic cassette is positioned perpendicular to the calves and the beam is oriented 30° downward from the horizontal and centered below the patella. Both knees are examined simultaneously. This provides a consistent image that can be used to measure outcomes after treatment as well as determine indication and plan for surgery. It captures the relationship of the patella to the trochlear groove in early flexion (15–20°) where it is most useful to evaluate pathologic conditions. It allows for many determinations to be made: the trochlear groove angle (the sulcus angle, normal under 145°), the patellar tilt. In addition, it offers details on the patella shape (Wiberg classification), the degree of dislocation and lateral overhang as well as patello-femoral arthritis. The Merchant view is still used today in determining patello-femoral congruity, although many measurements can be obtained from computed tomography (CT) or magnetic resonance imaging (MRI) (Fig. 8.9).

The Wiberg classification of patellar shape [11, 24]:

- Type I: the medial and the lateral facets are both concave and closely equivalent in size
- Type II: the medial facet is smaller than the lateral facet and has a flat or concave surface. The lateral facet has a concave contour.
- Type III: the medial facet is very small, nearly inexistent, describing a right angle in relation to the lateral facet.

H. Dejour described the 'crossing sign' on lateral X-rays, which is found with high prevalence among patients with trochlear dysplasia. This condition makes the trochlear groove move anteriorly and the medial and lateral facets posteriorly, creating a 'bump' which is pathognomonic for trochlear dysplasia.

Four factors were found relevant in knees with symptomatic patellar instability [7]:

- Trochlear dysplasia (85 %), as defined by the crossing sign (96 %) and quantitatively expressed by the trochlear bump, pathological above 3 mm or more (66 %), and the trochlear depth, pathologic at 4 mm or less.
- Quadriceps dysplasia (83 %), present when the patellar tilt in extension is more than 20° on the CT scans.
- Patella alta (Caton-Deschamps) index greater than or equal to 1.2 (24 %).
- Tibial tuberosity-trochlear groove (TT-TG) greater or equal to 20 mm (56 %).

Later, D. Dejour used CT scanning to develop the current 4 grade classification of trochlear dysplasia, although more recently, MRI scans have proved to be just as reliable [8].

The Dejour classification for trochlear dysplasia [24]:

- Type A: crossing sign present with trochlear morphology preserved (trochlea >145°)
- Type B: crossing sign present with supratrochlear spur and a flat or convex trochlea
- Type C: crossing sign present with double contour (a hypoplastic medial facet on the lateral view)
- Type D: crossing sign present with a supratrochlear spur, double contour, asymmetry of trochlear facets and a vertical link between the medial and lateral facets (cliff pattern)

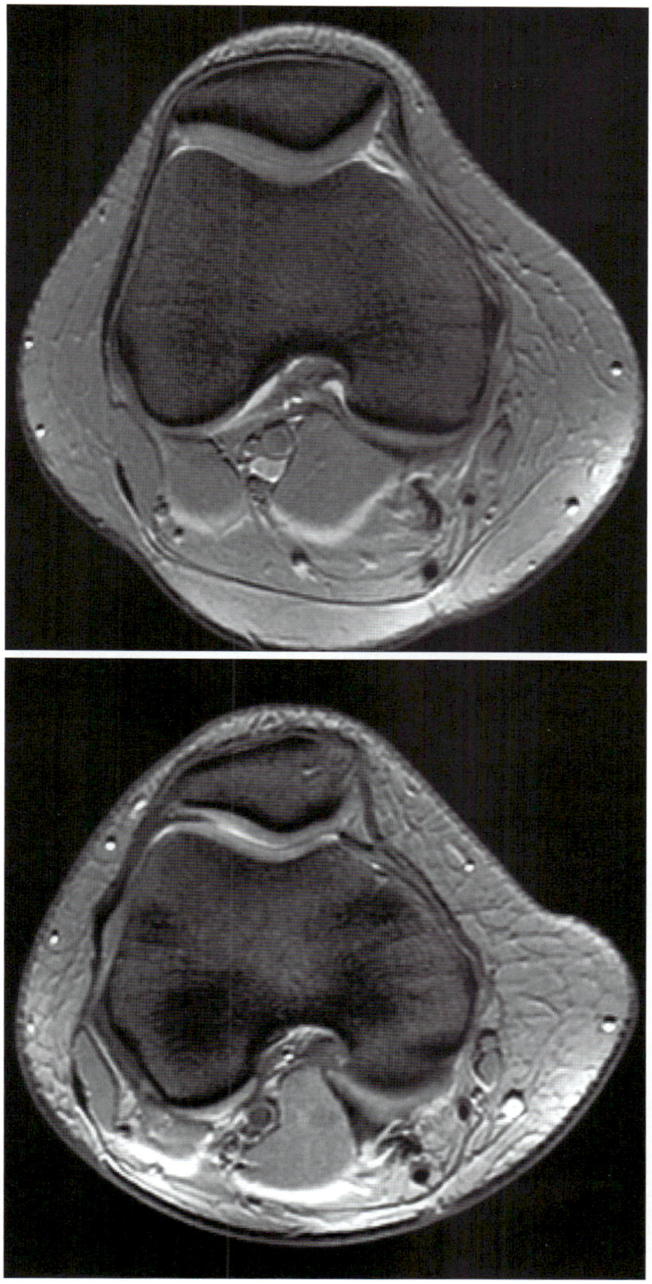

Fig. 8.9 Axial MRI views of a type I and II Wiberg patella shape

8.3.4 Clinical Case

A young male patient with a history of recurrent patellar dislocations with minimal trauma after, persisting after an initial sporting injury. In addition, the patient complained of little to no pain between the dislocation episodes but moderate articular effusion was almost always present. The clinical examination revealed a positive apprehension test, an excessive lateral patellar glide, a normal patellar tracking after 30° of flexion and likewise ranges of motion. The CT revealed increased patellar tilt, abnormally shaped patella with lateral facet degenerative arthritis and overhang, dysplastic short trochlea, increased TT-TG distance and patella alta (Fig. 8.10). The MRI did not show any additional pathology. We performed a Fulkerson osteotomy to move the tibial tuberosity in a more medial, anterior and distal position. This normalized the patellar height, reduced the pressures in the lateral patellofemoral compartment and improved the TT-TG alignment (Figs. 8.11 and 8.12). A partial external patelectomy and lateral release were performed to improve -trochlear congruity and reduce patellar tilt. The MPFL was reconstructed using the medial third of the quadriceps tendon. Postoperatively the patient was immobilized for 6 weeks followed by physical therapy (Fig. 8.13).

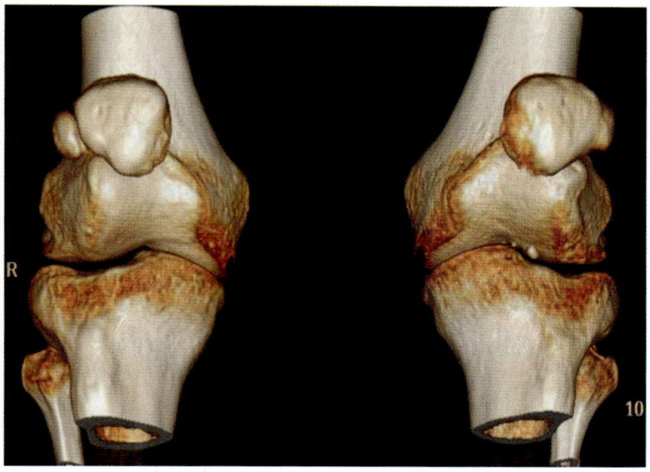

Fig. 8.10 3D CT reconstruction shows abnormal patellar shape, increased tibial external rotation and a short, dysplastic trochlea

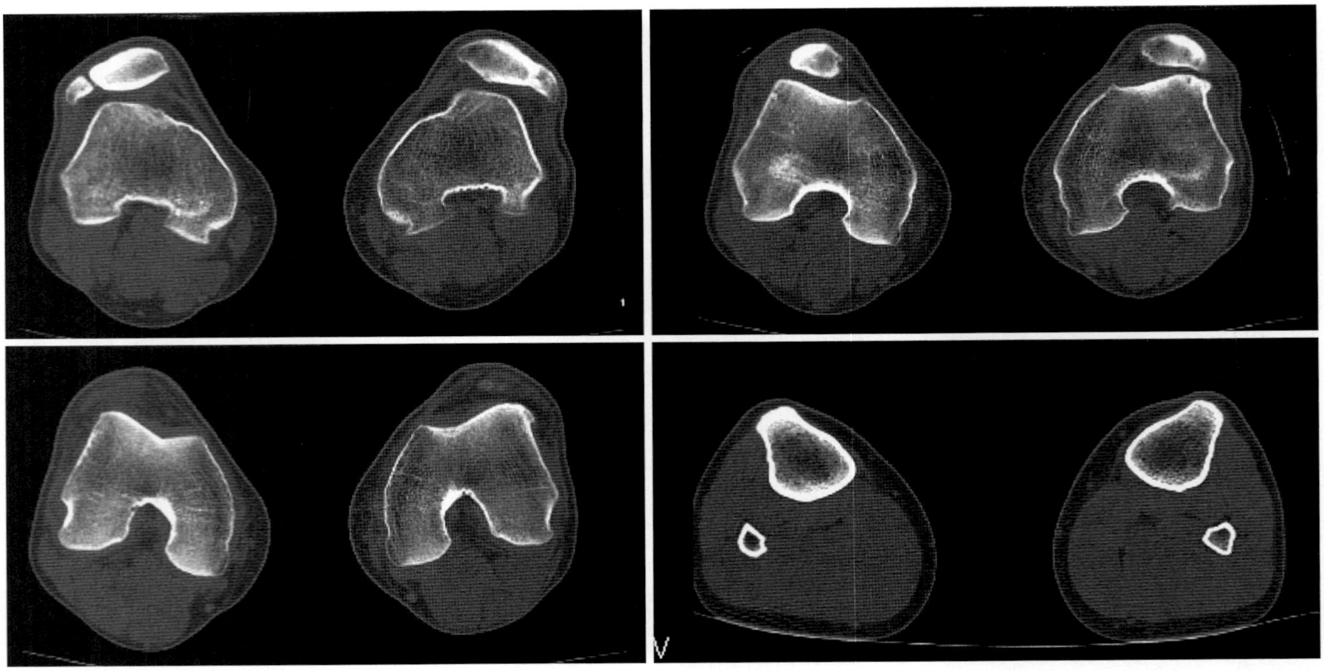

Fig. 8.11 Proximal to distal bilateral axial CT cuts showing increased patellar tilt, abnormally shaped patella with lateral facet arthritis and overhang, dysplastic short trochlea and increased TT-TG distance

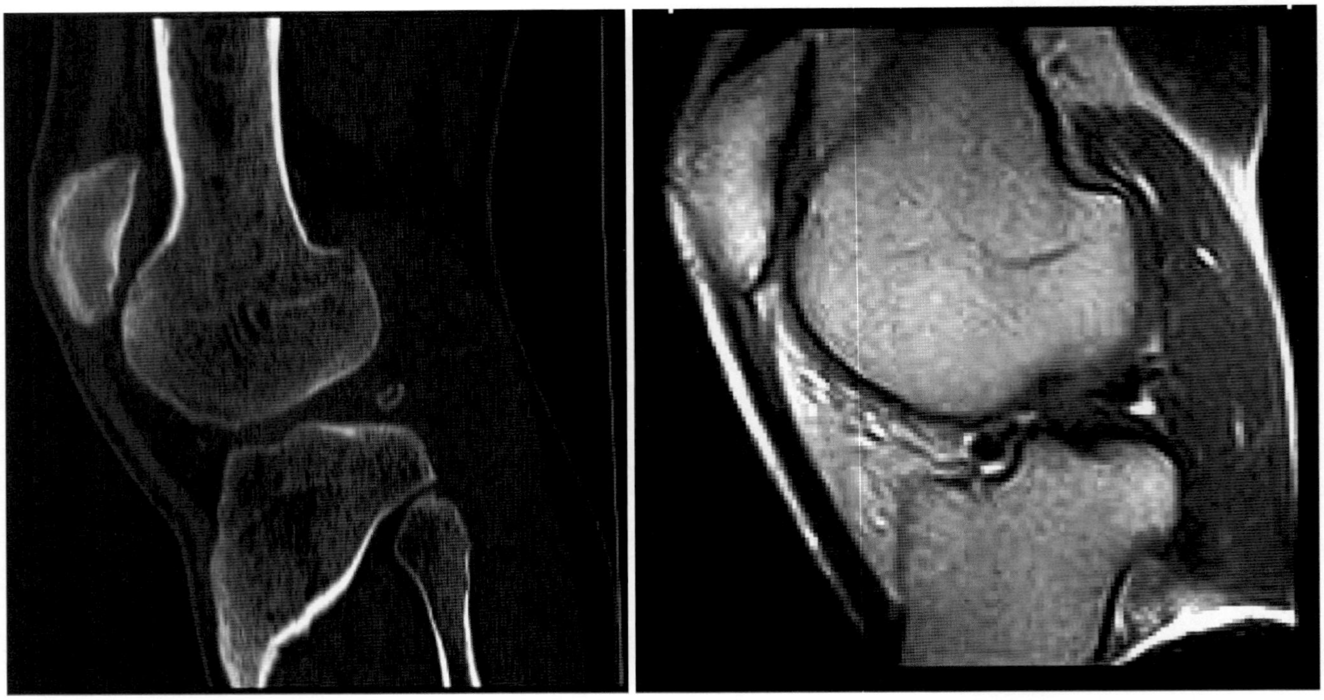

Fig. 8.12 Sagittal CT and T2 MRI of the same case with patella alta

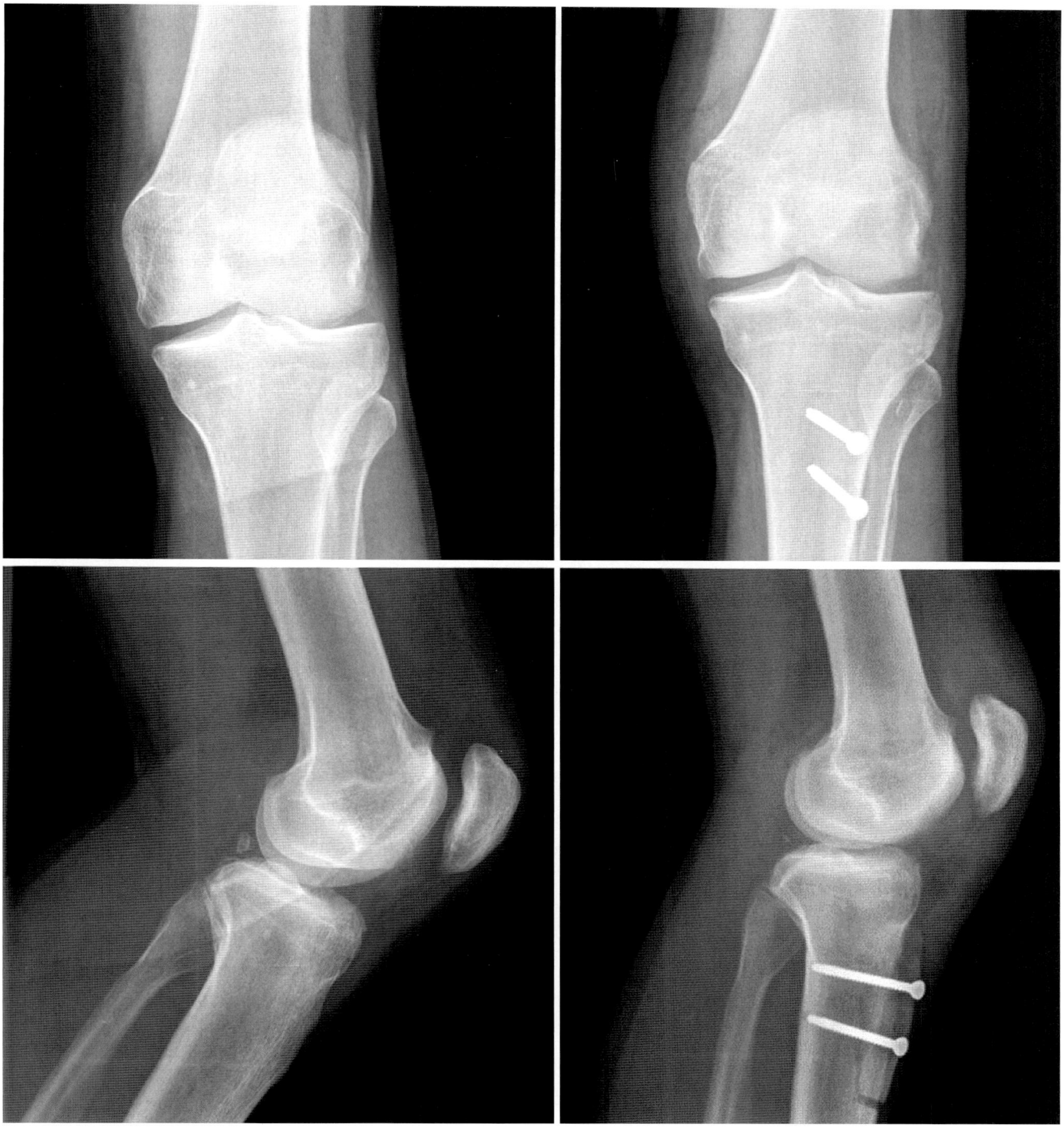

Fig. 8.13 Pre and postoperative AP and lateral x-ray views showing dysplastic trochlea and patella alta reduced after tibial tubercle distalization

8.3.5 Trochleoplasty

Several techniques to restore the shape of the trochlea have been described. They all aim at deepening the groove and raising the lateral facet by subtraction and addition of the subchondral bone. The surgery is commonly performed open, through a parapatellar arthrotomy, although arthroscopic procedures are possible. Indications for isolated trochleoplasty are very rare and the procedure requires a high degree of skill and experience.

8.3.6 Clinical Case

A 24 years old young female with Dejour type 4 bilateral trochlear dysplasia and habitual dislocations with marked instability especially in early flexion when the patella engages. Clinical examination found positive apprehension test, excessive lateral glide and requirement for manual centration of the patella in order to achieve flexion. Intraoperative images show the flattened trochlear groove deepened by open trochleoplasty using a modified Dejour technique (Fig. 8.14) [24]. A thin (less than 5 mm) osteochondral flap was elevated using chisels and bone was removed with a burr. The trochleea was then reattached and stabilized with a central band (Fibertape, Arthrex) and 3 anchors (SwiveLock, Arthrex). Lateral release was performed for the contracted retinaculum. Open MPFL reconstruction using autologus ipsilateral gracilis tendon fixed with 2 anchors on the patella and an interference screw in the femoral canal (see above for technique description) (Fig. 8.15).

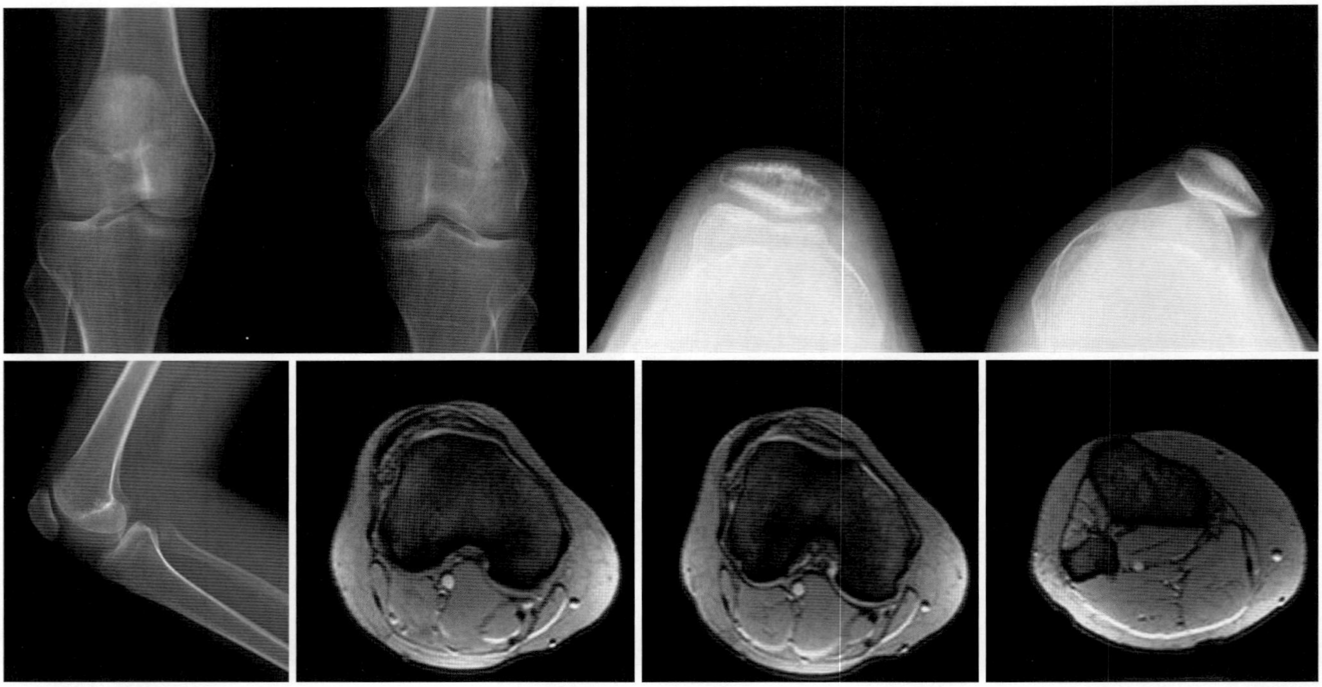

Fig. 8.14 Preoperative AP and lateral X-rays, as well as axial T2 MRI of the right knee, showing a dysplastic trochleea; 3 months postoperative axial 30 degrees X-ray after deepening trohleoplasty and MPFL reconstruction of the right knee

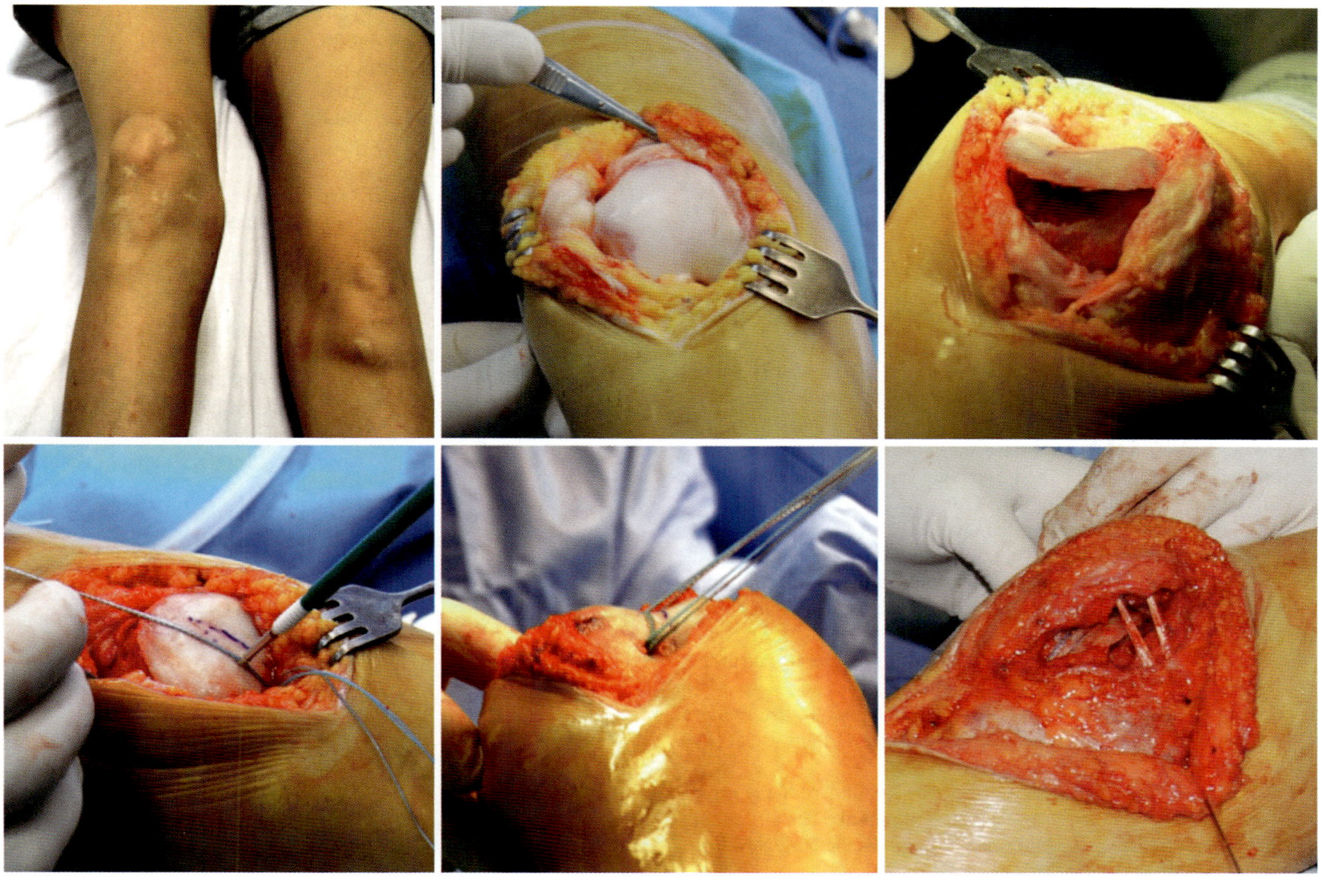

Fig. 8.15 Habitual dislocations with marked instability especially in early flexion when the patella engages. Intraoperative images show the flattened trochlear groove. A thin osteochondral flap was elevated using chisels and bone was removed with a burr. The trochleea was then reattached and stabilized with a central band and anchors. MPFL reconstruction using autologus ipsilateral gracilis tendon fixed with two anchors on the patella and an interference screw in the femoral canal

References

1. Warren LA, Marshall JL, Girgis F. The prime static stabilizer of the medical side of the knee. J Bone Joint Surg Am. 1974;56(4):665–74.
2. Desio SM, Burks RT, Bachus KN. Soft tissue restraints to lateral patellar translation in the human knee. Am J Sports Med. 1998;26(1):59–65.
3. Senavongse W, Amis AA. The effects of articular, retinacular, or muscular deficiencies on patellofemoral joint stability: a biomechanical study in vitro. J Bone Joint Surg Br. 2005;87(4):577–82.
4. Insall J, Salvati E. Patella position in the normal knee joint. Radiology. 1971;101(1):101–4.
5. Blackburne JS, Peel TE. A new method of measuring patellar height. J Bone Joint Surg Br. 1977;59(2):241–2.
6. Caton J, Deschamps G, Chambat P, Lerat JL, Dejour H. Patella infera. Apropos of 128 cases. Rev Chir Orthop Reparatrice Appar Mot. 1982;68(5):317–25.
7. Dejour H, Walch G, Nove-Josserand L, Guier C. Factors of patellar instability: an anatomic radiographic study. Knee Surg Sports Traumatol Arthrosc. 1994;2(1):19–26.
8. Lippacher S, Dejour D, Elsharkawi M, Dornacher D, Ring C, Dreyhaupt J, Reichel H, Nelitz M. Observer agreement on the Dejour trochlear dysplasia classification: a comparison of true lateral radiographs and axial magnetic resonance images. Am J Sports Med. 2012;40(4):837–43.
9. Merchant AC. Classification of patellofemoral disorders. Arthroscopy. 1988;4(4):235–40.
10. Eckhoff DG, Montgomery WK, Kilcoyne RF, Stamm ER. Femoral morphometry and anterior knee pain. Clin Orthop Relat Res. 1994;302:64–8.
11. Dejour D, Saggin PR, Meyer X, Tavernier T. Standard X-ray examination: patellofemoral disorders. In: Zaffagnini S et al., editors. Patellofemoral pain, instability, and arthritis. Heidelberg/New York: Springer; 2010.
12. Christoforakis J, Bull AM, Strachan RK, Shymkiw R, Senavongse W, Amis AA. Effects of lateral retinacular release on the lateral stability of the patella. Knee Surg Sports Traumatol Arthrosc. 2006;14(3):273–7.
13. LaPrade RF, Engebretsen AH, Ly TV, Johansen S, Wentorf FA, Engebretsen L. The anatomy of the medial part of the knee. J Bone Joint Surg Am. 2007;89(9):2000–10.
14. Muneta T, Sekiya I, Tsuchiya M, Shinomiya K. A technique for reconstruction of the medial patellofemoral ligament. Clin Orthop Relat Res. 1999;359:151–5.
15. Schöttle PB, Fucentese SF, Romero J. Clinical and radiological outcome of medial patellofemoral ligament reconstruction with a semitendinosus autograft for patella instability. Knee Surg Sports Traumatol Arthrosc. 2005;13(7):516–21.
16. Matsushita T, Kuroda R, Oka S, Matsumoto T, Takayama K, Kurosaka M. Clinical outcomes of medial patellofemoral ligament reconstruction in patients with an increased tibial tuberosity-trochlear groove distance. Knee Surg Sports Traumatol Arthrosc. 2014. [Epub ahead of print].
17. Vavken P, Wimmer MD, Camathias C, Quidde J, Valderrabano V, Pagenstert G. Treating patella instability in skeletally immature patients. Arthroscopy. 2013;29(8):1410–22.
18. Magnussen RA, De Simone V, Lustig S, Neyret P, Flanigan DC. Treatment of patella alta in patients with episodic patellar dislocation: a systematic review. Knee Surg Sports Traumatol Arthrosc. 2013. doi: 10.1007/s00167-013-2445-8
19. Siebold R, Sartory N. Arthroscopic medial reefing in acute patellar dislocation. In: Zaffagnini S et al., editors. Patellofemoral pain, instability, and arthritis. Heidelberg/New York: Springer; 2010.
20. Schöttle PB, Schmeling A, Rosenstiel N, Weiler A. Radiographic landmarks for femoral tunnel placement in medial patellofemoral ligament reconstruction. Am J Sports Med. 2007;35(5):801–4.
21. Marcacci M, Zaffagnini S, Lo Presti M, Vascellari A, Iacono F, Russo A. Treatment of chronic patellar dislocation with a modified Elmslie-Trillat procedure. Arch Orthop Trauma Surg. 2004;124(4):250–7.
22. Carney JR, Mologne TS, Muldoon M, Cox JS. Long-term evaluation of the Roux-Elmslie-Trillat procedure for patellar instability: a 26-year follow-up. Am J Sports Med. 2005;33(8):1220–3.
23. Fulkerson JP. Anteromedialization of the tibial tuberosity for patellofemoral malalignment. Clin Orthop Relat Res. 1983;(177):176–81.
24. Dejour D, Byn P, Saggin PR. Deepening trochleoplasty for patellar instability. In: Zaffagnini S et al., editors. Patellofemoral pain, instability, and arthritis. Heidelberg/New York: Springer; 2010.

Synovial Pathology

9

Dinu Vermesan and Dan Crisan

9.1 Synovial Plicae of the Knee

The synovial plicae represent a physiological structure of the knee joint that forms during the embryonic phase of development [1]. Multiple morphological variations exist, but only one has a clinical significance the medial synovial plica that, while an infrequent occurrence as a pathological entity it is one of extreme importance in the differential diagnosis of such pathological overlapping entities as anterior knee pain and the patellofemoral pain syndrome.

Two theories exist regarding the formation of the knee and the development of plicae. The first, which is widely accepted, suggests that the knee is formed into three separate compartments (medial, lateral, suprapatellar) that are divided by membranes of mesenchymal tissue. These membranes fuse together during weeks 9–12 to create a joint cavity. Plicae are remnants of the compartment-separating membranes that have not been reabsorbed. The second theory suggests that at 8 weeks into embryo development, mesenchymal tissue fills the space between the distal femur and the proximal tibia epiphyses. After this two processes take place. The first is the condensation of the mesenchymal tissue in areas that will become the menisci and cruciate ligaments, and resorption of the tissue in other areas to form patellofemoral, femoromeniscal and meniscotibial cavitations. After approximately 2 weeks these cavities converge into a single cavity with synovial lining. Where resorption of the mesenchymal tissue fails and cavitation is incomplete, plicae form, signifying that the plicae develop when the joint space is formed [1–3].

Because synovial plicae are normal structures usually found in asymptomatic knees they can be sometimes overlooked as the primary cause of knee pain and other structures such as meniscal injuries be more thoroughly investigated.

There are four variations of the position of the plicae in the knee joint cavity that have been described in literature. The superior and the inferior plicae are the most common (50–65 %) but have extremely little clinical relevance. Each variation may be of many various morphological types. The lateral plica is rare (1–3 %). The medial plica is present at autopsies in one of every three or four knees, while some authors report incidences as high as 80 % of the population, depending on race the highest number of medial synovial plicae can be found in those of Asian ethnicity and their incidence lower in patients of Caucasian ethnicity [4, 5]. It also is of various types, wide and thick in one of every 15 knees. Albeit not the most common the medial plica is the most relevant from a clinical perspective, and so it's the most studied and reported in specialty literature. The incidence of the medial plica syndrome varies between 3.5 and 5.8 % [2, 3, 6].

The infrapatellar synovial plica (also known as "ligamentum mucosum") can of various morphotypes:

I. separated from the ACL
II. some connections with the ACL, may impede in arthroscopic evaluation
III. pre-ACL septum that divides the anterior knee in a medial and a lateral compartment.

Wempfing has classified the suprapatellar synovial plica in five grades:

I. complete septum that separates the suprapatellar bursa from the femuropatellar compartment
II. suprapatellar septum with or without central orifice
III. suprapatellar septum with a lateral orifice

D. Vermesan, MD, PhD • D. Crisan, MD (✉)
Department of Orthopedics and Trauma,
University of Medicine and Pharmacy 'Victor Babes' Timisoara,
2 Eftimie Murgu Square, Timisoara 300041, Romania

I-st Clinic of Orthopedics and Trauma,
Emergency Clinical County Hospital Timisoara,
10 Iosif Bulbuca Blvd, Timisoara 300736, Romania
e-mail: vermesan@gmail.com; crisan.dan@gmail.com

R. Prejbeanu (ed.), *Atlas of Knee Arthroscopy*,
DOI 10.1007/978-1-4471-6593-4_9, © Springer-Verlag London 2015

IV. suprapatellar septum with lateral or medial perforation
V. small, rudimentary plica on the medial side

Munzinger classified the mediopatellar plica into four types based on appearance:

I. Cordlike
II. Shelf like, does not cover medial femoral condyle
III. Does cover medial femoral condyle
IV. Double insertion

Detection of these intra articular structures can be done routinely trough a number of imaging techniques. Arthrography, both classic and CT arthrography are very good methods but they have the disadvantage of being invasive. So the most readily available and widely accepted techniques by both physicians and patient alike that investigate soft tissues of the knee are MRI and ultrasonography. Both have their respective advantages and disadvantages. MR imaging provides a very detailed image of the knee and has proved a very useful tool in the investigation of the synovial plicae, together with the other structures of the knee. The disadvantage consists in the static nature of the image, making very hard to evaluate the dynamic behavior of the plica. Special attention should be taken when investigating an infrapatellar plica (ligamentum mucosum), which, because of its structure and orientation, can be confused with an intact ACL (in ACL deficient knees). Also the cost factor should be taken into account, MRI's are expensive investigations [7–10] (Fig. 9.1).

Ultrasonography is another well-accepted investigation method of the knee. It has several advantages over MRI, such as cost, reproducibility and investigation time. Dynamic sonography allows for the examination of the internal structures of the knee in movement relying not only on different tissue echogenicity but also on tissue adhesion in the dynamic state. Coupled with sonopalpation (tissue recognition under transducer pressure and pain perception when passing a transducer over the affected part), allows more accurate diagnosis. The main disadvantage of this technique consists in the need of specially trained personnel in performing and interpreting musculo-skeletal ultrasonography [11]. Arthroscopy still remains the most accurate mean of identifying synovial plicas of the knee [12], but there is no definitive indication to perform a diagnostic arthroscopy in order to confirm the presence of a synovial plica [13].

There is a syndrome that is caused by the irritation and resultant inflammatory reaction of the relic of the synovial plica of the knee that is known as "pathological synovial plica syndrome" (PSPS). It is characterized by supra- and mid-patellar pain with knee extension as well as the presence of audible cracking noises with knee flexion and extension. Contraction of the quadriceps associated with compression of the supra-patellar pouch also causes pain. In addition, patients often experience a sensation of instability when they are walking up or down stairs or slopes. These symptoms have been correlated with recent changes in the intensity or quality of patients' athletic activities. It appears especially in individuals who practice sports infrequently and subject higher stresses on untrained, unfit joints. Clinically a young active patient will present with dull, aching pain usually situated in the proximal medial aspect of the knee or in the infrapatellar aspect [13, 14].

The diagnosis of PSPS is mainly a clinical one, and in most patients conservative treatment will yield very good results. The classical clinical test used for the detection of a symptomatic medial plica is the Hughson plica test To perform this test the patient has to be lying in dorsal decubitus with the affected knee flexed at 90° while the examiner is internally rotating the tibia while passively moving the patella from lateral to medial all the while they are extending the affected leg to a straight position and then flexing it back to 90°. A positive Hughson test produces a sharp pain as the inflamed plica is caught between the articulate surfaces of the femur and the patella during knee flexion and/or a palpable clicking. A symptomatic plica will usually have a combination of these signs, as the clicking sensation caused by the interaction between the plica and the articular surfaces will usually produce pain or at least a sensation of local discomfort.

Plica pain is usually exacerbated by active quadriceps contraction. Other symptoms such as acute lateral pain or a giving away sensation can also be present at physical examination. MRI's are routinely performed in patients complaining of knee pain or instability, but they don't always show a clear image of synovial plicae, presumably because its static nature. The synovial plica syndrome is thus, despite advances in MRI imaging technique and advanced image interpretation, mostly an intraoperative diagnosis as it takes into account the clinically painful knee and the lack of other intraarticular pathology.

If diagnosed preoperatively, unassociated with other lesions, the routine treatment is conservative. Nonsurgical therapeutic modalities include rest from strenuous activities (such as prolonged running, sports, squatting), NSAID's. Anti-inflammatory medication can be administered orally, with limited efficacy, locally via topical applications or a local subsynovial, extraarticular, corticosteroid infiltration in the mediopatellar region [4] that can be guided ultrasonographically as well and intraarticular corticosteroid infiltration [6]. A physical rehabilitation program should be prescribed and it should include closed chain kinetic quadriceps exercises and hamstring stretching. Improved outcomes are obtained if the hamstring-stretching program is performed several times a day [15].

Open chain kinetic exercises such as knee extensions especially those that are done under added weights add stress to an already painful plica, can often cause a further increase in the symptoms.

The duration of the rehabilitation program should vary depending on patient specific response. About half of the patients have a positive response to 6 weeks of physical therapy noticing the resolution of or a significant improvement in their symptoms. A further 6 weeks of physical therapy provide relief of symptoms in the majority of the patients [16].

If the conservative treatment fails or a medial synovial plica is detected during knee arthroscopy that is performed for an unrelated pathology (such as a suspected meniscal tear), if the pathology that was suspected based on the clinical examination and preoperative imaging investigations is confirmed by arthroscopic visualization, it is recommended that it should be left in place by most authors. This treatment indication of plicae surgery is still controversial and some authors still advocate the resection of an asymptomatic medial plica even in conjunction with other associated intraarticular pathology in order to prevent the development of a subsequent plica syndrome [17].

But if after thorough examination of the knee no pathology is found and the presence of a synovial plica is detected we have found that the arthroscopic resection of the plica provides full relief of the symptoms in most cases [2].

There is a discussion in literature regarding the best way to treat a PSPS, either by totally resecting the involved mediopatellar plica to the capsular junction, a partial resection of the plica or just a incision, detensioning the synovial fold and allowing it to slide over the medial condyle into the recess during knee flexion. While some immediate relief of the painful symptoms may exist, just by arthroscopic incision and detensioning of the synovial plica there are no studies to demonstrate a long-term benefit and therefore this procedure is not considered to be advisable in treating a pathological mediopatellar synovial plica in the authors opinion, the risk of recurrence being significant. As the main complication of surgical treatment of a synovial plica is the persistence of symptoms we can conclude by saying that a complete arthroscopic resection of the plica should be performed if the decision to address the plica is made, either pre- or intraoperative. The resection should be extensive, up to the junction with the synovial membrane but care must be taken to avoid over resecting the plica because that could lead to iatrogenic injury to the capsular structures, rendering the medial retinaculum insufficient with subsequent patellar instability or it could cause iatrogenic vascular injury to the medial geniculate artery with subsequent hemarthrosis. Plica resection should therefore be performed with the arthroscope looking from the anterolateral portal and the working tool (this must include a shaver and preferably a radiofrequency probe apart from the regular arthroscopic punch) in the anteromedial portal. More so, as this is a technically difficult procedure because of the position of the plica and the viewing angles that are involved a medial suprapatellar portal can be used to facilitate access in the mediopatellar region of the joint [4, 18].

Postoperative management should begin with a period of relative rest. No knee immobilization is necessary in our experience and full weightbearing can be resumed as tolerated. However there should be a delay in initiating postoperative rehabilitation of around 2 weeks to minimize the risk of symptom recurrence due to the scarring of the synovial membrane in the area of the resected plica and to prevent secondary synovitis.

Arthroscopic resection proves a successful therapeutic tool for symptomatic synovial plicae in cases where conservative treatment has failed. Recurrence of symptoms is usually associated with residual intraarticular pathology that was left untreated during surgery [6, 13, 15, 19] (Fig. 9.2).

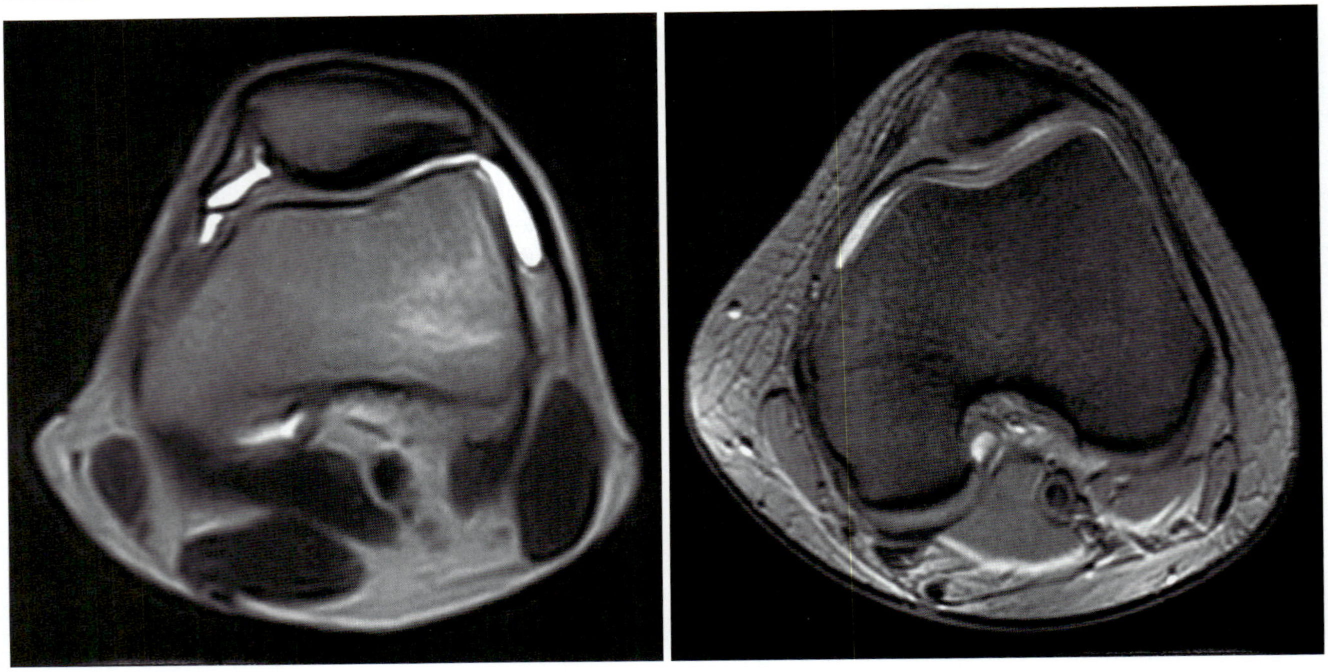

Fig. 9.1 Show the MRI appearance of a mediopatellar synovial plica

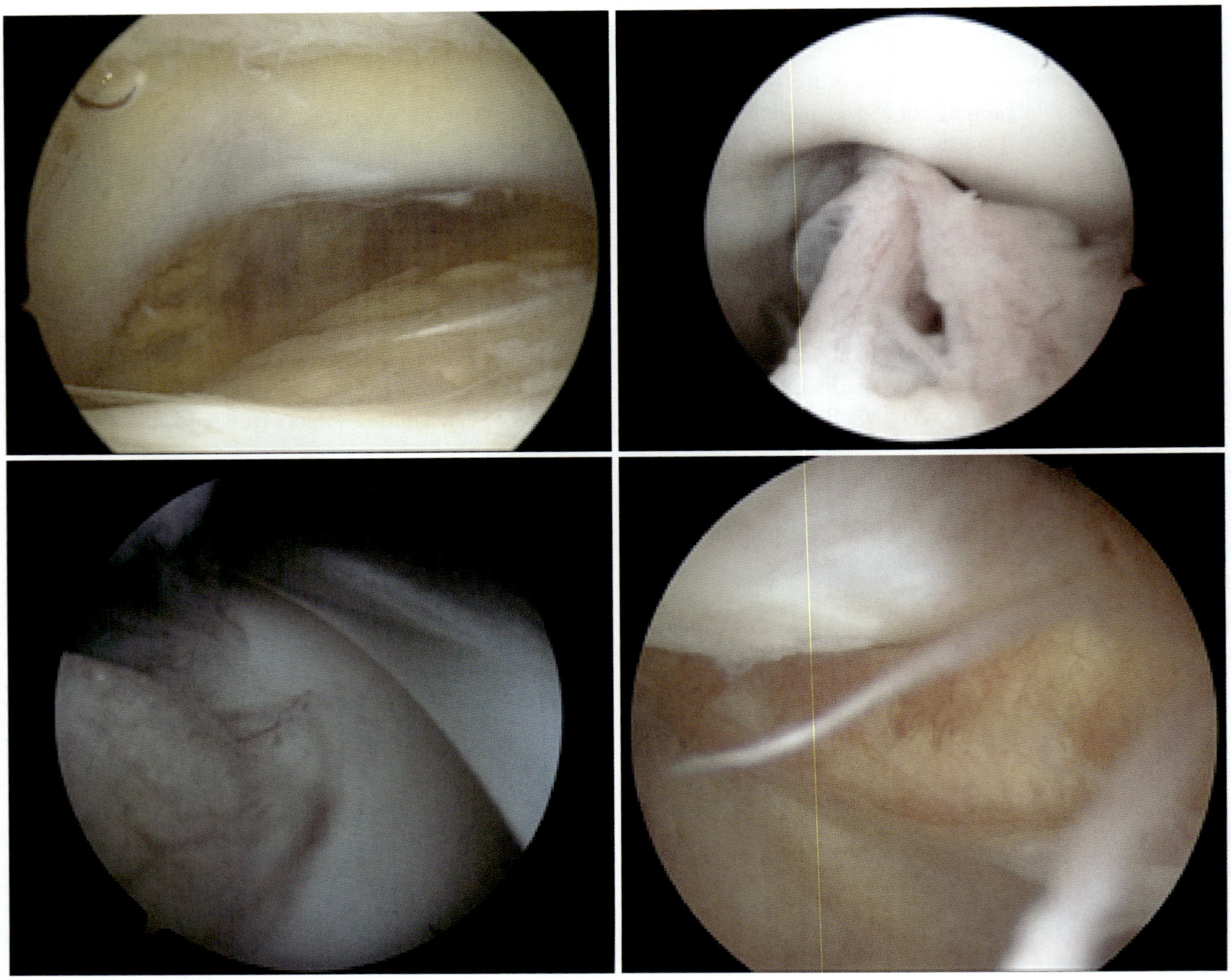

Fig. 9.2 Examples of supra, infra and mediopatellar plicae

9.2 Synovitis

The term "synovitis" depicts the inflammation of the synovial membrane that either acute or chronic. This can be caused by different underlying pathology such as rheumatoid arthritis (RA) or spondylarthropathy, lupus, gout or osteoarthritis being the most common causes of chronic synovitis, while acute synovitis follows a knee trauma or it can occur after a neglected meniscal injury. Pigmented villonodular synovitis (PVNS) of the knee is a proliferative disorder of the synovial membrane. It forms benign villi and nodules with large amounts of intracellular haemosiderin. The highest prevalence is in young adults between their twenties and their forties and although it affects other joints, the knee is the most frequently involved [20]. Two forms exist, localized PVNS and diffuse PVNS. Diagnosing PVNS is initially done with articular aspiration and confirmed with the help of MRI studies [20, 21], arthroscopic views confirm the disease but the positive diagnosis is made by histological exploration that makes the differential diagnosis with other synovial disorders such as chronic synovitis or RA. Increasing evidence supports the role of chronic synovial inflammation in the pathogenesis and structural progression of osteoarthritis (OA) a reciprocity has been created between the severity of synovial inflammation and the chondral joint degeneration and the number and size of osteophytes [1–3]. The hemophiliacs represent another group of patients prone to synovial inflammation and recurrent spontaneous hemarthrosis even during gentle manouvers. Arthroscopic synovectomy can be performed if the conservative treatment fails. It is usually performed as a two portal technique [22, 23] (Fig. 9.3).

Initial treatment for chronic synovitis should be conservative, rest, ice, oral antiinflamatories, cortisone injections if the symptoms are severe and the diagnostic resolution as to what the underlying cause of the synovitis is, either a joint related cause or a systemic disease. Repeated corticosteroid injections should be avoided due to several factors such as increased chondrotoxicity and the increased risk of post injection septic arthritis (Figs. 9.4, 9.5 and 9.6).

Regardless of the etiology of synovitis the present chapter aims at treating the arthroscopic aspects and the surgical treatment of synovitis. Synovectomy, the surgical removal of an inflamed synovial membrane in the knee joint can be done either arthroscopically or by open surgery. While each of these has their advantages local synovitis is usually treated with arthroscopic and the diffuse form is excised completely by open synovectomy [24]. Arthroscopic surgery has the advantage of being minimally invasive [25], but access is

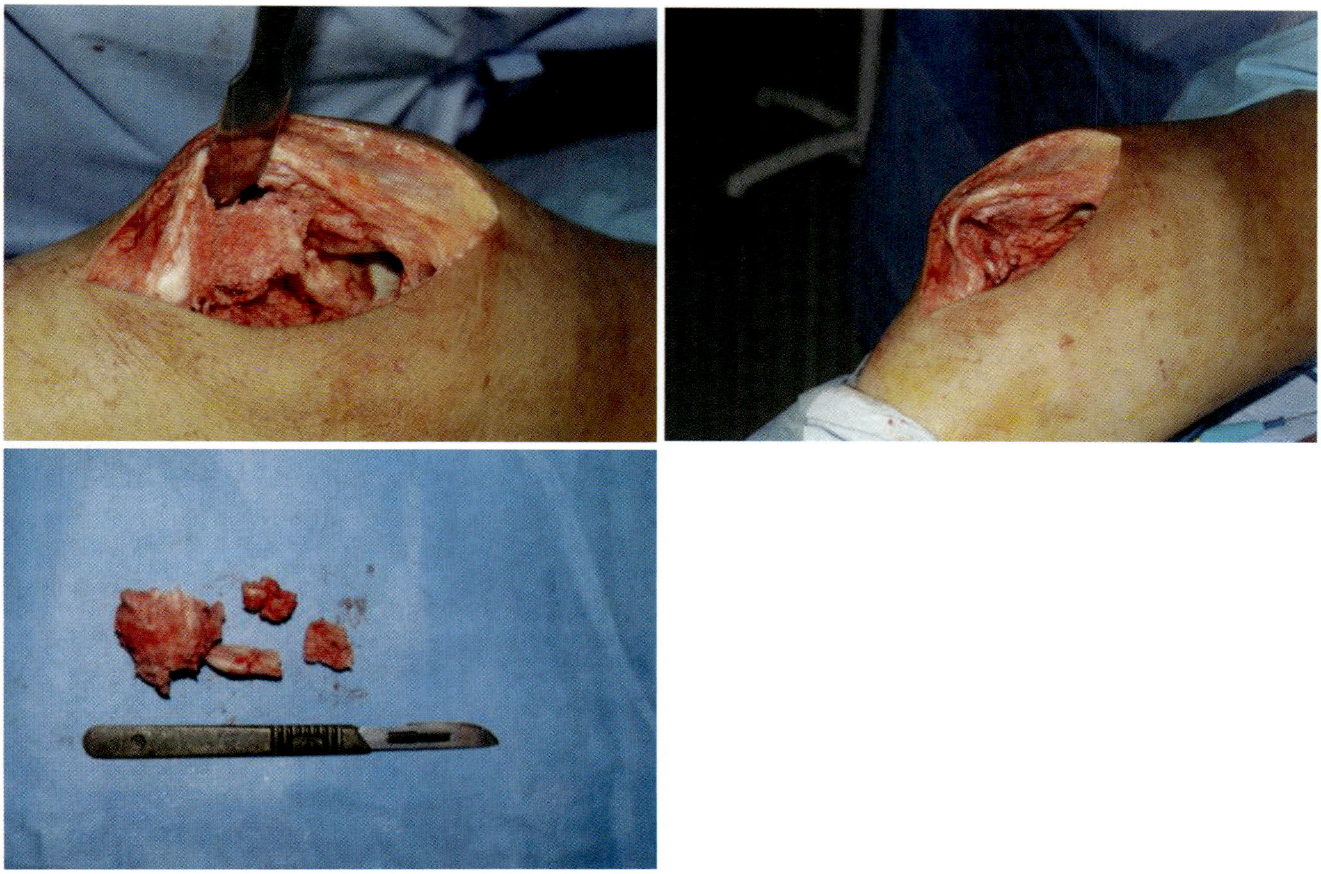

Fig. 9.3 Open synovectomy and the removed synovial membrane

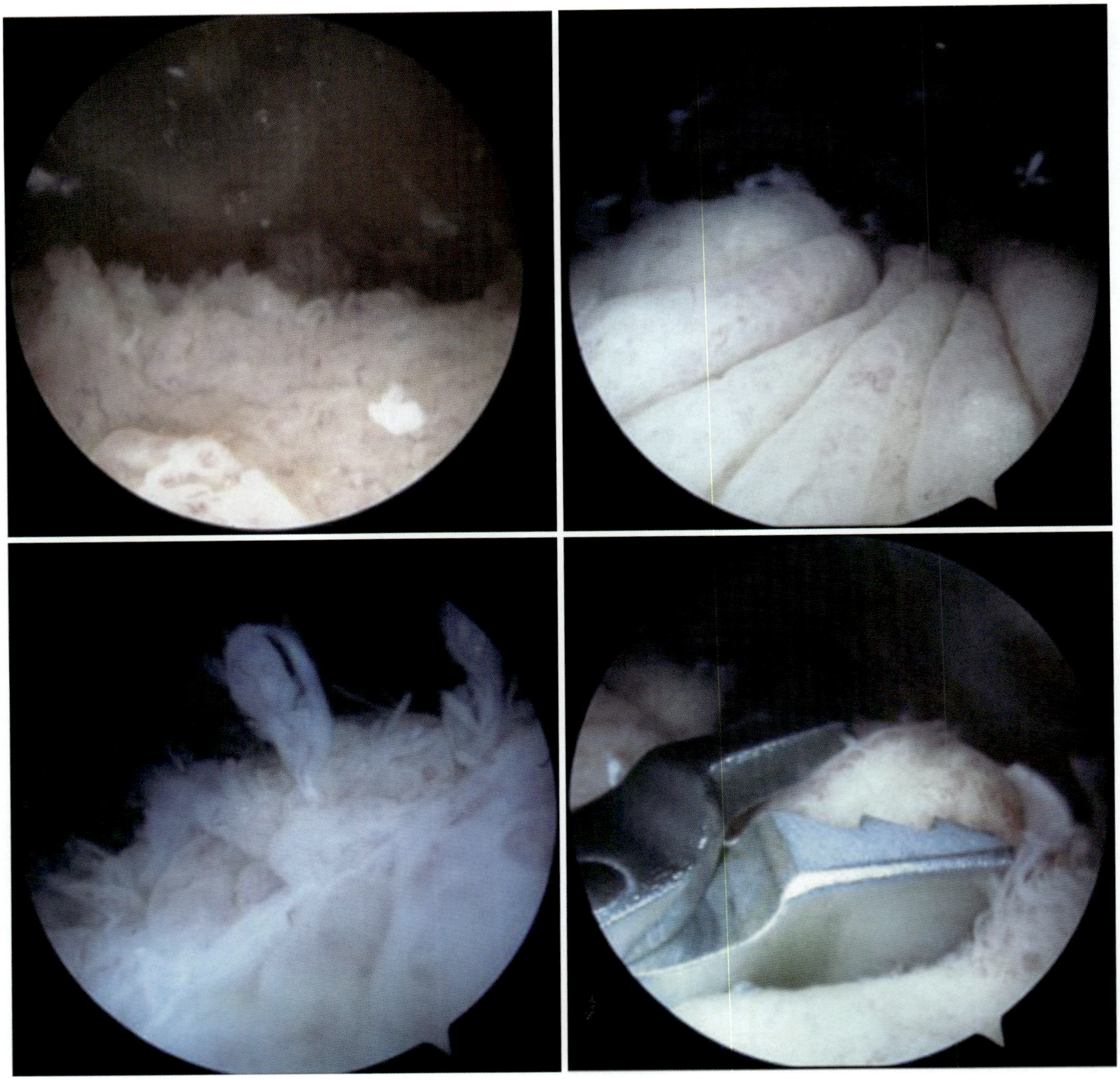

Fig. 9.4 Arthroscopic views of localized PVNS in the suprapatellar compartment of the knee. Figure 9.7 shows a arthroscopic punch taking synovial fragments for anatomopathological study (biopsy)

restricted to the more exposed areas of the knee joint. With open surgery, albeit more traumatizing, there is greater access and the recurrence rate is lower so open surgery it is still considered the gold standard for diffuse synovitis [26, 27]. Kubat et al. show that five portal arthroscopic total synovectomy can be just as effective as open synovectomy for diffuse PVNS data that is supported by other authors [28–32]. A study by Colman et al. found that a combination of arthroscopic and open simultaneous approaches appeared to have a significant reduction in the recurrence rate [33] (Fig. 9.7).

Recurrent synovitis is a more difficult situation to address, a combination of open or arthroscopic synovectomy with radiation synovectomy with yttrium 90 has been advocated by some authors [34, 35].

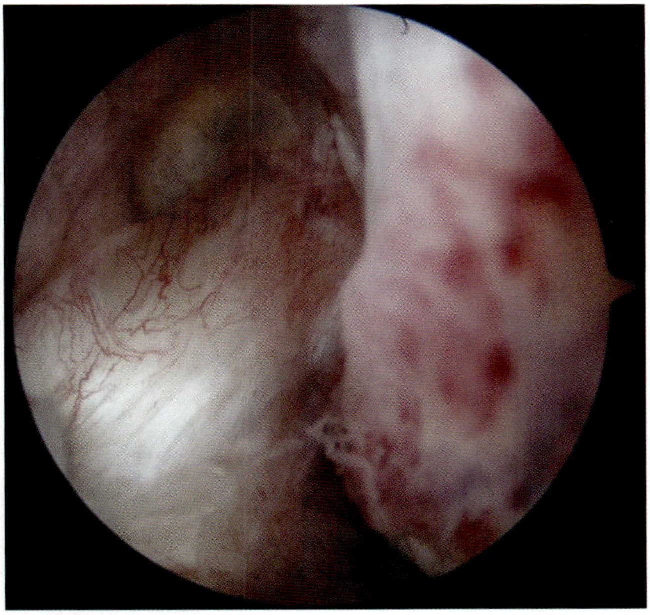

Fig. 9.5 Arthroscopic view of the notch showing hemorrhagic effusions in the synovial membrane

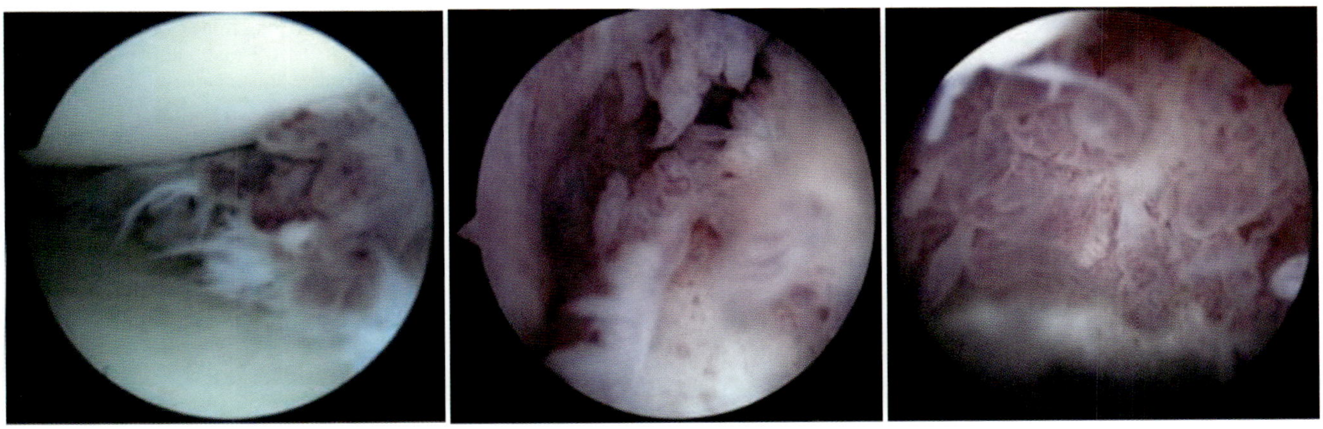

Fig. 9.6 Showing diffuse knee PVNS in the medial compartment (*left*), notch (*middle*) and suprapatellar compartment (*right*)

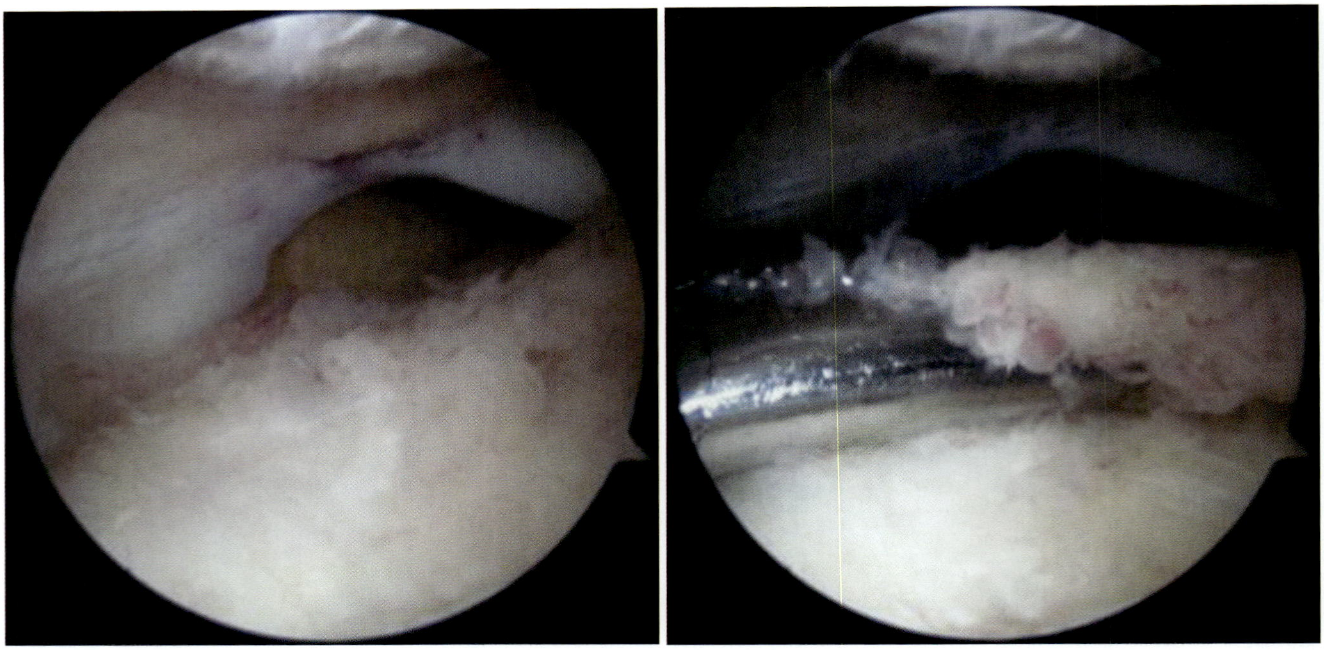

Fig. 9.7 Diffuse PVNS in the suprapatellar compartment and biopsy with a arthroscopic grasper

References

1. Vahlensieck M. Synovial lesions around the knee joint. Radiologe. 2006;46:65–70.
2. Poenaru DV, Petrescu H, Prejbeanu R. Plica sinoviala – rezectie sau nu? ASORIS. 2001;3:3–9.
3. Ogata S, Uhthoff HK. The development of synovial plicae in human knee joints: an embryologic study. Arthroscopy. 1990;6(4):315–21.
4. McKeon BP, Bono JV, Richmond JC. Knee arthroscopy. New York: Springer Science + Business Media, LLC; 2009.
5. Hayashi D, Xu L, Guermazi A, Kwoh CK, Hannon MJ, Jarraya M, Green SM, Jakicic JM, Moore CE, Roemer FW. Prevalence of MRI-detected mediopatellar plica in subjects with knee pain and the association with MRI-detected patellofemoral cartilage damage and bone marrow lesions: data from the Joints On Glucosamine study. BMC Musculoskelet Disord. 2013;14(1):292.
6. Griffith CJ, Laprade RF. Medial plica irritation: diagnosis and treatment. Curr Rev Musculoskelet Med. 2008;1(1):53–60. doi:10.1007/s12178-007-9006-z.
7. Kosarek FJ, Helms CA. The MR appearance of the infrapatellar plica. AJR Am J Roentgenol. 1999;172(2):481–4.
8. Vanhoenacker FM, Vanhoenacker P, Crevits I, Bracke P, De Schepper AM. MR imaging anatomy of the knee. Magn Reson Imaging Clin N Am. 2001;84(1):10–5.
9. Tasker T, Waugh W. Articular changes associated with internal derangement of the knee. J Bone Joint Surg Br. 1982;64(4):486–8.
10. O'Keeffe SA, Hogan BA, Eustace SJ, Kavanagh EC. Overuse injuries of the knee. Magn Reson Imaging Clin N Am. 2009;17(4):725–39, vii. doi:10.1016/j.mric.2009.06.010.
11. Paczesny L, Kruczynski J. Medial plica syndrome of the knee: diagnosis with dynamic sonography. Radiology. 2009;251:439–46.
12. Kent M, Khanduja V. Synovial plicae around the knee. Knee. 2010;17:97–102.
13. Sznajderman T, Smorgick Y, Lindner D, Beer Y, Agar G. Medial plica syndrome. Isr Med Assoc J. 2009;11(1):54–7.
14. Thomeé R, Augustsson J, Karlsson J. Patellofemoral pain syndrome: a review of current issues. Sports Med. 1999;28(4):245–62.
15. Al-Hadithy N, Gikas P, Mahapatra AM. Review article: plica syndrome of the knee. J Orthop Surg (Hong Kong). 2011;19(3):354–8.
16. Amatuzzi MM, Fazzi A, Varella MH. Pathologic synovial plica of the knee. Results of conservative treatment. Am J Sports Med. 1990;18:466–9.
17. Lyu S-R, Chiang J-K, Tseng C-E. Medial plica in patients with knee osteoarthritis: a histomorphological study. Knee Surg Sports Traumatol Arthrosc. 2010;18:769–76.
18. Schindler OS. "The Sneaky Plica" revisited: morphology, pathophysiology and treatment of synovial plicae of the knee. Knee Surg Sports Traumatol Arthrosc. 2014;22(2):247–62. doi:10.1007/s00167-013-2368-4.
19. Schindler OS. Synovial plicae of the knee. Curr Orthop. 2004;18:210–9.
20. Barile A, Sabatini M, Iannessi F, Di Cesare E, Splendiani A, Calvisi V, et al. Pigmented villonodular synovitis (PVNS) of the knee joint: magnetic resonance imaging (MRI) using standard and dynamic paramagnetic contrast media. Report of 52 cases surgically and histologically controlled. Radiol Med. 2004;107(4):356–66.
21. Coutinho M, Laranjo A, Casanova J. Pigmented Villonodular Synovitis: a diagnostic challenge. Review of 28 cases. Acta Reumatol Port. 2012;37(4):335–41.
22. Verma N, Valentino LA, Chawla A. Arthroscopic synovectomy in haemophilia: indications, technique and results. Haemophilia. 2007;13 Suppl 3:38–44.
23. de Almeida AM, de Rezende MU, Cordeiro FG, Villaça PR, D'Amico EA, Hernandez AJ, Camanho GL. Arthroscopic partial anterior synovectomy of the knee on patients with haemophilia. Knee Surg Sports Traumatol Arthrosc. 2013;1–7. doi: 10.1007/s00167-013-2706-6.
24. Oliva F, Frizziero A. One step open synovectomy without adjuvant therapy for diffuse pigmented villonodular synovitis of the knee in a soccer player. Muscles Ligaments Tendons J. 2011;1:36–9.
25. Loriaut P, Djian P, Boyer T, Bonvarlet J-P, Delin C, Makridis KG. Arthroscopic treatment of localized pigmented villonodular synovitis of the knee. Knee Surg Sports Traumatol Arthrosc. 2012;20:1550–3.

26. Akinci O, Akalin Y, İncesu M, Eren A. Long-term results of surgical treatment of pigmented villonodular synovitis of the knee. Acta Orthop Traumatol Turc. 2011;45(3):149–55.
27. Nakahara H, Matsuda S, Harimaya K, Sakamoto A, Matsumoto Y, Okazaki K, et al. Clinical results of open synovectomy for treatment of diffuse pigmented villonodular synovitis of the knee: case series and review of literature. Elsevier. 2012;19(5):684–7.
28. Kubat O, Mahnik A, Smoljanović T, Bojanić I. Arthroscopic treatment of localized and diffuse pigmented villonodular synovitis of the knee. Coll Antropol. 2010;34(4):1467–72.
29. Gu H-F, Zhang S-J, Zhao C, Chen Y, Bi Q. A comparison of open and arthroscopic surgery for treatment of diffuse pigmented villonodular synovitis of the knee. Berlin/Heidelberg: Springer; 2014. p. 1–7.
30. Jain JK, Vidyasagar JVS, Sagar R, Patel H, Chetan ML, Bajaj A. Arthroscopic synovectomy in pigmented villonodular synovitis of the knee: clinical series and outcome. Int Orthop. 2013;37(12):2363–9.
31. Pan X, Zhang X, Liu Z, Wen H, Mao X. Treatment for chronic synovitis of knee: arthroscopic or open synovectomy. Rheumatol Int. 2012;32(6):1733–6.
32. Aurégan JC, Bohu Y, Lefevre N, Klouche S, Naouri JF, Herman S, et al. Primary arthroscopic synovectomy for pigmented villo-nodular synovitis of the knee: recurrence rate and functional outcomes after a mean follow-up of seven years. Orthop Traumatol Surg Res. 2013;99(8):937–43.
33. Colman MW, Ye J, Weiss KR, Goodman MA, McGough RL. Does combined open and arthroscopic synovectomy for diffuse PVNS of the knee improve recurrence rates? Clin Orthop Relat Res. 2013;471:883–90.
34. Oztürk H, Bulut O, Oztemür Z, Bulut S. Pigmented villonodular synovitis managed by Yttrium 90 after debulking surgery. Saudi Med J. 2008;29:1197–200.
35. Oztemür Z, Bulut O, Korkmaz M, Gölge UH, Oztürk H, Tezeren G, Günaydın I. Surgical synovectomy combined with yttrium 90 in patients with recurrent joint synovitis. Rheumatol Int. 2013;33:1321–6.

Index

R. Prejbeanu (ed.), *Atlas of Knee Arthroscopy*,
DOI 10.1007/978-1-4471-6593-4, © Springer-Verlag London 2015